Praise for Steven Masley's

THE BETTER BRAIN SOLUTION

"In *The Better Brain Solution*, Dr. Masley shows us how brain and heart health are intimately connected and gives us the tools to correct insulin resistance, which will enhance brain function, prevent memory loss, and protect the heart. An important, essential, and welcome book." —Daniel G. Amen, M.D., author of *Change Your Brain, Change Your Life*

"Alzheimer's, dementia, and cognitive decline are all relentlessly gaining ground. Our brains are under constant attack—what to do? Take control! Dr. Masley expertly shows you how in this important new book." —Dr. Joseph Pizzorno, N.D., author of *The Toxin Solution*

"In this smart, well-researched, and urgently needed book, Dr. Masley gives us a clear, realistic plan to correct blood sugar, cope with insulin resistance in the brain, and boost cognitive function. Whatever your age, you need this book." —JJ Virgin, C.N.S., C.H.F.S., author of *JJ Virgin's Sugar Impact Diet*

"Well-done . . . awesome . . . superb—just a few adjectives to describe Dr. Masley's *The Better Brain Solution*! A timely book in the toxic times we live in, it astutely portrays proven remedies and solutions that will help support and protect the delicate and vulnerable tissues of your brain and even your heart. I loved reading *The Better Brain Solution* and totally agree with its insightful messages." —Stephen T. Sinatra, M.D., cardiologist and coauthor of *Health Revelations from Heaven and Earth*

"A well-substantiated guide to mental health." —*Publishers Weekly*

"In a world facing an epidemic of early-onset dementias, anyone over forty should protect their brain. Dr. Steven Masley's command of the scientific literature is easy for a layperson to understand, and the plan he lays out is revolutionary, and it works!" —Robyn Openshaw, author of *Vibe: Unlock the Energetic Frequencies of Limitless Health, Love & Success*

"Superb. . . . Dr. Masley's elegant book just may save your life!" —Howard Markel, author of *The Kelloggs: The Battling Brothers of Battle Creek*

STEVEN MASLEY, M.D.

THE
BETTER BRAIN
SOLUTION

Steven Masley, M.D., is the author of *The 30-Day Heart Tune-Up*, *Ten Years Younger*, and *Smart Fat*. He is a fellow of the American Heart Association, the American College of Nutrition, and the American Academy of Family Physicians. He has helped many patients improve their cognitive function and prevent or reverse type 2 diabetes and heart disease.

Masley's scientific articles have appeared in the *Journal of the American College of Nutrition*, *Journal of the American Medical Association*, and *American Family Physician*. His health programs have been seen on PBS, Discovery, and the *Today* show.

Dr. Masley is an affiliate clinical associate professor with the University of South Florida. He lives with his wife in St. Petersburg, Florida, where he heads the Masley Optimal Health Center.

www.drmasley.com

THE
BETTER BRAIN
SOLUTION

How to Sharpen Cognitive Function

and Prevent Memory Loss at Any Age

STEVEN MASLEY, M.D.

VINTAGE BOOKS
A Division of Penguin Random House LLC
New York

FIRST VINTAGE BOOKS EDITION, DECEMBER 2018

Copyright © 2018 by Steven Masley, M.D.

All rights reserved. Published in the United States by Vintage Books, a division of Penguin Random House LLC, New York, and distributed in Canada by Random House of Canada, a division of Penguin Random House Canada Limited, Toronto. Originally published in hardcover in the United States by Alfred A. Knopf, a division of Penguin Random House LLC, New York, in 2018.

Vintage and colophon are registered trademarks of Penguin Random House LLC.

The Library of Congress has cataloged the Knopf edition as follows:
Name: Masley, Steven, author.
Title: The better brain solution : how to start now—at any age—to reverse and prevent insulin resistance of the brain, sharpen cognitive function, and avoid memory loss / Steven Masley, M.D.
Description: New York : Alfred A. Knopf, 2018.
Identifiers: LCCN 2017016326
Subjects: LCSH: Brain—Popular works. | Nutrition—Popular works. | Mental health—Popular works. | Self-care, Health—Popular works. | BISAC: HEALTH & FITNESS / Diseases / Diabetes. | HEALTH & FITNESS / Diseases / Nervous System (incl. Brain). | HEALTH & FITNESS / Diseases / Alzheimer's & Dementia.
Classification: LCC QP376 .M368 2018 | DDC 612.8/2—dc23
LC record available at https://lccn.loc.gov/2017016326

Vintage Books Trade Paperback ISBN: 978-0-525-43324-8
eBook ISBN: 978-1-5247-3239-4

Book design by Iris Weinstein

www.vintagebooks.com

Printed in the United States of America
1 2 3 4 5 6 7 8 9 10

I dedicate this book to my patients at the Masley Optimal Health Center, who teach me each day that the best way to prevent memory loss is through lifestyle changes that improve cognitive function and enrich quality of life.

CONTENTS

I f you could protect yourself from the illness you fear most, what would it be?

Cancer? Heart disease? When I ask my patients this question, I almost always get the same answer: memory loss.

The brain is the very essence of your being. Every day it fires up all your senses, brings you pleasure (and yes, pain), catalogues a lifetime of memories, solves an array of problems, and connects you to the world around you. It makes you human. You can live with a mechanical joint, without kidneys on dialysis, with a transplanted heart, liver, or other organ, but nothing can substitute for a healthy brain. Without memory, we require constant care from family, friends, or total strangers, and we become a burden on the people we love the most. Like many other physicians, I put memory loss at the top of the list of conditions I wish we could permanently vanquish.

Despite billions of dollars of research, we've had no significant cures for medical problems such as dementia and Alzheimer's disease (the most common form of memory loss). In the United States, we now have nearly 6 million people diagnosed with Alzheimer's disease, and the annual bill for dementia care now tops $215 billion, more than is spent on cancer or heart disease. The number of victims is predicted to increase 200 percent by 2030, and to increase 400 percent by 2050—that's 24 million Americans with this disease—when the cost of Alzheimer's care will exceed $1.5 trillion yearly. On a global level, the numbers are even more staggering. In 2010 there were 36 million people with Alzheimer's; in 2050, at its current rate, there will be 115 million men and women worldwide with disabling memory loss—a 320 percent increase.

On a more personal level, if you have experienced a loved one struggling with dementia, you will undoubtedly agree it's a disease that unravels the life of the sufferer and upends the lives of family and friends as well. Its costs are far more than financial, and it can last for years. With Alzheimer's disease, which accounts for up to 70 percent of all dementias, the end result has been the same. Up until now, it has always been fatal, as we have not had any effective treatments or cures.

In fact, we're facing two urgent epidemics right now: escalating rates of disabling memory loss, and rapidly increasing rates of diabetes and pre-diabetes. As research has now proven, these conditions are intimately connected. But here is a life-changing fact: *Diabetes and memory loss are largely preventable.*

Before I tell you more, let me explain how my work as a heart guy led me to the brain. I don't think of myself that way, but because I'm known for my work in preventing and reversing heart disease, some people do. (I'm the author of *The 30-Day Heart Tune-Up* and created one of the all-time most popular health programs created for PBS, called *30 Days to a Younger Heart*.) It's true that as a physician and a nutritionist, I've dedicated much of my professional life to showing people how to stop and reverse heart disease. Now I want to help prevent another looming health crisis.

Thirty years ago as a medical resident, I focused on cardiovascular research, though I ultimately chose to become a family physician. I wanted to help heal the *whole person,* not just the heart, and I was more interested in preventing people from developing heart disease than in treating heart disease itself. Decades later, when I designed my medical clinic, the Masley Optimal Health Center, to assess and optimize aging, I knew that cardiovascular disease was—and still is—the #1 killer of Americans. I wanted to create treatments that would help with its prevention, and in some cases, its complete reversal.

We've come a long way in our fight against heart disease, and today it's possible to prevent 90 percent of all heart attacks and strokes, if people follow a simple plan like mine. If someone comes to me with existing heart disease, I've also been able to help shrink their arterial plaque, the dangerous inflammatory substance that builds up in the arteries as a result of diet and other lifestyle factors—and in the process prevent memory loss.

I've studied arterial plaque growth and its connection to various lifestyle factors that accelerate or reverse this deadly condition. I've presented my data to the American Heart Association, the American

College of Nutrition, and the American Academy of Family Physicians, and my book and PBS program are based on my findings.

Simply put, arterial plaque growth leads to heart attacks, strokes, and sudden death. We know it causes heart disease, but it belongs in this discussion about the brain because it has emerged as one of the most powerful predictors of memory loss and cognitive dysfunction, including Alzheimer's disease. Longitudinal data collected in my clinic powerfully illustrates this link between arterial plaque growth and the loss of cognitive function and brain speed.

Here's another key connection between arterial plaque growth and brain health decline: both are closely linked to poor blood sugar control, which is triggered not only by diet but by a variety of lifestyle choices. Uncontrolled blood sugar isn't just an issue for those with diagnosed diabetes. Many people with abnormal blood sugar levels, including those who are insulin resistant and pre-diabetic, seek a doctor's care only when they're in crisis. (Insulin resistance is the body's inability to respond to insulin, the hormone that regulates blood sugar levels.) But tens of millions of Americans are utterly unaware of their elevated blood sugar levels, caused by diet and lifestyle, and they are at much greater risk for advanced memory loss.

The risk of dementia is escalating at epidemic proportions precisely because of the insulin resistance, pre-diabetes, and diabetes that results from out-of-control blood sugar, brought on by the Standard American Diet (known as SAD, high in sugar and bad fats, making it sad indeed). Nearly 30 million Americans have diabetes (1.2 million have type 1 diabetes, an autoimmune disorder); another whopping 86 million have pre-diabetes, meaning they are at risk for full-blown diabetes (plus accelerated memory loss and heart disease) unless they adopt healthier diets and lifestyles. On top of that, likely one-third of the U.S. adult population has undiagnosed insulin resistance, and if you are a baby boomer, there is a 50 percent chance that you are afflicted.

Our brain function hinges on normal insulin activity, but when we make diet and lifestyle choices that impede insulin from regulating our blood sugar, we seriously damage our cognitive function and starve our brain's nerve cells. We actually kill off a part of our brain as these cells shrink and die. That is how poor blood sugar control can lead to memory loss and dementia. The connection between these conditions is now irrefutable. The evidence is overwhelming that if we want to prevent memory loss and disability, we need to achieve better blood sugar control.

Having insulin resistance or pre-diabetes can make you up to 60 percent more likely to develop Alzheimer's—the most common cause of dementia—than someone with normal blood sugar and insulin levels. And our current health care system is set up to intervene and "help" only those who suffer from advanced dementia; those treatments, for the most part, are limited to drug therapies that have shown no meaningful success.

Unfortunately, none of the current drugs used to treat advanced memory loss actually stop the progression of the disease. (As of this writing, about 200 drugs have received approval from the Food and Drug Administration for fighting memory loss, but none seem to do so effectively.) The only solution, therefore, is to focus on methods that can enhance our cognitive performance *now* and to either stop or slow early cognitive decline before it's too late. That is precisely why my results with my clinic patients are very good news for *anyone* with a brain.

For more than a decade, I have been measuring brain function and more than one hundred aspects of aging in my clinic, plus I have watched thousands of patients who follow my program become mentally sharper and quicker and turn back the clock on aging. I have the published results to prove it: the men and women who follow my Better Brain Solution—the same plan I'm going to share with you—experience on average a 25 percent improvement in executive brain function, improve their heart health, shrink arterial plaque, get their blood sugar under control, and have much more energy than before. In many cases, weight loss is a beneficial side effect. And these improvements aren't fleeting. In patients I've tracked over the years, the changes are lasting.

The key is identifying memory loss ten, twenty, or even thirty years in advance, well before you even notice that you forgot why you walked into the dining room, what your neighbor's name is, or where you parked the car. With my early intervention to slowing and preventing memory loss and cognitive decline, you too can experience a major boost in brain function, heart health, and energy and a whole host of other benefits.

What to Expect, Brain and Body

My Better Brain Solution provides all the tools you will need to protect your brain, but it's up to you to use them. If you do, you can expect some fantastic results—including being mentally sharper and more physically fit and drastically reducing your risks for memory loss and heart disease. I will be asking you to move your body a little more and say goodbye to SAD, the Standard American Diet (filled with everyday foods like juice, cereal, and toast for breakfast; sandwiches and chips or fast food for lunch; candy or soda for a pick-me-up; pizza or burgers and fries for dinner). Whether we're talking about diet or lifestyle, if your current comfort foods and old habits set you up for serious health problems and decrease your performance at work and at play (even in the bedroom), it's time to find a new path. You may have to take some things off your plate, but you will be adding some delicious alternatives, including specific nutrients that will boost your health and performance.

It all comes down to change. I want to help you change how you feel, for the better. I want to change our health-care system from its current focus on end-stage therapy to prevention, and I want to change how we as a society think about food and health.

The information in the book will be backed by the most current research, as well as compelling data from my own clinical practice, and include fifty nourishing recipes. (If you're concerned that these brain- and heart-healthy meals will taste like cardboard, fear not. As a physician, a nutritionist, and someone who completed a chef internship at the Four Seasons Restaurant in Seattle, I can assure you that this food will be easy to prepare and delicious, and that your family and friends will love it.)

No matter how old you are or what your state of health may be, ask yourself: Who among us wouldn't benefit from being 25 percent mentally sharper and quicker? If you follow the Better Brain Solution, you can look forward to feeling focused and getting more work done in less time, and growing trimmer and fitter, while preventing heart disease and protecting against memory loss. Your stamina will increase, and you will have more fun, including better romantic function. You can look forward to the pleasures of a long, rich life, made possible by a healthy brain and strong body.

When it comes to brain health, it's not too late to reverse damage, and it's never too early to prevent it. (And the same can be said for heart health as well.)

Promises

Here are my promises to you. I will offer you:

- An easy-to-understand connection between blood sugar control, heart disease, and memory loss
- A practical way to assess your cognitive function
- A list of factors that increase your risk for memory loss and tips to stop them in their tracks
- A medically sound program to improve your brain function
- A scientifically proven plan to help prevent memory loss
- Recipes that are easy to prepare, with foods that are great for your brain and body, and that your family and friends will love to eat
- Activities that will tune up your brain, rev your metabolism, and help you get trim and sexy
- A program that you can share with your partner, spouse, children, and/or parents, that is safe for all ages
- A plan that is realistic if you have a busy schedule
- Results that you can feel and measure within thirty days

PART I

Save Your Brain

CHAPTER I

Origins of Memory Loss: The Brain–Blood Sugar–Heart Connection

Your heart gives you circulation and blood flow, bringing your physical body to life.

Your brain gives you cognition, igniting your mind and your spirit.

Cognition is the act of knowing or thinking, and having optimal brain function means being capable of properly inputting information, processing the information, responding appropriately and in a timely fashion, and remembering that activity. But should the heart fail, the brain may also decline. And while the heart can sometimes be repaired, in many cases the brain will not recover.

As a physician, I've met many families who've lived through a relative's struggles with memory loss, but I have also experienced it on a personal level and know how very painful it can be.

I met Chuck Odegaard, the man who'd become my stepfather, when I was in high school, after my parents had divorced. I remember encouraging my mom to marry this really nice guy, who was so kind to me and such a loving, supportive partner to her. She did, they had a wonderful marriage, and Chuck—always there when I needed him—would go on to become a terrific grandfather to my two sons.

Chuck had been both a Washington State and regional national park director. A few days after he retired, he was walking down a street, on his way to a meeting where he'd be volunteering for the city of Seattle, when he developed serious chest pains. He was taken to the hospital, and as a result of a cardiac procedure that dislodged a section of arterial plaque, he suffered a severe stroke that triggered immediate, profound dementia.

That is when I saw, firsthand, what dementia truly means and how it impacts loved ones. Chuck couldn't get dressed, shower, shave, or make himself a snack or cup of coffee. He couldn't remember what he'd eaten twenty minutes before. Unlike someone with Alzheimer's disease, he could recognize people he knew, but he couldn't learn anything new. He wandered around the condo where he lived with my mother as if in a fog, bewildered and lost. This once energetic, sharp, and thoughtful man, so professionally accomplished and looking forward to a happy retirement with my mom, lost it all in an instant. About seven years later, as he became increasingly confused, he fell and broke his hip. In terrible pain, he stopped eating and drinking. Chuck was dying, and I came home to say goodbye.

By the time I arrived, others told me I was probably too late—he had not opened his eyes all day and was no longer speaking. But upon hearing my voice, Chuck actually sat up and grasped my hand. "Don't let what happened to me happen to others," he said. I sobbed and told him I'd do my best.

That was twenty years ago. More recently my wife, Nicole, faced a similar situation with a parent. Her late mother, Joy, whom I knew for three decades, had always seemed cheerful and was rarely sick, but she experienced a serious health crisis that spiraled into dementia. Her family has a history of early-onset Alzheimer's disease. (Joy's own mother had it, and now both of her younger brothers have it as well.) Joy, who did not always eat well, eventually began a struggle with heart disease; she underwent heart procedures that caused additional injury to her brain. In fact, a brain scan from years back showed brain shrinkage (due to Alzheimer's) as well as vascular injury (signs of mini-strokes); Joy had a mixture of Alzheimer's disease and vascular dementia.

When Joy first began to lose her memory, she would become agitated and angry, clearly frustrated at losing normal cognitive function and the independence that comes with it. Over time, as she grew more forgetful, she grew more passive. The sad reality is that we lost Joy many years ago, well before she died, as she didn't know who she was or who was with her. Despite having been a wonderful mother-in-law, wife, mother, and grandmother—that person had vanished.

I watched my own mother try her best to care for Chuck, a challenge that aged her tremendously, although in the years since he died, she has recovered and regained much of her health and vitality. Now I appreciate firsthand what it is like to care for a loved one with Alzheimer's disease, having watched my wife, her siblings, and her father do their best to care for Joy. It's been beautiful to see such love in action, but at the same time it has been profoundly painful to witness how hard this disease is on everyone involved. I have felt all their angst and tears, especially the toll it has taken on my father-in-law, Jean, as the stress of the situation has ruined his health as well. And so I think about what Chuck said to me—*Don't let this happen to other people.*

It doesn't necessarily have to happen to you or to anyone you love. The fact is that we can prevent most dementias right now—including Alzheimer's—and we don't need to wait around praying for someone to develop a new drug or other intervention. It starts with all of us making the right choices in our daily lives, and once we have a fundamental understanding of the clear connection between the brain, blood sugar, and the heart, those changes will become easier to make.

The Path to Better Brain Function

When I am explaining cognition, I focus on two primary areas: memory and processing. Memory is our ability to encode, store, retain, and recall past information and experiences. Processing is getting things done, focusing, and handling information. Though memory and processing are two separate cognitive functions, you need them both for your brain to work properly. It's like a computer. You can have one with tons of memory, but if you have a slow or damaged internal processor chip, it becomes increasingly difficult to access and use all that information.

Executive function is the part of processing that helps us plan and achieve goals, focus, and manage our tasks. If you are familiar with how the brains of babies and children develop as they grow into adulthood, you know that under normal circumstances, executive function continues to mature and improve throughout a young person's teens and twenties. I consider executive function and mental sharpness to be the same thing, and I use the terms interchangeably. When we're mentally sharp—that is, when our executive function is optimal—we can jump from one task to another quickly. We can refocus our attention and recall information as needed.

When executive function is impaired or in decline, memory lags as well—like a slowing computer when the processor chip isn't working at the speed it should. If you need to replace an aging or damaged computer, it's simple. But if the brain slows down or "crashes," you can't just order up a new one.

How the Better Brain Solution Can Prevent Memory Loss: The Proof

Changing your lifestyle probably won't impact your intelligence or your IQ. However, making the right lifestyle changes—in areas like diet and exercise and even how you spend your leisure time—will improve your mental sharpness and overall executive function, and these same changes will ultimately help you to prevent memory loss. I've read thousands of medical articles, and reviewed hundreds of clinical trials that show just that—and I've also conducted and published my own peer-reviewed research.

The idea of improving brain function through lifestyle changes isn't just theoretical. It works in real life, and it will work for you. As a physician, I have strived to improve cognitive function in my patients every day, as part of improving their overall health and reducing their risk of disease; as a researcher, I have measured these cognitive improvements, and I know *this program works.* The evidence is there: You can improve your brain function if you make the right choices.

At my clinic, we work with patients to stop accelerated aging in its tracks and detect early signs of disease before problems set in. Our goal is to educate and empower ordinary men and women to make lifestyle changes that optimize their overall health and wellness for the rest of their lives. Over fifteen years, we've seen amazing and inspiring results, including reversals of heart disease and other conditions. We begin by taking a baseline physical assessment, from head to toe, and a major component of that evaluation is measuring cognition.

We administer a thirty-minute computerized battery of seven tests, which generate ten independent scores. For instance, patients are asked to remember shapes and words for as little as one minute or as long as thirty minutes. They process colors, digits, and symbols, performing a variety of simple tasks designed to evaluate cognition and test visual and verbal memory. In the end, we obtain scores for overall complex information processing, memory, attention, motor speed, and processing speed—the executive function measures that are so important in predicting brain health. (I'll give you more information on this assessment, known as the Central Nervous System Vital Signs, or CNS VS, in Chapter 2, where I explain cognitive testing and provide a simple test where you can interpret your own performance.)

When patients enter our program and follow our recommendations, they tune up not only their hearts but all their organ systems (including the brain) that depend on healthy cardiovascular function. They wind up with better brain function. Our average patient loses weight and sees improvements in blood pressure, cholesterol, and blood sugar level. Their arterial plaque—from my research, a powerful predictor of memory loss—shrinks instead of grows, and they are mentally sharper.

Rather than start my patients on new medications, I often wind up weaning people off drugs they no longer require. Many medications have harmful side effects. For instance, statins are often the first line of defense against heart disease and are indeed a lifesaver for some. (No one should stop a medication without their doctor's consent.) But it turns out that statins also cause a rise in blood sugar levels (moderate, but still an increase), as well as memory loss. An increase in blood sugar is a major risk factor for dementia. However, if you make the right lifestyle changes to improve your executive function, you'll naturally improve your cholesterol profile, shrinking your arterial plaque—and you may no longer need a medication that might decrease your memory and cognitive performance.

I knew the improvement that I was seeing among my regular patients was real, yet I wanted to get scientific proof that my program could work for anyone, including you. I received permission from my local hospital research committee to perform a clinical trial to test my recommendations with an intervention group randomized to follow my plan, and a control group that continued their same lifestyle without any changes.

The average person entering the study had a fairly typical American lifestyle. He or she exercised at most once per week, ate a low-fiber diet with too many refined carbs, and was moderately overweight. We tested cognition, fitness, nutrient intake, and we measured body composition both before and after the study. My ten-week program primarily involved making simple modifications in diet (increasing fiber from vegetables, fruits, beans, and nuts, plus eating more smart fats), increasing weekly exercise, and engaging in stress management.

After ten weeks the participants were retested; the control group showed no improvements. The intervention group, however, improved their overall complex information processing and executive function by 25 percent, an amazing improvement that made them feel mentally sharper and able to accomplish more in their day. Their attention and focus improved 40 percent. They were also trimmer (having lost ten pounds of body fat in ten weeks) and fitter, and they reported feeling better, too.

I have now published nearly a dozen studies from my clinic reflecting similar positive results. If you follow the same path as my patients and those who've participated in these studies, there's no reason you can't see the same dramatic results—in both body and brain.

Without doubt, it is possible to prevent memory loss. The first step is to improve your mental sharpness and executive function. That is what this book is all about.

Understanding Memory Loss: From Mild Cognitive Impairment to Dementia and Alzheimer's Disease

One of the very earliest signs that you are losing memory over time *isn't* that your memory fails.

Let's say, for instance, you go into a meeting at work and are sitting across the table from a business associate you've met before, but you have totally forgotten her name, and professionally speaking, you really should be able to remember that information. You get through the meeting without having to say her name or introduce her to a colleague (thankfully). Then, as you are walking back to your office, you suddenly remember her name—as well as her phone number and where her son goes to college. Usually you're so good with names and faces. *Is this,* you wonder, *the beginning of a serious problem?* Probably not.

Here's what just happened: your internal processor—your executive function—was sluggish. You were able to access your memory but not as quickly as you wanted to. Maybe you were sleep deprived, you had eaten poorly, and/or you were stressed. That kind of memory mishap is not uncommon, and it doesn't mean you're heading toward severe memory loss. (It does, however, mean that you should make some changes to stop your executive function from sliding.)

But the first true sign of memory loss is that sharpness and executive function decrease *gradually* over time. Some of that decline may be due to normal aging—but even that process can be slowed. Now, instead of occasionally forgetting a name or two in a meeting, you experience a steady decline in your ability to hold on to important information, on a regular basis. (You can't recall that colleague's name, you also can't focus on the content of the meeting, and you are unclear about what tasks you're supposed to carry out as a result of the meeting.) That pattern of memory loss is more worrisome, but once again, by making the right lifestyle changes, you can reverse your decline or slow it significantly.

There is a wide spectrum of brain function that varies from optimal, to normal, to sluggish, to having mild cognitive impairment, to becoming disabled and dependent upon others for daily function, which we call dementia. Seventy percent of dementias are caused by Alzheimer's disease, a state where brain cells gradually die and the whole brain volume shrinks (with the formation of unusual brain proteins, called beta-amyloids, and neurofibrillary tangles). Most of us, when we think of extreme memory loss and dementia, think of Alzheimer's disease—but it's not the only cause.

By the time the brain reaches full-blown dementia—shrinking from a plump grape to a shriveled raisin—and the victim is fully disabled, the damage is likely permanent. At this time, I know of no treatments or lifestyle changes that will reverse the death of healthy brain cells, which is why we must do more early on to prevent it entirely.

I've indicated that lifestyle changes are key, and we'll explore them in depth—but one lifestyle factor in particular deserves your attention now, starting with your next meal or snack. If you follow the Standard American Diet (with its "sad" lack of healthy fiber and its abundance of bad fats and refined carbohydrates), then you are very likely decreasing your brain performance. In a moment, I'll explain why that is, but first let's look at how SAD gradually impacts memory and processing.

When you eat the SAD way, instead of optimal brain function your mental performance is a bit sluggish. Over time, as your brain cells show signs of dysfunction and brain cells die, you may feel what we call "brain fog." You're forgetful, and your friends, family, and co-workers think of you as absentminded. You repeatedly lose your keys, cellphone, and glasses. You forget about meetings and deadlines at work, and you lose track of important e-mails or files on your computer. You get lost even in familiar environments, and you forget names. This forgetful state is what is called subjective cognitive impairment (SCI). If this worsens further and your performance begins to decline in a measurable way, you reach the diagnosis of mild cognitive impairment (MCI).

With MCI, you are not disabled, and you can still perform your day-to-day activities safely, but you are struggling with memory and processing information, and likely your friends and family have noted that this is becoming a problem. Perhaps you go to a full-time job every day, but you're no longer working to capacity. Once MCI occurs, most people progress to dementia and disability within five to eight years, converting to Alzheimer's disease at about 15 to 20 percent per year. MCI is frightening and sadly is very common in older adults. My aim is to help prevent people from acquiring a diagnosis of MCI and to help them avoid progressing to dementia.

Fortunately, Alzheimer's disease doesn't happen overnight. Think of it as a twenty-year progression. You typically have five years of early cognitive decline without symptoms, then ten years of subjective cognitive impairment (SCI), followed by five years of being impaired but not disabled (MCI), and finally progressing to being disabled with dementia. The longer you wait, the harder it is to stop the decline and to reverse the symptoms.

There are several types of dementia (many of which overlap). Sixty to 70 percent of dementias are related to Alzheimer's. Fifteen percent are related to vascular dementia, which is caused by a stroke or insufficient blood flow to the brain; vascular dementia tends to occur in a stepwise fashion following mini-stroke after mini-stroke, instead of a gradual decline. Other less common forms include frontal temporal dementia, Lewy body dementia, and those related to other neurological diseases, such as Parkinson's disease, Huntington's disease, and Creutzfeldt-Jakob disease.

Ultimately, though, it's less important than you may think to divide up, rank, or label the various types. That's because most dementias—including Alzheimer's—can be delayed or prevented with a healthier lifestyle that reduces its number one cause: uncontrolled blood sugar. Let's look closer at why this one factor plays such a major role in brain health.

The Real Cost of Alzheimer's Disease

Alzheimer's is a devastating, progressive disease, and it is always fatal. It is often harder on the patients' families and caregivers than on the patients themselves. Early in the disease process, people with memory loss may be agitated and sometimes even aggressive, but over time they typically become more passive and withdrawn. They often quit speaking, and many become physically inactive, even wheelchair bound or bedridden. The impact on their families can be devastating and exhausting.

Technically, we confirm the diagnosis of Alzheimer's at autopsy, after a person has died, in a brain biopsy. The classic signs of the disease include the formation of beta-amyloid protein (an inflammatory protein substance) and of neuro-fibrillary tangles. Yet for physicians and patients, it is not practical to wait until somebody has died to get a firm confirmation of the disease, so we make a diagnosis based upon clinical signs. First and foremost, we diagnose Alzheimer's when someone shows a gradual decline in brain function that has rendered them mentally disabled. We then confirm it by testing for increased beta-amyloid protein in the spinal fluid or in deposits on the brain, using sophisticated brain scan studies that also show brain shrinkage. (There is intense debate within the scientific community as to whether beta-amyloid is the cause or a by-product of Alzheimer's disease. So far there is no definitive proof either way.)

In 2014 the direct cost of treating Alzheimer's disease was

$214 billion, and most of this expense was not for drugs or doctor visits; instead, most went to nursing home care and home care. If we added the indirect cost associated with family and caregivers providing care to those with dementia, the cost would double. By 2050, the total cost of care for Alzheimer's disease is expected to exceed $1.5 trillion per year. This disease has the potential to bankrupt our health care system and our government if we don't do more to prevent it.

The emotional impact on loved ones of people with dementia goes far beyond the financial cost. Spouses and children become exhausted from caring for their disabled loved one night and day. People with dementia lose track of time, they stop sleeping at night, and they often wander and need constant assistance. I've watched husbands, wives, sons, daughters, and other close family members ruin their own health caring for someone with dementia. Not only should we want to avoid memory loss ourselves; we should have a profound motivation to prevent it so it doesn't impact those whom we love most.

What Really Causes Dementia

In my thirty years as a physician, I've encountered many patients with dementia. Years ago we were told we couldn't do anything to prevent it, but now we know better. We really can prevent nearly two-thirds of all dementias. Even better, we can do it through simple choices we make each day, as we go about our lives—we don't have to hope for a miracle drug or a complicated treatment. But the trick is to do something about it right now, before it's too late.

Let's start by looking at ten factors that can decrease your cognitive function and accelerate your risk for memory loss. We're going to pay particularly close attention to number one in this chapter, and we'll address the other risk factors in the following chapters.

1. Insulin resistance and elevated blood sugar levels
2. Cardiovascular disease

3. Inactivity
4. Nutrient deficiencies
5. Toxins
6. Unmanaged stress
7. Inflammation
8. Hormonal imbalance (as a result of menopause and andropause)
9. Depression and anxiety
10. Genetics

You can modify all ten of these risk factors with the Better Brain Solution. (For those of you who may be especially concerned about the tenth factor—genetics—here is a key fact to consider now: while certain genes can increase your risk for memory loss, they don't have the last word. You can influence the outcome with lifestyle. I'll talk more about the role of genes, and useful genetic testing, in Chapter 2.)

The most important risk factor sits at the top of the list, and you will benefit more from correcting this one factor than from addressing the others: blood sugar regulation and insulin resistance. Though it's the number one target on our enemies list, you'll see that it's closely related to the next item—cardiovascular disease. Once you understand the role that blood sugar plays, we'll address how cardiovascular disease impacts brain function.

Seven Myths about Memory Loss and Alzheimer's Disease

1. It only happens to old people. Alzheimer's disease can strike people in their thirties, forties, and fifties. In the United States, there are 200,000 people younger than sixty-five with "younger-onset" Alzheimer's disease.
2. Memory loss is a normal part of aging. In reality, as people age, occasionally forgetting a name or a fact is pretty common, but being disabled by memory loss is not normal. Getting lost in your own apartment, being unable to care for yourself, and not knowing the names of your loved ones

is not a normal part of aging. This is a disease we need to prevent.

3. <u>Memory loss is caused by vaccines and flu shots.</u> People who are vaccinated against diseases such as diphtheria, tetanus, polio, or influenza, studies show, have a lower risk of developing Alzheimer's disease than people who are not vaccinated.

4. <u>Memory loss is caused by using aluminum cans and pots.</u> I discourage people from using aluminum pans, as aluminum has no known health benefits and may be linked to some health concerns. But the idea, arising in the 1970s, that it caused Alzheimer's never bore fruit. There is no solid evidence it does.

5. <u>You can't improve your mental performance or prevent memory loss, so don't bother trying. Brain cells can't be repaired.</u> Fortunately, hundreds of scientific studies show that you can improve cognitive performance and memory and in some cases prevent or postpone memory loss. The Better Brain Solution gives you the strategies to do this.

6. <u>Alzheimer's won't kill you.</u> Alzheimer's disease destroys brain cells and in its advanced form is always fatal. It is a progressive disease that leads to profound memory loss, disruptive behavior, and loss of body function, such as bladder and bowel control.

7. <u>There are treatments for Alzheimer's disease.</u> At this time, there are no medical treatments to cure or to stop the progression of Alzheimer's disease. Once diagnosed with advanced Alzheimer's, people will lose their ability to eat, talk, and walk. They cannot dress themselves, and they become incontinent, usually forced to wear diapers. In time they will die. FDA-approved drugs temporarily slow some of the symptoms (like anxiety) but only for six to twelve months. Furthermore, only about half of the individuals who take these drugs experience this limited benefit. There is no current effective treatment for Alzheimer's, so our focus should be on preventing it.

Blood Sugar and the Brain

There was a time when ordinary people didn't pay attention to blood sugar unless they were diabetic. Now we know that blood sugar is something everyone, regardless of their physical condition, should keep tabs on.

Blood sugar regulation is an essential aspect of health and overall wellness, and it can mean the difference between being fat and thin—or between life and death. Poor blood sugar control, in addition to ultimately leading to diabetes, is also the number one risk factor for developing dementia and heart disease. Unhealthy blood sugar levels bring on obesity, nonalcoholic fatty liver disease, kidney disease, and cancer. There are, obviously, lots of reasons to avoid uncontrolled blood sugar, but nearly 100 million Americans fail to do so, as well as millions worldwide, even when we are educated about the risks.

I don't think of abnormal blood sugar control as a disease in and of itself, because it's not. It is, however, a combination of inappropriate lifestyle choices that clashes with our genetic makeup. Many people have a greater genetic risk of developing type 2 diabetes when they follow the blood-sugar-stoking Standard American Diet than others do, but ironically these same genes would probably help them survive famine.

In ancestral times, feast or famine was a way of life. When times were good, people ate well and fattened up. When times were bad, they conserved their physical energy by moving less and trying not to starve to death, using their bodies' reserves of stored fat. Their genetic makeup allowed for this up-and-down cycle of plentiful eating followed by relative (for them) inactivity. Nomadic people walked up to eighteen miles a day and ate mainly plants (fruits, nuts, seeds), with meat on an infrequent basis. Their foods were naturally unprocessed and clean. Fast-forward to modern times, where most of us no longer face famine nor do we need to call upon energy-storing (fat-storing) genes that help us do so. Therefore, when we eat the modern SAD way, consuming too much sugar and bad fat, then sit all day at a desk, this same genetic "advantage" will eventually kill us.

Another reason many of us don't address blood sugar control more aggressively is that we think of it as something only diabetics should worry about. Lots of my patients initially think of blood sugar control as a yes or no. Either they have diabetes or they don't—and therefore they either have to control blood sugar or they don't. But blood sugar control should be thought of as a continuum, with normal blood sugar and diabetes being at opposite ends.

What most people don't know is that insulin resistance starts years before blood sugar levels are even mildly elevated.

Insulin Resistance: Feeding the Body, Starving the Brain

To understand the connection between blood sugar and the brain, it's important to get a snapshot of how insulin works and what happens when we overload and damage its mechanisms through diet.

When you eat carbohydrates from *any* source—whether it's your breakfast of cereal and toast, or a glazed doughnut, or even that organic broccoli in your lunchtime stir-fry—your body naturally converts the carbs in these foods into glucose (a simple form of sugar), which passes from your intestinal tract to your bloodstream. Glucose is an energy source that every cell in your body can use, including your brain cells. Insulin is the hormone that regulates blood sugar (that is, glucose) levels; one of insulin's primary jobs is to push glucose into cells, either to be stored as energy or to be used as fuel. The more carbohydrates you eat, the more insulin you produce.

In a normal situation, our muscle cells, very sensitive to insulin's message, store glucose in long molecular chains, called glycogen. Meanwhile our fat cells convert any extra glucose into fat. During periods when we are active, our muscle cells burn the glycogen as fuel, and as glycogen stores become depleted, fat is then burned as fuel. This balance keeps glucose levels stable within the bloodstream. Problems set in when we take in more calories, especially those from refined carbs, than we burn, and more than our muscle cells can store.

When we eat too many refined carbs, particularly those in sugar and flour, we experience a rapid influx of glucose into the bloodstream; then blood glucose levels spike, and insulin levels jump to push more glucose into cells. But at some point, when the muscle cells become saturated, the body can't store more glucose as glycogen, and the muscle cells stop listening to insulin's message to store more glucose.

It's like a hotel with no more rooms; the phone is ringing (the glucose entourage is in town again and needs lots of rooms), but the front desk staff is ignoring the calls from guests trying to book in. The first cells to quit answering that phone are the muscle cells. If the muscle cells aren't getting much of a workout (due to a sedentary lifestyle) and therefore don't have a need for usable energy, the excess glucose will eventually be converted and stored as fat. No worries if this is a rare event, like feasting to end a fast, but if these spikes become a day-after-day (meal-after-meal) occurrence, not only muscle cells but cells body-wide become increasingly resistant to insulin's message to store glucose as a usable energy source.

Insulin is often called the "weight gain" hormone because it helps you to retain body fat to prepare for some future famine. Unfortunately, too many of us are following a diet that contains more calories than we need, resulting in more insulin production than we want. The cells stop listening to insulin's message, a condition called insulin resistance. Over years, as your insulin response becomes less and less effective, your blood sugar levels will become modestly elevated, and if uncorrected, they will continue to rise until you qualify for a diagnosis of diabetes. The average time to progress from insulin resistance to diabetes is about ten years.

Why Insulin Resistance Is a Brain Killer

When brain cells become insulin resistant, they are unable to absorb glucose from the bloodstream or to use their own stores of glucose as energy. A recent study of insulin-resistant adults with an average age just over sixty confirmed that those with the highest levels of insulin resistance had the lowest levels of brain cell glucose metabolism. Insulin resistance literally stops you from using your brain. Think of the brain as a motor requiring fuel. With insulin resistance, it's almost as if someone has put dirt in the gas, and the brain-cell-energy-burning motor won't work.

Normal insulin activity is essential to nerve cell health, especially in the brain, but impaired insulin activity results in a cascade of neurodegenerative related problems, including nerve inflammation, oxidative stress (explained on page 18), and damaged nerve cells, which subsequently die. When blood sugar is out of control and insulin is unable to do its job, the brain's nerve cells are "starved" for the right kind of energy, and they show a broad range of dysfunction, causing cognitive decline. Ironically, at a time of glucose excess, brain cells don't receive enough glucose, and because of insulin resistance, they can't use the glucose they have. Over time this leads to brain cell death, shrinking brain volume, and dementia. This explains, in part, why uncontrolled blood sugar leads to memory loss and dementia.

Here is another way to envision this process. Consider that every brain cell draws on an energy-producing factory called mitochondria. Mitochondria are like tiny, special bacteria that live within every cell in the body, and they produce energy for each cell the way a power plant produces electricity for a city, burning energy and making some exhaust in the process. Now, consider a steamship from the nineteenth century. The energy-producing area of the steamship was the furnace. A man positioned inside the furnace room would shovel coal into the furnace to produce energy to run the ship. Here the man acts as the mitochondria, making energy for the ship, the way mitochondria make energy for cells.

If you can't get food (energy) to the man shoveling the coal, he weakens, and the energy production for the whole ship decreases. The problem is that the energy from the furnace also runs the fans that ventilate the room, and as the energy drops, the exhaust builds up, and the furnace room grows smoky. The man coughs and sputters, growing weaker as his food supply dwindles even further. The smoke gets worse, no food ever arrives, and the man sickens and will eventually die. Then the ship catches fire, burns, and sinks. Yet even in the later stages, this could have been prevented. We could have gotten food to the man, restored energy flow, ventilated the room, stopped the fire, and prevented the ship from sinking.

When insulin resistance occurs, your brain cells don't get the energy they need, they don't function well, and the mitochondria malfunction and produce abnormal free radicals and inflammatory compounds (exhaust and smoke). This is the meaning of oxidative stress, the dysfunction that occurs within a cell from dirty energy production. The longer this condition persists, the more likely your brain cell function will decline, and cells will eventually die. It is, however, possible to reverse insulin resistance, restore energy flow to the brain, and regain optimal cognitive performance.

Insulin Resistance and Alzheimer's Disease

More than half of all diagnosed cases of Alzheimer's disease may be directly related to insulin resistance. Not only does insulin resistance impact energy usage, but high insulin levels appear to cause an entirely different problem as well. Keep in mind: to compensate for insulin resistance, your body makes more insulin, meaning that people with insulin resistance have elevated insulin levels. In a person with normal insulin sensitivity, their fasting insulin level is usually less than 5 μIU/mL (micro units per milliliter). When they have insulin resistance, their fasting insulin level is often over 10 and sometimes over 20 μIU/mL. As glucose levels go up and down, insulin levels also go up and down—you don't want elevated insulin levels pushing energy into cells when your blood sugar levels are low, or you'd potentially pass out and have a seizure from low blood sugar levels. Therefore, keeping insulin levels in balance is a very high priority.

Melissa Schilling, a professor at New York University, noticed that the same enzyme (insulin-degrading enzyme) that breaks down insulin is also required to break down beta-amyloid, the inflammatory protein that is present in Alzheimer's patients (in spinal fluid or brain deposits). In her 2016 research, she hypothesized that when insulin levels are elevated, much of the enzyme activity that could prevent amyloid accumulation is diverted to remove insulin instead. When people secrete too much insulin due to a poor diet, obesity, and diabetes (a triple-threat condition called hyperinsulinemia), the enzymes are too busy breaking down insulin to break down beta-amyloid, causing beta-amyloid to accumulate.

Schilling's work has raised an amazing point: more than half of all Alzheimer's disease cases in the United States are likely due to insulin resistance and hyperinsulinemia. Fortunately, both are preventable and treatable using simple lifestyle changes that are part of the Better Brain Solution. And this gives us hope: if we could reverse insulin resistance and blood sugar regulation problems, we could simultaneously eliminate up to 60 percent of all Alzheimer's cases.

The problems outlined here aren't genetic and fixed, although admittedly some people are at more risk for insulin resistance than others. Rather, they're related to how we live, eat, move, and sleep, and dozens of studies highlight the relationship between insulin resistance, pre-diabetes, diabetes, and dementia.

The Maastricht Aging Study, which followed nearly thirteen hundred individuals aged forty and over, provides startling proof of this link between out-of-control blood sugar and dementia. The subjects' cognitive functions were tested three times over the course of twelve years (at the start, after six years, and then at twelve years). Those people with baseline type 2 diabetes had a staggering 300 percent decline in their information-processing speed compared to nondiabetics. Those with diabetes requiring insulin treatment fared even worse, with a 400 percent decline.

Type 1 diabetes (or "juvenile diabetes") is what happens, most often to children, when an autoimmune response damages the cells that make insulin. These children quickly develop a life-threatening illness, get hospitalized, and are treated with injectable insulin for the rest of their lives. Ninety-five percent of all people with diabetes have what we used to call "adult onset diabetes," as it used to occur in adults who ate too many refined carbs and sugar, gained weight, and became insulin resistant, but now this problem also occurs in childhood. We've seen an epidemic rise in insulin resistant diabetes in children, so we have started calling it "type 2 diabetes."

With type 2 diabetes, as blood sugar control worsens, patients are typically treated with oral medications to initially enhance insulin sensitivity, but these drugs are effective only in the short term, perhaps for one to three years. For that reason, and because our health care system generally fails to address the underlying lifestyle issues causing the problem, most of these patients worsen over time. Eventually the combination of multiple oral medications will not provide adequate control, forcing patients to resort to injectable insulin therapy. Many of these patients eventually develop end-stage complications of diabetes, including dementia, amputations, kidney failure, blindness, heart attack, and stroke.

Such outcomes are not inevitable. I have helped thousands of type 2 diabetic patients make the lifestyle changes to restore normal sugar and insulin control and to no longer qualify for blood pressure, blood sugar, statin, and other drug therapies. The medications themselves are not harmful, as they clearly provide more benefit than harm in high-risk patients. However, as people become healthier, the risks and side effects associated with drug therapies will eventually outweigh their benefits, and people no longer qualify to use them. My patients love it when I tell them they can stop a medication because they no longer need it.

Recently, one scientist began referring to Alzheimer's disease as "type 3 diabetes." It was researcher Suzanne de la Monte, M.D., M.P.H., a physician-scientist at Brown University, who coined the term. She and her team identified Alzheimer's disease as fundamentally a metabolic disorder, where the brain is unable to use glucose, a problem related to insulin resistance. In animal studies, they demonstrated that when a drug was used to block normal insulin activity in the brain, the animals immediately developed Alzheimer's disease. The drug they used resembles nitrosamines, chemical preservatives that are common in processed food, such as deli meats and bacon (and discussed in Chapter 8 as a brain toxin). Dr. de la Monte's work underscores my point that if we want to prevent Alzheimer's disease, we need to improve the food we eat, avoid insulin resistance, and eliminate toxins from our diet.

Many other studies also have consistently proved that diabetics (type 1 and 2) are much more likely to develop dementia, especially Alzheimer's disease and vascular dementia. That insulin resistance and elevated blood sugar are connected to memory loss and dementia is now undeniable, and it's clear that you don't have to have full-blown diabetes to be affected; the earliest signs of abnormal blood sugar regulation—even mildly elevated blood sugar levels—are implicated in this disease process. The evidence is overwhelming that if we want to prevent memory loss and disability, we need to achieve better blood sugar control.

With this in mind, consider that 30 percent of all adults and 50 percent of all baby boomers have insulin resistance. This troubling fact means that a huge portion of the American population is at increased risk for our most terrifying problem, Alzheimer's disease.

Metabolic Syndrome: When Insulin Resistance Takes over the Body

So how do you know if you are developing insulin resistance? While insulin resistance in the brain leads to brain cell dysfunction and eventually brain cell death, *body-wide* insulin resistance shows other signs of dysfunction as well and is commonly called *metabolic syndrome*. It is, essentially, accelerated aging of the body, especially the heart and brain. Also known as Syndrome X and pre-diabetes, metabolic syndrome is the number one cause of heart disease and also increases your risk for weight gain, diabetes, and cancer.

Metabolic syndrome reflects the body's abnormal energy utilization and metabolism. These inner dysfunctions may be outwardly visible when you look in the mirror, since the first sign is often weight gain. In addition to an expanding waistline, your blood pressure may increase, and your cholesterol profile may worsen. After several years, metabolic syndrome progresses through insulin resistance to a high blood sugar level (a fasting glucose level of 100 mg/dL or higher—that is, milligrams of glucose per deciliter of blood) and later to a diagnosis of type 2 diabetes (a fasting glucose level of 126 mg/dL or higher).

To qualify for a diagnosis of metabolic syndrome, as I detailed in my book *Ten Years Younger,* you must meet three of five criteria, per national standards in the medical community. I include a sixth criterion at my clinic: inflammation, measured with a high-sensitivity C-reactive protein (hs-CRP) blood test, and I believe you need only three of six items on the list below. If you meet one or two of these criteria, you may not qualify for the diagnosis of metabolic syndrome, but you should consider them to be early warning signs. They may well indicate that you are at elevated risk for memory loss and heart disease. Here are the six criteria:

1. Expanding waistline (more than 40 inches in men and more than 35 inches in women)
2. High blood pressure (higher than 130/85 mm Hg)
3. High triglycerides (equal to or higher than 150 mg/dL)
4. Low HDL cholesterol (lower than 40 mg/dL for men, and lower than 50 mg/dL for women)
5. High fasting blood sugar levels (equal to or higher than 100 mg/dl—note this is often the last sign to occur)
6. Elevated inflammation (hs-CRP higher than 1), as measured by a high-sensitivity C-reactive protein blood test

Thousands of people with metabolic syndrome have been helped to reverse it permanently. Not only have published clinical trials results showed that it can be done, I have the patients to prove it as well. And the Better Brain Solution gives you the strategies to do what they've done.

Now that you understand the connection between blood sugar control and brain function, there is one more major link in the chain to look at: cardiovascular health.

The Heart-Brain Connection

Poor blood sugar control sets off a series of events that, over time, can result in metabolic syndrome and its wide-ranging and detrimental impact on the body. Abnormal blood sugar regulation, with its ability to trigger everything from insulin resistance to mild blood sugar elevation to diabetes, is the main cause of memory loss. It can also lead to obesity, high blood pressure, arterial plaque growth, inflammation, and other conditions that dangerously overtax the body's cardiovascular system, resulting in heart disease, stroke, and sudden cardiac death.

A variety of studies have shown that people with heart and cardiovascular disease are much more likely to develop dementia and Alzheimer's disease than those who do not have heart problems. For instance, among people who have had a stroke: at one year 7 percent have dementia; by three years, 21 percent have it; and by 5 years, 32 percent of stroke sufferers have dementia.

Even elevated blood pressure (130/80 mm Hg), an obvious risk factor for heart disease, increases the risk for Alzheimer's. A 2005 Kaiser Permanente study showed that those with hypertension at midlife had a 24 percent greater risk for getting Alzheimer's disease. The Honolulu-Asia Aging study found in 2000 that with even borderline high blood pressure, their subjects had a threefold increased risk for Alzheimer's disease.

We know that irrefutable evidence suggests a strong link between cardiovascular disease (CVD) and dementia, but there is also dramatic proof that we can alter that relationship. Yes, they are two different diseases—but they have the same cause and the same solution.

The landmark Rotterdam Study tracked risk factors for over ten thousand people older than age fifty-five for up to two decades. The researchers measured and analyzed levels of CVD factors for each subject, including obesity, hypertension, diabetes, cholesterol, smoking, and education. The results, including follow-up studies as well as dozens of smaller studies, have been conclusive: addressing the risk factors for CVD (which includes all forms of heart disease, including stroke) through lifestyle changes dramatically reduces a person's chances for dementia. Just one example: when you increase blood supply to your brain through exercise, you produce more brain-derived neurotrophic factors, or compounds that help to regenerate brain cells.

Researchers in this study concluded that by modifying a few CVD risk factors, 25 to 33 percent of dementias can be prevented by making changes of the type found in the Better Brain Solution. As I've said earlier, physicians like me were once told we couldn't do much to prevent or slow dementia, but now we know that's not true.

Different Diseases but the Same Risk Factors

One reason we can draw a straight line between dementia and heart disease is that their risk factors overlap. If any of the following apply to you, you may well be at high risk for both problems:

- Insulin resistance, metabolic syndrome, and diabetes
- Smoking
- Inactivity (less than thirty minutes of aerobic activity, like brisk walking, a day)
- High blood pressure
- High LDL/HDL cholesterol ratios
- Obesity
- ApoE4 genotype (commonly associated with Alzheimer's and heart disease)

In my clinic, I explain that cardiovascular risk factors and cognitive function are both related to arterial plaque growth. Arterial plaque is an important predictor of memory loss. When arterial plaque builds up in the arteries, it narrows their diameter and reduces healthy blood flow. More dangerously, softer forms of plaque stick to the arterial lining in mounds, forming lesions called atheromas that can burst and cause blood clots to form, resulting in heart attack, stroke, and sudden death.

Our clinic database contains lab results from nearly a thousand patients who have undergone cognitive testing; at the same time, we measured their arterial plaque growth, nutrient intake, fitness, body composition (fat-to-muscle ratio and body fat percentage), and more. In total, we analyzed more than one hundred markers of health and aging to compare with cognition.

To measure arterial plaque growth, I performed a test known as carotid artery intimal media thickness, or carotid IMT. This high-resolution ultrasound technique measures the thickness of the lining of the carotid artery, the vital blood conduit between the heart and the brain. For each subject, we collected at least ten images from the right and left carotid arteries, with anterior, lateral, and posterior views. The results of this comprehensive imaging were then scored, based on average artery thickness. (Carotid IMTs are not as common as cardiac catheterization, which involves the insertion of a catheter and the injection of dye to check for arterial plaque blockage. Studies have shown, however, that patients who had a catheterization and a noninvasive carotid IMT on the same day had the same test results at least 95 percent of the time.)

Out of one hundred measures of aging, the carotid IMT score turned out to be one of the *best* predictors of complex information processing. Clearly less arterial plaque is strongly connected to optimal cognitive function, while increased arterial plaque is associated with cognitive dysfunction. (Later I'll expand upon other factors that helped predict better cognitive function, including greater fitness and superior nutrient intake—especially fiber, fish oil [long chain omega-3 fats], and B vitamins.)

Before you begin the Better Brain Solution, let's get a sense of how sharp your brain is right now. No doubt you'd like to assess your brain performance and your risk for memory loss, then separate out the differences between normal brain aging and faster-than-normal loss of brain performance. Even if you fall into the latter category, just remember this encouraging fact: the realistic changes I am asking you to make will improve your brain function and help reduce your risk for memory loss and heart disease.

CHAPTER 2

How Sharp Is Your Brain?

Your brain weighs, on average, a mere three pounds, yet it controls all the senses and functions of the body. It has a memory capacity capable of holding more information than all the reference materials in your local library—an astounding accomplishment for something that weighs the equivalent of just a few books. It is capable of holding an enormous trove of knowledge.

In order to understand how to improve brain function—including sharpness—let's take a closer look at how this sophisticated organ is structured and how it works with the rest of the body. Then we'll see how your brain stacks up with a simple self-test or two, and what kind of cognitive testing and other assessments you might find valuable, particularly if you're trying to determine if what you're feeling, brain-wise, is normal aging or something else.

Brain Power: Where It Comes From

Most likely you've seen cartoonish depictions of the brain in movies—think of *Frankenstein,* or other films, with the odd-looking, rounded, rippled organ suspended in a giant jar of liquid. Or perhaps you've watched a science documentary or seen high-resolution images of an actual human brain (which does resemble Frankenstein's after all). What *is* all that squiggly, wrinkled stuff, and what does it do? Let's take a tour of the brain to answer just those questions, so set aside the images—the ones you have stored in your brain, of course.

The brain is composed of a complex network of more than 100 billion neurons (also called nerve cells). Between every pair of neurons is a point of connection, called a synapse. Information travels from synapse to synapse through chemical neurotransmitters, naturally occurring chemicals that serve as nerve system messengers, like dopamine (the feel-good chemical released during moments of pleasure) and serotonin (which can control everything from appetite to mood). Each neurotransmitter is made from a specific amino acid through a series of steps that require specific nutrients, called cofactors.

There are trillions of synapses in the brain, and the brain's speed and sharpness depend upon these biochemical connections. The messages being sent along this route can be anything from "stop eating, you're full" to "hit the brakes" to "remember to call the plumber"—virtually all our thoughts and deeds travel across these channels. Because our body's biochemistry, which we can alter with diet, keeps this neuron-synapse-neuron assembly line moving, it shouldn't be surprising that nutrition plays a substantial role in brain performance.

The human brain experiences much of its growth after birth, reaching about 80 percent of its adult size by age two. But though its physical growth may level off early on, the brain's cognitive function continues to grow and improve throughout childhood and well into adulthood. (By contrast, a chimpanzee generally reaches its cognitive function by age three or four, consistent with when it becomes self-sufficient.) Your ability to process information quickly and to remember facts improves gradually from birth until age thirty.

At our peak, the brain's total memory capacity is amazing and exceeds that of a computer. Each year after thirty, most people have a natural, gradual drop in mental speed. This is normal, but it isn't always noticeable because as we gain experience and retain memories, we make up for it with knowledge. As you age (particularly after forty), it is almost as if you have to work with a slightly slower computer, but with experience, you don't need to rely as much on that computer.

Memory and attention also decrease over time, but these functions should decline more slowly than processing speed does. Many people are capable of maintaining their memory and attention into their eighties and nineties, even if it takes them more time to access the information; the knowledge may still be in their brains—it just requires a little longer to pluck that book off the shelf, so to speak, and look up the fact. Losing memory isn't a balanced process: typically we lose the ability to recall a name or fact before we lose the ability to recognize. Hence we are likely to forget someone's name before we forget who they are.

Executive function or mental sharpness is different from memory—it is the ability to problem-solve and jump from one task to another. The better your executive function, the more complex work you can accomplish in a given amount of time. (For patients in my clinic, executive function seems to be the most important aspect of cognitive function that makes them successful in their work and personal lives; we'll look at how it impacts productivity shortly.) If your executive function is sluggish or impaired, however, your memory will underperform as well.

Brain Structure Basics

The brain and its functions can be divided into three major parts: the forebrain, the midbrain, and the hindbrain.

The hindbrain, which some scientists call the reptilian brain, is the primitive part of the brain that controls the basic "automated" body functions we don't think about every time they occur: the beating of our hearts, breathing, and blood circulation. The hindbrain, which all animals have, evolved from the brains of our earliest reptilian ancestors— hence its name.

Higher on the evolution tree is the midbrain, which regulates what we sense and controls basic instincts, such as seeking food and reproducing—aspects related to basic survival. It has a broad range of duties as it regulates motor control, hearing, vision, body temperature, thyroid and adrenal function, fertility, libido, and our wake and sleep cycles. It controls involuntary processes, such as coughing, swallowing, sneezing, and vomiting. An alligator has only a mid- and hindbrain (though at least it moved beyond its original reptilian brain). When it sees food, it eats. When it sees danger, it flees.

The midbrain doesn't compel you to think about whether the food is healthy or junk (the alligator definitely won't stop to think); it wants you to eat to avoid famine, period. The midbrain has another important responsibility: it sends us into survival mode. When we are stressed, this part of the brain tends to take over, whether we're escaping from a burning building or are sleep deprived and juggling multiple deadlines at work.

The forebrain (also called the neocortex) is what makes humans different from animals. It is responsible for processing sensory information from vision (eyes), smell (nose), sound (ears), taste (tongue), and touch (skin). The forebrain's frontal lobes allow humans to process complex information and problem-solve, while the temporal lobes hold memories and process language.

Brain Action ▶ *Body Reaction*

The neocortex also allows you to inhibit impulses. When someone puts food in front of you, this part of the brain can say, "Stop, I don't need to eat now, and I certainly don't need to eat junk." That is under normal circumstances. But when stress is introduced, the brain reacts accordingly. When you are stressed, it's as if an internal alarm goes off; blood is shunted away from the inhibitory neocortex to the midbrain so "survival mode" can kick in. For example, if a lion is chasing you, you want to divert blood flow and energy to the midbrain and hindbrain, which helps you to escape.

Diverting blood supply from the neocortex fires up your midbrain appetite center. If there is food around, unless you're running from a beast, you'll eat it. This is how chronic stress results in prolonged impulsive eating. Willpower resides in the forebrain, and you need peace and calm for willpower to overcome survival mode.

When we're really stressed out, it's easy to settle for the quick-and-easy fix, particularly if we're on the go and racing from one crisis to another. That's when we're most likely to hit the drive-through or reach for candy, pretzels, or even a "healthy" granola bar (which is likely just a candy bar with healthy-sounding packaging).

For every food action, there is a brain reaction. When we eat the wrong foods, hormonal shifts blunt our satiety—that important sense of feeling satisfied and full so that we put the fork down—and appetite-regulating hormones (like leptin and ghrelin) ultimately go haywire, which make us instantly hungry. This powerful, hormone-induced hunger message sends an alert to the midbrain ("avoid famine, store calories!"), which in turn creates cravings as blood is shunted from the forebrain to mid- and hindbrain.

Cravings win out over willpower. This is one of the reasons calorie counting is so ineffective. Eventually, the longer we are stressed, the more the midbrain will dominate over the forebrain, and we'll be overwhelmed by hunger. Now that you know what abnormal blood sugar is capable of doing to the brain, you can appreciate why managing stress is so important. (When we discuss foods to eat and to avoid, I'll focus on those that prevent hormonal swings, provide satiety, and prevent hunger, even when you follow a partial fast.)

Why We Should Diffuse Stress, the Brain Bomb

When our more thoughtful forebrain is running the show, we make healthier decisions (not just about what we eat) and are less stressed. For instance, when researchers examine MRIs that capture images of the brain during meditation, they can actually see the increased blood flow to the neocortex, a healthy circulation pattern that makes us less impulsive. When we're less impulsive, we think before we act and make better choices about how we treat our bodies. It becomes a positive feedback loop. So reducing stress and learning to manage it effectively, such as with some form of daily meditation, is an important part of the Better Brain Solution.

The male and female brains are nearly identical in structure, but certain hormones can impact behavior and even cognitive function. (I'll explore this more thoroughly in Chapter 9.) One interesting midbrain difference between men and women affects the choices we make when we're stressed. When men are stressed, the midbrain takes over to "feed and breed." They'll eat and have sex even if disaster is looming. That's because men don't have to be concerned about being pregnant, giving birth, and lactating. When women become stressed, it's yes to feed but no to breed. If a famine is coming, a woman doesn't want to become pregnant. This ancient survival mechanism has a modern application as a clear incentive for men to keep their female partners happy, not stressed.

Where Memories Come From and Where They Go

Memories begin when an experience is imprinted on the brain. That experience can range from learning how to cook or drive a car, reading a newspaper or book, meeting a person and learning their name, or going on a vacation and taking in the sights. All these experiences, great and small, are ultimately stored in our brains as memories, information that we can access at will when our executive function is working properly.

Memories are scattered in different parts of the brain. Memorized facts are typically processed first in the frontal lobe cortex and then encoded in a region of the temporal lobe called the hippocampus, which is often referred to as the brain's memory center. *Hippocampus* is the Greek word for "seahorse," so named because its structure has a seahorse-like shape.

Habits and motor skills, like riding a bicycle, are stored in the basal ganglia and putamen of the midbrain. Emotional memories, like fear of a snarling dog or joy in celebrating a special holiday, are stored in the amygdala, also in the temporal lobe and near the hippocampus. The amygdala also acts as the fight-or-flight center and, in response to a high degree of fear, can generate instantaneous unrestrained responses. In Greek, *amygdala* means "almond," and this part of the brain has an almond shape. Thus with a stroke or a head injury, different types of memories may be lost or retained, depending upon the location of the damage itself.

When you see a word (think of when you learned to read the word *cat*), you perceive the image in the back of the eye along the retina. Then information is transmitted to the midbrain, processed in the frontal lobes, and stored in the temporal lobe memory center. Thousands of neurons are involved in this type of simple task.

Imagine how many times that has happened over a lifetime, second by second, in an organ that weighs barely three pounds. Now consider the astonishing level of neuron and synapse activity that goes on in your brain when you're engaged in complicated problem solving, courtesy of your executive function. Is it any wonder that the human brain requires 20 percent of the total energy we obtain through the food we consume? (All the more reason to feed it the right food.)

Entire books have been written on brain structure, and neurologists and other brain experts train for years to learn about every nook and cranny of this complex and nuanced organ. The brain and its many functions is a fascinating topic, and I highly recommend you dive into it and learn more, if you're so inclined. Researchers are constantly uncovering new facts about neurological structure and performance.

What you've just read is by no means a comprehensive guide, but it is meant to provide you with some brain basics, so that you can better understand how lifestyle choices can impact your cognitive function, for better or worse. Now that you have a grasp on what parts of the brain control various aspects of cognitive function, let's turn to some ways to measure its performance.

Assessing Mental Sharpness

It would be wonderful if all of us could take a single test that would accurately measure brain health and cognitive function, taking into account factors like age and overall wellness, predicting problems and noting risks, and highlighting areas that require improvement. We can take blood samples, listen to the heart, perform MRIs, and do other diagnostic testing and preventive screening, but unfortunately, there is no single, fail-safe way to precisely measure normal brain function.

That is, in part, because the most common brain testing tools focus on end-stage memory loss, when it's too late to reverse damage and strengthen cognition; tools that assess greater levels of function are less standardized and are used infrequently. How best to measure brain function is a controversial topic among experts. The controversy is compounded by the fact that our current health care system focuses on diagnosing and treating diseases, not on improving brain function and performance or taking preventive measures against memory loss. Furthermore, medical insurance usually will not cover the handful of tests that do measure function.

Today the most common tool in use to detect memory loss is the Mini-Mental State Examination, known as the MMSE.

MMSE: Testing for Dementia

The Mini-Mental State Examination, used extensively in clinics and hospital settings, is essentially a thirty-point questionnaire. It is used so widely that nearly everyone in the health care field understands its scoring system. It takes only five to ten minutes to perform, and it doesn't require any fancy equipment.

The primary function of the MMSE is to screen for dementia, which turns out to be a disadvantage for some people. It is not designed to distinguish between being mentally sharp and being mentally dull, and it likely won't identify the very first signs of cognitive loss. Sample questions include

- "What is the year? Season? Date? Day? Month?"
- "Where are we now? State? County? Town/city? Hospital? Floor?"
- "Count backward from 100 by sevens." (93, 86, 79, 72, 65 . . .)
- "Repeat the phrase: 'No ifs, ands, or buts.'"

If you have an elderly parent or other relative or friend with dementia and have accompanied them on doctors' appointments, perhaps you've been with them when this type of test was administered. Given the types of questions, it's obviously most useful for screening for dementia, and in fact by the time some patients take (and sadly fail) it, they are often mentally disabled and have become dependent upon others for care.

On the 30-point MMSE scale, a score greater than 27 is generally considered normal, although it may reflect subjective cognitive impairment. Depending upon one's education, many scientists would consider a score of less than 26 or 27 as mild cognitive impairment, and a score below 23 to 25 as dementia.

There is another concern with using the MMSE. A person who is hearing-impaired or has another physical disability may score low on the MMSE, even though their cognitive function is healthy. The MMSE is not designed to account for such variables and is a guide only for dementia diagnosis. It must be combined with clinical savvy. A health-care professional should not make a diagnosis of dementia based solely on the MMSE.

Though it is widely administered—and it may well be the test you are given if you go to your own physician concerned about memory loss—the MMSE is of little value to someone experiencing the onset of reversible memory loss, or simply wanting to know *How sharp is my brain?*

The Brain Symptom Score:
Testing for Early Signs of Memory Loss

For the last decade, if a patient in my clinic has early symptoms of cognitive dysfunction, we use our own Brain Symptom Score questionnaire. It is a far less standardized tool (it hasn't been used on hundreds of thousands of patients by thousands of doctors, like the MMSE). But it aims to assess whether a person is suffering not from dementia or mild cognitive impairment but rather from cognitive dysfunction fairly early on in the process, To take our test, ask yourself the following questions.

1. Do I lose things (keys, pens, cellphone, glasses) more often?
2. Is it harder to find my car in a big parking area?
3. Is it difficult to remember a bank password and enter it, or a seven-digit phone number and dial it?
4. Do I find myself writing lists to help my memory more than I used to?
5. Am I forgetting names of movie and sports stars or other well-known figures I once knew well?
6. Is it easier to remember an event from twenty years ago than two days ago?
7. Do I have trouble dealing with everyday math problems, like reviewing personal finances, working with numbers at my job, calculating percentages for tipping, and performing household measurements?
8. Am I challenged when I have to learn a software program or assemble a piece of furniture?
9. If I'm in a meeting at work or listening to a detailed lecture, does my mind start drifting sooner than it used to?
10. When I'm working on a project, do I find it hard to get back into the groove after being interrupted by a phone call, text/e-mail, or an office visitor?

How did you do? Score your responses based on the number of questions you answered yes to.

- 0 questions: You're doing great! I'd suggest you ask yourself this battery of questions yearly.
- 1–2 questions: You're likely fine, but you should watch for further cognitive loss. Some people have never been good with names or finding their car in a large parking lot. Others may work in an environment that's chaotic beyond their control. If your company is about to be sold and everyone is constantly interrupting you with the latest gossip, it is probably difficult to return to what you were doing. Not being able to remember names, find objects, or refocus on a task isn't worrisome, unless these blips are new and worsening with time.
- 3–4 questions: This would be a cause for concern. Check in with your doctor.
- 5 or more questions: Clearly, further mental function testing guided by your doctor would be suggested.

Don't be discouraged if you scored higher than you'd hoped. The Better Brain Solution can help you improve your results over time. And if you scored zero, that's a perfect reason to preserve your cognitive function!

In addition to the Brain Symptom Score questionnaire, my clinic uses a tool called Central Nervous System Vital Signs (CNS VS). It is a computerized tool to assess memory, brain speed, attention, and executive function. It takes about thirty minutes to perform. I use it with my patients every year or two to monitor their cognitive function over time. I've occasionally repeated this test after four to six weeks when the person scored poorly and has a major medical issue such as poorly controlled blood sugar.

Another cognitive testing system that also includes brain training is BrainHQ. This system is used worldwide and its developers have published results showing an improvement in cognitive function over time.

The aim with my patients, and now with you, is to identify a drop in cognitive performance ten to twenty years before it becomes significant and to try a variety of interventions to prevent that decline. Some of my patients love the challenge of taking this test, and honestly, some of them dread it and ask to skip it. Sometimes I have to remind them that the point is to identify and prevent cognitive decline, as it becomes harder and harder to reverse the loss, and the earlier we identify the process, the easier it is to get better and prevent further loss.

Ask your physician about the CNS VS, particularly if you're concerned about your score on the test above. Medical insurance generally does not cover tests for optimal cognitive performance, but ironically testing such as I do in my clinic is often covered *only* if you have real symptoms of memory loss and a medical diagnosis for some type of cognitive dysfunction. The CNS VS test provides a detailed picture of cognitive function and is vastly more useful than the MMSE.

Unhelpful Reminders

For people with established, advanced dementia, a challenging cognitive test like the CNS VS is far too complicated. It can bring people to tears, a frustrating reminder to them of their mental decline. There is little point in subjecting a person already diagnosed with disabling memory loss to such a comprehensive test.

This brings me to another point. A person with dementia doesn't want or need to be told that they can't remember things. Such reminders from friends, family members, or caregivers may be done with the best intentions, but telling someone, "You already asked me that question—don't you remember the answer?" or "I've already told you that four times," verges on cruelty. If they truly have established cognitive impairment, there is no sense in responding this way to their condition. They may no longer be able to remember things, but at a certain fundamental level, they know that their brain function is in deep decline, and it's extremely painful for them. As my loving mother-in-law Joy once said, "I know I'm losing my memory, but I want to maintain my dignity. Please don't point out that I'm forgetting things. It's humiliating."

Normal Signs of Brain Aging
vs. Accelerated Cognitive Loss

Cognitive testing shows that after age forty, brain speed and reaction time gradually decrease. Attention and memory also typically decrease but at a slower rate. Like graying hair or perhaps weakened vision, some of this slowdown is a normal part of aging. *Accelerated* cognitive loss, however, is different.

One of the first symptoms of accelerated or advanced cognitive loss is a drop in short-term memory. You remember things from years ago clearly, but you can't quite remember what happened in a meeting one hour ago. *I was supposed to do three things when I walked out of the conference room,* you think. *First, call John . . . but what were the other two?* Sound familiar? Maybe you didn't get enough sleep last night, or you were distracted during the meeting, but if such episodes are becoming a familiar pattern, that is worrisome.

Another sign of accelerated cognitive loss is that it takes you longer to react to and process information—because your brain speed has decreased. Let's say you're driving on the highway and check your rearview mirror. You see a truck is coming up behind you at a fast speed. If your brain is working normally, you instantly know to switch lanes. But if you're experiencing cognitive loss, it takes longer for you to register the need to take immediate action and to move to the other lane—and that's a problem. On a more mundane level, perhaps you find yourself rereading a piece of information before you finally comprehend its meaning. In addition, you're slower to jump from one task to another, an ability that is a marker of executive function. If you work in an environment where you're required to do just that, accelerated cognitive loss will throw you off your game.

When a Work Slowdown Isn't on Purpose

Accelerated cognitive loss can impact job performance in a significant, quantifiable way. Take the average high-level professional who might be interrupted by a random thought, phone call, or office mate up to 120 times per day. Each time she is interrupted, it might take her, on average, an extra 15 seconds to get back to work and fully engage with her tasks. That's 15 seconds × 120 interruptions = 1,800 seconds, or 30 minutes every day, potentially lost. Now suppose she is also experiencing accelerated cognitive loss and functions only at half-speed for the first minute after being interrupted and therefore loses another 30 seconds. That's an additional 30 seconds × 120 interruptions = 3,600 seconds, or 60 minutes every day. She is losing up to 90 minutes of work time; over a week, that is practically a full eight-hour workday. Let's make sure this doesn't happen to you.

With long-term cognitive decline, brain cells are not only functioning more slowly; they are dying. Over time the brain shrinks in volume. Once it has shrunk dramatically, I don't know of any realistic way to bring it back to normal. That's why the Better Brain Solution is so important, because it gives you the tools to optimize your current performance and slow or prevent further cognitive decline.

What Kind of Testing Should You Have If You Notice Cognitive Decline?

Start by making an appointment with your own physician, who knows you and your medical history. This book can't and shouldn't try to replace that relationship, but let's focus on areas of testing that you and your doctor should consider.

Many physicians will look at standard factors that clarify your risks for developing Alzheimer's disease. To use the table, see if you have any of the conditions listed, then check to see how much they increase your risk and discuss your concerns with your doctor.

Note that one of the greatest risk factors listed here—diabetes—is also highly preventable, particularly if you follow the Better Brain Solution.

CONDITION:	RISK INCREASE COMPARED TO HEALTHY IS:
Age	At age 65, 7–10% of people have dementia At ≥65, 13% have Alzheimer's At age 80, 17–25% have dementia At ≥ 85, 40% have Alzheimer's
Elevated fasting glucose (≥100 mg/dL)	Up to a 60% greater risk (which is now 30% of the adult population and 50% of baby boomers)
Diabetes, not using insulin therapy	300% greater risk
Diabetes, using insulin therapy	400% greater risk
Hypertension (> than 140/90 mm Hg)	24% at midlife, up to 300% increased risk late in life
Tobacco use	50% greater risk for Alzheimer's
Obesity	70–100% greater risk
History of depression	Increases risk for dementia 200% in women Increases risk for dementia 400% in men
Severe head injury	450% increased risk
ApoE4 genotype	• 1 of 2 alleles increases the risk for Alzheimer's disease 3-fold (300%) • 2 of 2 alleles increases the risk for Alzheimer's disease 15-fold (1500% increase)

If you don't have any of these risk factors or signs of cognitive decline and don't need or want testing, jump ahead to Part II and get started with the plan.

If you have any of these risk factors, read on for an overview of testing that you and your doctor should consider.

A Physical Examination

When I started medical training back in the 1970s, we didn't have much ability to scan brains. We were forced to use a physical exam to determine various neurological diseases. The reality is that we can still identify a variety of neurological problems with just a detailed examination. Testing for balance, light touch sensation, vibratory sensation, fine motion and tremor, strength, and agility tells a capable physician a great deal. Such testing often will identify a critical nutrient deficiency: a decreased sense of vibration, for example, is a sign of B12 deficiency, which can cause irreversible nerve injury and memory loss. A detailed conversation—the doctor asking questions and listening to what a patient has to say, from the straightforward yes-no responses to the more nuanced answers—can also provide much helpful information.

Sadly, as the demands of our insurance industry force many physicians to see more and more patients per day, these conversations about a person's medical history and current state of mind are becoming a lost art. I love seeing only one or two patients a day and having time to chat with them and learn about their lives. Doctors can't do this when they see thirty to fifty patients per day. In many ways, I'm old school. I still like to try to figure out what might be going on by taking a detailed history and doing a comprehensive physical examination before I jump to imaging and laboratory testing.

Assessment for Depression

Depression is one of the most common medical problems that primary care providers encounter. The combination of chronically high stress levels, limited activity, a low-fat diet, and poor nutrient intake are a perfect storm for causing depressed brain function, which leads to clinical depression. (Yes, I said low-fat—and I'll explain why in Chapter 3.)

Depression can mimic the signs and symptoms of memory loss and cognitive decline, and it is a major risk factor for memory loss, increasing the risk for dementia 200 percent for women and 400 percent for men.

Certain assessment tools are very helpful, such as the Beck's Depression Inventory, which you can ask your doctor about. Asking some basic questions, such as the following, can suggest a true medical form of depression with depressed brain chemistry. If a number of these conditions are occurring every day for at least two to four weeks, that could indicate depression.

1. Do you have trouble sleeping? Can you not get to sleep or are you constantly sleepy and can't wake up?
2. Do you have trouble with concentration?
3. Do you have decreased energy and drive for exercise, sex, and work?
4. Do you have feelings of sadness and pain?
5. Do you lack enjoyment? Do you go about your daily activities and do things with others because you should, but nothing feels like fun anymore?

Depression is easily confused with memory loss, but it's not the same. Still, if it's not properly identified and effectively treated, it becomes a risk for dementia. (I'll offer recommendations for avoiding and reversing depression in Chapter 9.)

Head Injury and Dementia Risk

Just one incident of serious head trauma can increase a person's risk of Alzheimer's by 450 percent. As adults grow older, the effect of even a single traumatic brain injury is cause for concern. In one study researchers compared data from patients in their seventies and eighties who had suffered a traumatic brain injury with others who had been injured (such as a leg fracture) as a result of falling, an unfortunate but common accident among elderly people with balance issues. Those who had traumatic brain injury had a 26 percent higher risk for dementia than those who had other fall-related injuries. A broken hip, arm, or leg is difficult enough, but hitting one's head is particularly dangerous and puts cognitive function at risk. That is a compelling reason for people to maintain fitness—and balance—especially later in life.

Chronic traumatic encephalopathy (CTE) is a degenerative brain disease that eventually can lead to dementia and death. It is brought on by a history of repetitive brain trauma, including concussions, both with and without symptoms. Athletes who engage in hard contact sports taking blows to the head, such as boxers, as well as football and hockey players, have succumbed to CTE, but this disease is not limited to them. Any person who sustains repeated head trauma is at high risk for CTE. Yet just a single head injury is enough to cause concussion, which has also been linked to dementia.

If you have had one or more serious head injuries, it is essential that you take steps to protect and nourish your brain. When you discuss concerns about memory and cognitive function with your physician, make sure he or she is aware of any head trauma history, even if the injury happened years ago.

Laboratory Testing

If you aren't depressed but are having troubles with memory and cognitive function, some useful laboratory tests can identify problems that are generally treatable. If such issues are missed, some of them can result in permanent memory loss.

A chemistry profile (also called Chem 20, or CMP) blood test is a good start. If it's done while you are fasting, it will give you a fasting blood sugar (glucose) level, which is absolutely essential. Given the connection between abnormal blood sugar and dementia, you should know your own fasting blood sugar level, and I hope it is less than 95 mg/dL. This test can also identify low sodium, which impacts memory, liver and kidney disease, and other basic illnesses that impact cognition.

In addition to fasting blood sugar, if I'm assessing for cognitive decline or assessing elevated blood sugar, I will also measure a fasting insulin level, to identify people with insulin resistance who still have normal blood sugar levels. A level greater than 5 µIU/mL suggests early signs of insulin resistance, and clearly an insulin level greater than 10 µIU/mL shows signs of insulin resistance. Some laboratories don't consider insulin to be elevated until the levels exceed 20 µIU/mL, but that is for diagnosing diabetes, a disease, rather than looking for signs of insulin resistance.

Thyroid testing is essential to identify a treatable cause of cognitive dysfunction, as low thyroid function can be effectively addressed with the right medication. Most endocrinologists suggest a simple thyroid-stimulating hormone (TSH) test to assess basic thyroid function, but I'm concerned that it misses up to 20 percent of people with low thyroid function. In my clinic, for someone with cognitive dysfunction, I always include, in addition to a TSH test, free T3 and free T4 thyroid hormone levels and sometimes thyroid antibodies as well.

I always want to assess inflammation, and the easiest test is for **high-sensitivity C-reactive protein (hs-CRP)**, a marker for systemic inflammation. A major limitation is that if you have been injured or sick thirty days prior to an hs-CRP test, the results won't be valid, as hs-CRP will be appropriately elevated short term. You should be well and fully healed for at least thirty days before taking this test, to get an accurate result.

Adequate **nutrient levels** are essential for protecting brain health, but during a regular physician evaluation, nutritional needs are often not addressed, and nutrient levels are not tested. I'll discuss these specific nutrients in detail in Chapter 5, but keep in mind that vitamin D deficiency will increase your risk for memory loss. Vitamin B12 deficiency can cause serious, irreversible dementia and neurological problems. Omega-3 fatty acids are essential for proper brain function. And homocysteine is a marker for B vitamin deficiencies and predicts an increased risk for dementia.

Testing for toxins is an essential part of cognitive function testing. In particular, **lead** and **mercury** can impact brain function.

The tragic events in Flint, Michigan, made lead poisoning a national issue, not only for children but for the whole population. Even in minute quantities, lead is a brain toxin, causing permanent harm. If you live in a house or work in an office that was built prior to 1978, lead paint may have been used that can contaminate the building. Lead pipes, another common source of lead exposure, were used through the 1960s. I recommend lead testing for all children and adults who live in a home or work in an office built before 1978, especially those who have any symptoms of cognitive dysfunction. Your lead level should be zero. (Lead is discussed in more detail in Chapter 8.)

Mercury toxicity is far more common and is associated mostly with large-mouth fish intake. Rising up the food chain from plankton to tiny copepods, to shrimp, to small fish, to bigger fish, to large-mouth fish (like tuna, grouper, bass, kingfish, and swordfish), mercury levels increase exponentially. The larger and older the fish, the higher the mercury levels. Still, seafood, safely consumed, is an excellent source of brain-healthy nutrients, especially omega-3 fatty acids, and it should be a part of your diet. If you eat more than three to four servings of big-mouth fish per month, ask your doctor to measure your mercury level with a "whole blood" mercury test, not just a serum level. I'll lay out the relationship between fish consumption, mercury levels, and cognitive function in Chapter 8, including how to reduce your risk of mercury exposure.

The final laboratory testing I consider for people with cognitive dys-function is **sex hormone testing**, looking at **DHEA-S and total and free testosterone for men,** and **total testosterone, estradiol, progesterone, and DHEA for women.** Women going through menopause can have major brain fog, though it is different for every woman. Men going through andropause can have depression, anxiety, and decreased cog-nitive performance when their testosterone levels drop, and how they feel varies significantly. I'll discuss assessment and treatment issues for menopause and andropause in detail in Chapter 9.

Artery Plaque Testing (Carotid IMT)

As you know by now, brain health and cardiovascular health are strongly connected. If you are growing plaque in your arteries, your brain is likely shrinking too. In 2014, I published a paper in *The Journal of the American College of Nutrition* based on my patient database, to show how cardiovascular risk factors impact cognitive function. My coau-thors and I noted that several cardiovascular risk factors—including fitness, and dietary intake of fiber, B vitamins, and fish oil—impacted cognitive scores. By far the strongest predictor of cognitive function was carotid intimal media thickness, which can be determined through carotid IMT testing (see Chapter 1). If you are growing plaque in your arteries, your cognitive function is declining.

This test is different from the typical carotid ultrasound performed in most hospitals and clinics. A carotid Doppler test measures flow through the carotid arteries; a high-velocity flow shows signs of arterial blockage, qualifying somebody for surgery. Long before we can note this advanced state with the Doppler test, we can measure the thickness of the lining of the artery with simple ultrasound testing. No radiation or needles are involved in a carotid IMT test—just a ten-minute procedure to measure the age of arteries. The challenge is that this type of testing is considered age management, not disease testing, so typically it isn't covered by insurance. The vast majority of medical centers don't offer this type of testing, but check the resource center at www.DrMas ley.com/resources for more information on carotid IMT testing.

Fitness Testing

Aerobic fitness is one of the strongest predictors of better brain performance and executive function. The gold standard for testing aerobic fitness is to measure the maximum amount of oxygen that you can burn with peak exercise, usually on a treadmill or stationary bike. The resulting score is called your VO2max, as in maximum oxygen volume burn rate per minute per your weight in kilograms.

Much easier and more practical is to use a gym treadmill or elliptical machine to measure your metabolic equivalency (MET) level. If you belong to a gym, seek out an exercise physiologist on staff who does fitness testing and ask them to assess your maximum MET level achieved. Most people with proper training can increase their MET level by one or two points, which will decrease their risk of a cardiovascular-related death by 12.5 to 25 percent. The training also helps them improve mental sharpness and overall cognitive function.

I'll go over the best activities to improve your brain performance—those that can actually cause the memory portion of your brain to grow in size—in Chapter 6.

Sleep Study

As you age, you've likely noticed that you don't feel as sharp after a poor night's sleep. However, several other aspects of sleep also impact your mental performance, including how much time you spend in deep restorative sleep, such as REM sleep, and whether sleep apnea causes your oxygen levels to drop during the night. A lack of oxygen supply to the brain can lead to brain cell death. Clearly anyone with a history of waking up gasping during the night, having headaches in the morning, and sleeping during the day needs **testing for sleep apnea.** But most cases are not that dramatic. Key signs of sleep apnea are afternoon sleepiness, or a partner who says you stop breathing during the night. (Some people with sleep apnea are also very loud snorers because their breathing is obstructed.)

When people with poor sleep—whatever its cause—improve its quality, they see a big improvement in cognitive performance. We'll explore more sleep issues in Chapter 7. If you are considering some form of a sleep study and are on the fence, note that many of my patients were not even aware, before their testing, that they had terrible sleep!

In the past, to have a sleep assessment and check for sleep apnea, you needed to spend a night in a hospital for overnight monitoring and observation. But now a simple device can be used at home—it consists of a headband with a recording feature. (We use it at my clinic.) If you have a mild case of sleep apnea, you can wear a mandibular device— basically a fancy mouthpiece—to keep the airway open at night. For more advanced cases, we recommend treatment with a CPAP, a machine that blows pressurized air into your mouth or nose to keep the airway open. It requires overnight testing at a hospital and careful adjustments to the pressure levels to ensure the open airway is maintained.

Cognitive Testing

Computerized cognitive testing was originally designed for pharmaceutical studies that were treating such conditions as head injuries, attention-deficit hyperactivity disorder (ADHD), memory loss, or Parkinson's disease. As the databases have grown, we now have far more applications to assess cognitive function. We can use these tests to assess response to a treatment and clarify whether brain processing or memory has improved. Many tools are available—CNS VS (pages 35–36) is an example of such a test. Clinics specializing in neurocognitive testing frequently offer these tests, but they are typically not available in a primary care medical office. The website www.BrainHQ.com also offers forms of cognitive testing and training.

Structural Brain Imaging

- A simple **brain scan**, such as computed tomography (CT) or magnetic resonance imaging (MRI), looks at structure, not function. The images it produces can identify a blood clot on the brain, increased fluid in the brain, and other treatable problems. These tests are expensive, but if a person has real memory loss, the price of treatment and care becomes so astronomical that most insurance companies will cover some form of brain scan.
- **Amyloid plaque brain scans** are used primarily to assess for beta-amyloid plaque formation, which, as we have seen, is highly suggestive for Alzheimer's disease. These scans (usually not covered by insurance) have been available since 2013–14. There is a major limitation in trying to draw conclusions from amyloid screening. Thus far, drugs that block amyloid production don't seem to be working nearly as well as we had hoped and sometimes even cause harm. It may be that amyloid production is a marker for Alzheimer's disease, such as protecting the brain from an infection, but not the cause of memory loss itself. Amyloid production might even be a protective adaption by the brain to avoid loss in volume and damage.

Functional Brain Imaging

Functional brain imaging reveals how well cells in various brain regions are working by showing how actively they use glucose or oxygen. Examples include positron emission tomography (**PET**) and functional MRI (**fMRI**), which measure glucose uptake in specific regions. Radiotracers are also used to detect cellular and chemical changes linked to specific diseases, as in single photon emission computed tomography (**SPECT**). The mainstream medical community is not ready to advocate these types of functional brain testing for everyday patients, and medical insurance generally does not cover them. But a variety of clinics provide these services, and some individuals will gain tremendous insight from this type of evaluation.

Genetic Testing

Genetic factors can increase your risk for memory loss, but they don't determine whether it actually happens. Most genes are pleomorphic, meaning that lifestyle choices modify how and whether we express those genetic features. If your brain is a target, and your genes are the gun, your lifestyle is the trigger that may or may not fire the gun. Some genetic tests won't change your outcome, like testing for the dreaded Huntington's disease, which has no cure and, for the moment, no clear path to prevention. But some more common genetic testing options do have an impact and have action plans that should reduce your risk.

If you have a family history of dementia, or you are concerned about decreased cognitive function, then you should address at least two genes. The first is the ApoE gene; the second is the gene associated with converting folic acid into biologically active forms of folate.

ApoE

Apolipoprotein E (ApoE) is a gene that has consistently been associated with longevity. It is a complex plasma protein that plays an important role in cholesterol metabolism and inflammation. In humans, ApoE has three major forms: ApoE2, ApoE3, and ApoE4. All early humans and primates had the ApoE4 gene; 220,000 years ago a mutation occurred and the ApoE3 gene emerged, and 80,000 years ago the ApoE2 gene occurred. Now, only 20 percent of people have the ApoE4 gene.

Each person has two of these genes, be they a double of E2, E3, or E4 or a mixture of E2, E3, and E4. Of these three, ApoE3 is now the most common. The ApoE2 genotype is associated with people living to one hundred, and ApoE4 has been shown to be associated with age-related diseases, including heart and Alzheimer's disease. To clarify the different risk for Alzheimer's disease based upon the ApoE4 genotype, consider that:

- For 80 percent of the population with either the ApoE2 or 3 genotypes, 9 percent get Alzheimer's disease in their lifetime.

- For 75 million Americans (20 percent of the population) with a single ApoE4 gene (heterozygotes for the gene), 30 percent get Alzheimer's disease in their lifetime.
- For 7 million Americans (2–3 percent of the population) with two ApoE4 genes (homozygotes for the gene), 90 percent get Alzheimer's disease in their lifetime.

If you are among the 20 percent of the population that has an ApoE4 gene, your risk for Alzheimer's disease increases threefold. If you have two ApoE4 genes, your risk is fifteenfold higher than someone who has ApoE2 and ApoE3 genes. A single ApoE4 gene also increases the risk for heart disease by 42 percent compared to people without it.

People with a single ApoE4 gene have increased inflammation pathways to fight infections, but decreased brain and artery protection mechanisms and decreased brain repair mechanisms, so it is absolutely critical that they follow an optimal-health lifestyle, like the one outlined here. (For those with the ApoE4 gene, see Chapter 10 for tips on lowering the risk of cognitive decline.)

Genetic Methylation Testing

Methylation is a process that helps repair damaged DNA. If you can't protect your DNA with methylation, then you have an increased risk for memory loss, cancer, and heart disease.

Methylenetetrahydrofolate reductase (MTHFR) is a very important enzyme in the body, responsible for converting basic folic acid from our diets to a usable form of folate called 5-methylenetetrahydrofolate. If you don't have this enzyme, you tend to form a toxic compound, homocysteine, that is an indicator of poor methylation.

Many foods, like flour, are fortified with basic folic acid, and many supplements contain it as well. The challenge is that nearly 40 percent of people have a genetic defect and lack this special enzyme, so they cannot make this conversion.

Genetic testing can clarify whether a person has the ability to make this folate conversion. For my own patients, I always recommend a multivitamin with activated forms of folate (including adequate 5-MTHF) instead of inexpensive folic acid; the genetic testing seems less important when one is already treating for this condition. Be aware that if you are taking a standard, inexpensive multivitamin from a pharmacy or grocery store; if you have a family history of dementia; or if you're wondering if poor methylation might be a factor for you, you should discuss testing and treatment options with your doctor. (I'll clarify how to find a multivitamin with the best forms of folate in Chapter 5.)

Educating yourself about tests like these is important. At the very least, start with a baseline physical exam, and then, depending on your history, ask your doctor about the value of these other assessments.

Whatever results you may get from all those lab reports, facts, and figures, the biggest takeaway remains this: controlling blood sugar, remaining or becoming active, stopping smoking, managing stress, reversing nutrient deficiencies, and eating the right foods can prevent up to 60 percent of all dementias. And since we can't totally prevent dementia—it typically occurs at the end of life—simply delaying its onset by just five years could decrease its prevalence by nearly 50 percent.

Let's begin with my easy-to-follow Better Brain Solution, the plan that will improve your cognitive function and prevent future memory loss.

PART II

The Better Brain Solution

I n Part II, we will discuss the Better Brain Solution:

- A diet rich in brain-boosting foods
- Nutrients that fuel cognitive function
- Physical activity that reverses insulin resistance and energizes mind and body
- Stress management to calm and focus the brain

At first glance, each of the four pillars that make up the Better Brain Solution could seem to stand on its own as a smart approach to overall wellness. But they won't be as effective individually as they would be when combined, especially when it comes to brain health and preventing memory loss.

You can, for instance, improve the quality of the food you eat, but if you have unaddressed nutritional deficiencies, or if you consume all those healthy meals while sitting at your desk or lounging in front of the TV, your efforts to eat more healthfully will yield less of a lasting benefit. You may follow a perfect diet and exercise religiously, but if your stress levels are too high, you are undoing that work. You may look great on the outside, but on the inside you're hurting, and your brain health is suffering as well.

That's why the best approach to a better brain is a comprehensive one—following all four of my recommended strategies together. If that sounds like too much to tackle at once, rest assured that it is doable.

Scientists like to study one action at a time, such as a trial of fish oil supplements or a specific exercise routine, to gauge its effectiveness. In the past, researchers have criticized my programs because I prefer to use multiple interventions, simultaneously, for the greatest benefit to my patients—combining food, nutrients, exercise, and stress management tools—and it works. The program's measurable benefits include a 25 percent improvement in executive brain function. But the researchers who reviewed my results were frustrated because they couldn't pinpoint which single aspect of my program created that result. The answer: it was the *combination* of tools—not one single aspect of the program.

Memory loss is related to not just one or two risk factors, but anywhere from ten to twenty-five, which include insulin sensitivity, nutrient deficiencies, a history of brain trauma, obesity, hypertension, smoking, diabetes, inflammation, depression, poor sleep, gut issues, toxin exposures, hormone imbalances, infections (like herpes, Lyme, and Zika), and elevated cholesterol levels. Likewise, our ability to decrease these risk factors and avoid dementia rests upon pursuing multiple approaches all at once. Focusing on a sole aspect will never be as effective as treating the whole person, and numerous scientific studies have proven this to be true.

I've analyzed thousands of scientific articles that reviewed single interventions to treat dementia—everything from adding a daily workout to adding a particular supplement. Often the conclusions are the same: stand-alone strategies such as adding vitamin B12, engaging in vigorous exercise, lowering mercury levels, or following other interventions showed mixed results. Some studies showed more benefits, and others showed none. Anyone in search of a single effective treatment for memory loss might find this field of research to be confusing, frustrating, and inconclusive.

However, when intervention trials use *multiple* treatments simultaneously, the outcomes are quite different. Such trials consistently show dramatic improvements in brain function and a decrease in cognitive decline. The FINGER study from Finland, for instance, conducted from 2009 to 2011, followed more than 2,600 individuals between the ages of sixty and seventy-seven, who had risk factors for heart disease and/or signs of early cognitive decline. In this randomized clinical trial, half the subjects were in a control group: they were given general health advice but no prescribed changes to their lifestyle. The other half were assigned to an intervention combining a Mediterranean-style diet (plant-based meals flavored with fresh herbs and spices; healthy fats like olive oil, nuts, and seeds; and small portions of animal protein—similar to what I recommend in the Better Brain Solution), exercise, cognitive training, and cardiovascular disease risk reduction.

Those in the multi-therapy intervention group showed improved baseline scores on overall cognitive function, and their cognitive decline was slowed. Also heartening was that the dropout rate was low, despite the researchers' initial concern. Combining multiple interventions seemed to improve compliance—perhaps because the men and women making these changes felt consistently better and were motivated to stick with it.

For those with early Alzheimer's disease, there is now hope that a multidimensional treatment plan will help them regain some lost function. Dale Bredesen, M.D., a professor of neurology and an expert on neurodegenerative disease, has described how a comprehensive program with up to fifteen to twenty-five lifestyle-focused interventions all at once, using nutritional supplements, brain-nourishing foods, blood sugar control, brain training, hormone therapies, and proper sleep, can help people with early Alzheimer's. He enrolled ten patients in his program, and nine of the ten displayed improvement in cognition within three to six months; the one failure was a patient with advanced Alzheimer's. Six of the patients, when they began Dr. Bredesen's program, had had to discontinue working or were struggling with their jobs; by the end, all were able to return to work or to continue working with improved performance. The improvements have been sustained, and two and a half years after the initial treatment, each person showed ongoing improvement, and his success with other patients continues to grow.

The nonprofit Alzheimer's Association, a global organization dedicated to Alzheimer's prevention, care, and research, has looked at the latest studies and science for multiple interventions, such as regular physical activity combined with the prevention/management of diabetes and obesity and cognitive training. It concluded that a varied approach shows the most promise in reducing the risk of dementia and improving brain function. The association also endorses food choices that are heart-healthy and beneficial to the brain, and advocates following a Mediterranean diet—recommendations consistent with the 12 Smart Foods discussed in Chapter 3.

Step by Step to a Better Brain: The Foundation

1. **Food** is the first pillar of the Better Brain Solution. Admittedly it's my favorite topic, as I love good food, but it's also of major importance for brain health. (In fact, the next two chapters are devoted to food and diet.) My focus is on adding—rather than taking away—beneficial, great-

tasting foods. I have made it easy for you to incorporate these changes into your daily life, no matter how busy you are or who else may be at your dinner table. Everyone will benefit from eating this way.

2. The second pillar is **nutrients**. Your diet will be adjusted for better brain health, but some specific key nutrients can be added to ensure you are getting everything you need.

3. **Exercise** is the third pillar. Physical activity benefits the heart, but it's also crucial when it comes to preventing insulin resistance and helping the brain grow rather than shrink. When you understand the powerful cognition-enhancing benefits of physical activity and you feel the amazing results, you will get—and stay—motivated!

4. The last pillar is **stress management**, which is important for keeping your brain young. Managing stress prevents memory loss and improves cognitive performance. It helps you regulate the stress hormone cortisol. From getting better sleep, to maintaining supportive relationships, to challenging yourself mentally, there are many pleasurable and simple paths to combating stress.

There is also a chapter on toxins—those substances that can be detrimental to your brain, from environmental hazards to everyday things that you may be exposed to; and a chapter on tools to improve your mood, with a special look at how hormonal imbalances—for both women and men—can impact cognitive function and be corrected. A final chapter features great-tasting recipes you can prepare for yourself and your whole family or guests.

So that everyone can use the Better Brain Solution, I have created three leveled steps for each of the four pillars, from easiest to hardest.

- Step 1 is essential and nonnegotiable for protecting your brain against memory loss.
- Step 2 reinforces Step 1, helping you reach optimal blood sugar levels and slow the cognitive decline that comes with normal aging.
- Step 3 is recommended for those most at risk for dementia and Alzheimer's.

Take food, for example, to see how the steps work. Step 1 involves adding certain foods to your diet; in Step 2, you'll replace certain foods with those that specifically help with blood sugar control. Step 3 offers advanced strategies like partial intermittent fasting—not easy but, for those who are most in need of blood sugar control, highly effective. For some of you, the first two steps may be all you need.

Work on all four pillars simultaneously—don't wait until you "master" food before you move on to adding nutrients, exercise, and stress management. Everyone is on a different timetable. Some of you may be able to get through the first two steps for each pillar within a few weeks, but for others it can take longer. The moment you begin to make even the simplest of changes, you are starting the process of saving your brain and feeling better each day—in mind, body, and soul. This is your opportunity to be mentally sharper and protect your health for years to come. Don't overthink it—just turn the page to get started.

CHAPTER 3

Boost Your Brain with 12 Smart Foods

P erhaps when you were in your teens and twenties, you rarely cooked and instead lived "off the land"—grabbing food on the run (even from drive-throughs) and consuming dorm cafeteria fare or whatever you could microwave. Despite making these poor food choices, you may have powered through whatever you were facing, whether it was a final exam, an athletic event, or early years at a first job. Over time you may have realized that you didn't perform well after eating junk. The pounds around your waistline started adding up, and you wanted to look and feel better. Perhaps you stopped eating fast food daily. You started to grocery-shop. You learned how to use the stove. Your behaviors changed and matured—in part, because your body was beginning to revolt!

You got a message from your brain, an old saying that turned out to be true: *You are what you eat.* When you eat well, you perform well, mentally and physically. When you eat poorly, you can't think sharply, and your energy plummets.

Whether your current diet is fairly healthy or in need of an upgrade, if you want to improve your brain performance and halt memory loss, you will benefit tremendously from eating the 12 Smart Foods. These heart-healthy foods help control blood sugar, the key to a better brain, and can easily form the basis of flavorful, nutrient-rich meals and snacks. Study after study, including results from my own clinic, has found that these foods are most closely associated with improved cognitive function.

Step 1: Aim to Eat These Foods Every Day

1. Green leafy vegetables
2. Other vegetables (except potatoes)
3. Omega-3-rich seafood (or a long-chain omega-3 supplement)
4. Olive oil and other healthy cooking oils
5. Nuts and other healthy fats
6. Berries and cherries
7. Cocoa and dark chocolate
8. Caffeine sources (green tea and coffee)
9. Red wine
10. Herbs and spices
11. Beans
12. Fermented foods

Ideally, you should eat each of these foods daily, but you may have good reasons for saying no to some of them. You may be allergic to dairy or tree nuts, or you may not tolerate beans well. Perhaps you have an aversion to the taste and smell of wild salmon and sardines. You may not like coffee or drink alcohol. The point is that you don't have to eat from all these groups every day, but try to **eat as many of these foods as you enjoy and can realistically fit into your lifestyle.**

1. Green Leafy Vegetables

If you want a younger brain, eat your greens (spinach, kale, broccoli, Brussels sprouts, Swiss chard).

Eating **one cup of green leafy vegetables** every day will make you, on average, eleven years physiologically younger than someone who skips them. These delicious greens are packed with fiber, vitamin K, folate, potassium, flavonoids (antioxidant and anti-inflammatory compounds), and carotenoids (valuable plant pigments). They decrease inflammation system-wide, and because they provide fiber with little to no sugar, they improve blood sugar control. Green leafy veggies are fantastic for your brain, arteries, bones, and waistline.

Plants create pigments (chemical compounds characterized by specific colors) in part to protect themselves from the damaging ultraviolet rays of the sun. When we consume these pigments, they offer us protective benefits that help decrease the biochemical process of oxidation (which results in aging) within our cells.

2. Other Vegetables (except potatoes)

Beyond leafy greens, other rainbow-colored vegetables are loaded with protective pigments (particularly nitrate-rich beets, as well as carrots, fennel, artichokes, peppers of all colors, red and yellow tomatoes, butternut squash, and more). Eating more of them will slow cellular aging (including brain cells), improve blood pressure, enhance cholesterol and blood sugar profiles, lower cancer risk, and improve gastrointestinal function. They are also good for your skin and bones. Aim to **eat at least 3 cups of vegetables** every day. (The recipes in Chapter 10 will make that easy.)

Plant *nitrates* are converted to *nitrites,* which form nitric oxide, the master regulator of blood flow control and artery inflammation. So vegetables rich in nitrates improve blood pressure and blood flow, boost aerobic athletic performance, and increase blood flow to the neocortex, which enhances cognitive performance. Vegetables that are particularly packed with nitrates include beets, arugula (also called rocket), spinach, celery, and most forms of lettuce. (An important note on terminology: Vegetable-based nitrates are not the same as nitrosamines, which are also commonly called nitrates and are added to deli meats and bacon to extend their shelf life. As I'll explain in Chapter 8, nitrosamines are toxins that can give you cancer and Alzheimer's disease, so don't confuse them.)

Fresh-pressed vegetable juices are popular, but if they are made with fruits (or with added sugar), they are not good choices. High-quality green juices made from pure, organic vegetables are a good source of vitamins and minerals, but whole vegetables are preferable because of their superior fiber content. Freshly prepared juices have higher nutrient content than bottled juices that are weeks or months old. Enjoy fresh-pressed, vegetable-only juices, but do not consider them a substitute for whole vegetables.

Beets Get Your Blood Pumping (in more ways than one)

Aphrodite, the Greek goddess of love, ate beets to increase her beauty and sexual appeal—which is why they came to be known as an aphrodisiac. The Romans agreed and ate them before going to battle and to the bedroom. (They even depicted beets in frescoes decorating the walls of a brothel preserved in Pompeii.) There is more to the secret potent power of beets than myth and legend; there is science. Beets are a particularly rich source of nitrates, and they are excellent for improving blood pressure and blood flow, including the all-important blood flow required for erectile function. I recommend them to my patients to enhance blood pressure as well as sexual function.

Savvy athletes, particularly elite runners and cyclists, binge on beet extract drinks to up their aerobic performance. In the future, beet juice and beet extract beverages could overshadow popular sports drinks at high-level sporting events! For non-athletes, beet juice provides more sugar than most people need, and the average person should rely on eating beets or taking more expensive beet extracts that don't contain sugar.

As for brain function, the news is very promising. Beets are reported to increase blood flow to the neocortex and have the potential to offset stressful events that shunt blood flow to the midbrain, the survival center. In a study performed in Australia, researchers randomly chose forty men and women for a placebo group and a group that consumed beet juice with 5.5 mmol of nitrate. Those in the nitrate-enriched group had a significant improvement in cerebral blood flow and modestly enhanced cognitive performance.

As generations of mothers have said, eat your beets! Try them roasted and tossed with fresh spinach, with a bit of organic goat cheese and walnuts. (See the recipes on pages 295 and 301.)

3. Omega-3-Rich Seafood (or a long-chain omega-3 supplement)

For more than 100,000 years, humans have eaten cold-water seafood from rivers, lakes, and oceans. Cold-water fish, shellfish, and seaweed have been an integral part of our nutrient and protein intake. One distinctive nutrient that comes uniquely from seafood, including fish, shellfish, and the algae and plankton they consume, is long-chain omega-3 fats. Studies in humans have shown that greater long-chain omega-3 intake correlates with better brain function, reduced risk for dementia, lower beta-amyloid levels, higher total brain and hippocampal volume, and lower carotid IMT scores. Based on this evidence, I recommend that you eat **a five-ounce serving of omega-3-rich seafood at least twice a week, or take a high-quality fish oil supplement.** I personally eat at least two to three servings of wild salmon or sardines each week, plus I take 1,000 mg of eicosapentaenoic acid (EPA) and docosahexaenoic acid (DHA) daily. (For more information on fish oil supplements, see Chapter 5.)

Like humans, fish can't produce these essential omega-3 fatty nutrients themselves, but plankton and algae can. Plankton and algae manufacture these highly flexible fats so that their cell walls remain supple when exposed to cold water. Mussels, oysters, and shrimp consume plankton and store more omega-3 fats, little fish eat the shrimp, and bigger and bigger fish consume smaller fish, accumulating these essential fats. Typically, the colder the water and the higher a species is on the food chain, the greater its omega-3 content.

There are different kinds of omega-3 fats, characterized by the length of their molecular "chain"—short, medium, or long. Medium-chain omega-3 fats come from land plants and are not the same as long-chain omega-3 fats from cold-water fish, although they are frequently marketed as the same substance. Medium-chain omega-3 fat sources—such as flaxseeds, soy products, and walnuts—are healthy, but the fats do not have the same anti-inflammatory properties and don't prevent cardiac arrhythmias. Nor are they concentrated in the brain, as long-chain omega-3 fats are. This last point is of particular importance with regard to brain health.

The brain consists mostly of fat, and nearly 40 percent of it is in the form of long-chain omega-3s. Most researchers estimate that we can convert 2 to 7 percent of medium-chain omega-3 fats into long-chain omega-3 forms, but that isn't nearly enough to meet what is recommended. The majority of health benefits related to omega-3 fats come solely from two long-chain sources.

The most studied and important long-chain omega-3 fats are DHA and EPA. DHA has more anti-inflammatory and triglyceride-lowering capacity than EPA, but both DHA and EPA are beneficial, and both forms occur in natural fish oil.

If you are a vegetarian and don't consume shellfish or fish, seaweed food sources have the same long-chain omega-3s. You will need to have a seaweed salad several times per week, or take a seaweed source of DHA, to meet your long-chain omega-3 needs.

If you do choose to supplement instead of eating seafood for omega-3, you should be aware that in most studies, eating fish consistently provides more benefits than supplements alone, though it is unclear why. It could be that fish provide protein as well as important minerals like selenium, or that the supplement quality is inferior to the omega-3 fats in fish.

In Chapter 5, I will tell you more about how to choose carefully from among the variety of fish oil supplements currently on the market, as well as how to choose a supplement with the right ratio of DHA to EPA. Much of what is mass-marketed and sold in drugstores or big-box chains is rancid (making it illegal in most European countries) and may be harmful to your health. Higher-quality pure supplements have been shown to benefit those with mild cognitive impairment and heart disease in multiple randomized clinical studies. (It can't be emphasized enough that quality matters when it comes to fish oil—and all other—supplements.)

Finally, the type of fish you eat matters. Total intake is less important than the variety of fish. **Choose fatty cold-water fish for maximum long-chain omega-3s**—think salmon and sardines, as opposed to white fish such as cod, grouper, or tilapia. There is nothing wrong with those varieties if they're responsibly sourced, but when it comes to omega-3 content, fatty cold-water fish are superior. Wild-caught usually contain more omega-3s than farm-raised and are less worrisome with regard to mercury and pesticide levels. (For a discussion of fish and mercury, a brain toxin, see Chapter 8.) In addition to salmon and sardines, excellent sources of long-chain omega-3 fats are herring, anchovies, mussels, oysters, sole/flounder, and trout.

If you're looking for another reason to serve fish to your family—

particularly to your children or grandchildren—keep this in mind: both adults and children experience cognitive benefits from consuming long-chain omega-3s. The lower the blood level of these special fats noted in children, the greater the benefit from consuming them—and children appear to benefit more from consuming omega-3 fats than adults. It's never too early to start protecting the brain.

4. Olive Oil and Other Healthy Cooking Oils

Olive Oil

Olive oil has been a culinary star for thousands of years, adding an irresistible layer of flavor to food. It's a staple in the Mediterranean diet—famous for decreasing the risk of stroke and heart attack and improving cholesterol profile—plus it's packed with antioxidant and anti-inflammatory compounds. Most people have heard about its heart-healthy attributes, but it's also well documented that people who consume more olive oil have lower rates of cognitive decline and better brain function. For this reason, I recommend **one or more tablespoons a day of extra virgin olive oil.**

The acclaimed Predimed-Navarra study, conducted in Spain, compared the health benefits of a standard low-fat diet with those of a Mediterranean-style diet featuring liberal amounts of olive oil (and is considered conclusive). It was designed to assess the impact of these diets on heart disease outcomes. The randomized trial assessed 522 participants for cognitive function with the Mini-Mental State Examination and a drawing test. Not only did the participants who followed the Mediterranean diet have fewer heart attacks and strokes, their brain health also improved. After 6.5 years of follow-up, more subjects in the low-fat diet group developed mild cognitive impairment and dementia than in the olive-oil-consuming group. Further, those who ate extra olive oil had higher cognitive scores than the low-fat eaters.

Like other foods that have developed well-deserved reputations for their health benefits, olive oil has become so popular that the market is now flooded with a confusing array of options, many of them bearing no resemblance to the genuine olive oil that is at the core of the true Mediterranean diet. Perhaps the biggest recent problem is that distributors are diluting or adulterating it with less healthy oils such as rapeseed or soybean oil. Make sure you buy your olive oil from a reliable vendor.

The most nutritious form of olive oil is **extra virgin olive oil**, the oil obtained from initially crushing the olives without damaging heat or chemicals. **Virgin olive oil** is obtained from crushing the olives again. Regular processed **olive oil**—which does not include the words *extra virgin* or *virgin* on the label—may be produced with heat or chemicals to pull out additional oil from the olives, processes that commonly damage the oil. That's why extra virgin and virgin olive oil are preferable.

Good olive oil is not inexpensive, but it's well worth it. If you are planning to cook with it, though, be aware of its smoke point, the temperature at which both flavor and nutrient value begin to degrade. Heat-damaged oils can also become oxidized and pro-inflammatory, undoing all the inherent health benefits. Extra virgin olive oil has a smoke point of 400°F, too low for most cooking, which is typically medium-high heat (425–475°F). Virgin olive oil will tolerate medium-high heat and is a good choice for most cooking. The difficulty is finding virgin olive oil, as most stores only carry extra virgin olive oil or regular processed olive oil.

I use extra virgin olive oil for salads, dressings, and low-heat cooking. I cook fish and vegetables with virgin olive oil at medium-high heat, not higher. Alternatively, you can use a high-heat stable oil, such as avocado oil, for the initial cooking, then reduce the heat to simmer and add extra virgin olive oil—providing flavor and nutrient value.

Other Healthy Cooking Oils

I've switched to using **avocado oil** for most of my medium-high-heat or high-heat cooking, which gives that sear effect to protein and vegetables. It has a pleasant neutral flavor and a high smoke point of 520°F. It is loaded with healthy monounsaturated fats. And it isn't packed with pesticides, unlike many grain and seed oils.

Nut oils are another solid choice for cooking. In particular, I like cooking with **almond oil** (smoke point 430°F) and **pecan oil** (smoke point 470°F); both have a light, nutty flavor. (For more information on cooking fats and oils, see my website, www.DrMasley.com.) As part of the Better Brain Solution, you can safely consume **a tablespoon a day of heat-stable cooking oil** in addition to olive oil.

There is a widespread myth that coconut oil is great for high-heat cooking, but in fact this fat—which can be beneficial for brain health—has a relatively low smoke point, at 350°F (considered medium-low for cooking). Heating the oil past 350°F damages its delicate fatty acids, converting it into a partially hydrogenated oil—the worst of all cooking oils. The scientific reality is that coconut oil should not be heated beyond medium-low heat.

Partially hydrogenated oils were designed by the food industry to extend the shelf life of food, but they will shorten your life if you consume them. For years they were packed into almost everything we ate (as old-fashioned margarine, Crisco, and the like). They are still commonly found in processed foods and baked goods. Consuming partially hydrogenated fats will worsen insulin resistance and cholesterol profiles, increase cancer risk, and accelerate memory loss. Avoid them.

5. Nuts and Other Healthy Fats

Nuts are back. After years of shying away from nuts while we overemphasized low-fat eating, we've restored their role as a healthy dietary fat. Nearly every study to assess the impact of nuts on health is positive. Nuts improve cholesterol and blood sugar profiles and curb hunger as they help with weight loss. One study showed that eating two ounces of almonds as a pre-dinner snack (about two handfuls) suppressed appetite and total calorie intake dropped; subjects who were asked to eat more almonds lost more weight than those who did not consume nuts. It is a myth that nuts are "fattening," a reputation they have because they are not a low-calorie food, but their ability to suppress hunger, plus their multiple health benefits, makes their calorie intake worthwhile.

The landmark Predimed-Navarra study (mentioned on page 64) followed subjects who were randomized to consume extra olive oil and more nuts, or to follow a low-fat diet. Those who ate two or more ounces of nuts (or olive oil) for 6.5 years had fewer heart attacks and strokes, lower rates of mild cognitive impairment and dementia, and better cognitive testing scores than those who followed the low-fat diet. Nuts are rich in fiber and smart fats. Since your brain is approximately 60 percent fat, you need good fat in your diet to nourish it, and nuts are one of the most brain-nourishing choices you can make.

Enjoy nuts as a snack, or chop and toss them in a salad. Put nut butters, such as almond butter, in a smoothie, and used slivered nuts as a garnish on a variety of dishes. They add flavor, a pleasant crunchy texture, and a powerful load of nutrients with each serving. Aim to enjoy **one or two handfuls (1–2 ounces) of nuts** every day. My favorite nuts, those with proven benefits, are **almonds, pistachios, pecans, hazelnuts, walnuts,** and **macadamias.** (You don't see peanuts in this line-up because peanuts are a legume—technically not a nut at all—and are, gram for gram, higher in omega-6 fats than nuts like almonds. In addition, for people with food allergies, peanuts are high on the allergen list. For those who eat enough long-chain omega-3 fats, peanuts can be a healthy, satisfying snack in moderation, but they don't have the same cognitive benefits as nuts.)

In a study of healthy college students on the campus of Andrews University in Michigan, researchers assessed the impact of daily walnut intake in 273 subjects during eight weeks. Students ate banana bread with or without walnuts; the group that ate the nuts showed a modest short-term improvement in reasoning, although without any improvement in memory. Walnuts in particular were selected as they are high in alpha linolenic acid (a building block for forming omega-3 fats), fiber, folate, vitamin E, and polyphenol antioxidants. The authors of the study think people with cognitive impairment might even have greater benefits than the students, though that has yet to be studied and confirmed.

Avocados are another of my favorite high-fat foods. They are loaded with fiber, potassium, and monounsaturated fats, and they have a delicate taste. Enjoy them a few times a week sliced into salads. Try mixing chunks of avocado with chickpeas, cucumbers, tomatoes, and shrimp, dressed with olive oil and lemon juice, for a refreshing and satisfying lunch or dinner. (See the recipes in Chapter 10 for more ways to incorporate healthy fats into your meals and snacks.)

6. Berries and Cherries

Many flavonoids, but especially blue, purple, and red plant pigments (anthocyanins) are associated with increased cerebral blood flow and a lower rate of cognitive decline. Berries and cherries are high in flavonoids as well as fiber. They satisfy a taste for sweetness, but without the damaging effects of increasing blood sugar levels, plus they reduce both oxidation and inflammation.

In particular, blueberries have been shown to improve cognition and to slow cognitive decline. Feeding children blueberry-rich meals improves memory and information processing, and older adults showed improved cognitive function after consuming blueberries daily for twelve weeks. Scientists have tried to clarify the mechanism in berries that improves brain function. In addition to their obvious anti-oxidant and anti-inflammatory properties, blueberries have been shown to reduce the production of beta-amyloid, the protein associated with Alzheimer's disease.

Enjoy one half to one cup of cherries or berries every day. The fresh ones are delectable, when you can get them in season, but frozen varieties are wonderfully convenient and equally beneficial.

7. Cocoa and Dark Chocolate

Another delicious source of dietary flavonoids is cocoa and dark chocolate. With functional MRI brain imaging, we can actually see how cocoa intake improves cerebral blood flow, in particular to the memory center of the brain, the hippocampus.

For years, I've recommended **daily cocoa or dark chocolate**, as it improves blood pressure levels as well as insulin sensitivity, and it decreases the oxidation of cholesterol into artery plaque. More recent research has also shown that eight weeks of daily cocoa intake improved cognitive testing results in older adults, especially for those with early cognitive decline. Subjects in this study drank about one cup of unsweetened cocoa daily. (If you need your cocoa at least slightly sweetened to consume it, consider adding stevia or xylitol.)

Dark, unprocessed cocoa will contain up to 10 percent of its weight as flavonoids. Be aware that Dutch processing (chemical processing by manufacturers to reduce the perceived harshness or acidity of cocoa) reduces flavonoid content. Studies measuring the benefits of cocoa for brain function carefully selected cocoa brands that provided at least 375–500 mg of cocoa flavonoids per serving, although smaller dosages still provided some benefit. (Look for brands labeled "natural" or "non-alkalized" to ensure maximum flavonoid content.)

When it comes to selecting chocolate for brain benefits, don't confuse milk chocolate with dark chocolate. A chocolate must contain at least 70 to 80 percent cocoa to qualify as what I'd call dark chocolate. Although some may worry that consuming chocolate will worsen blood sugar control, at least the Physicians' Health Study (which followed more than eighteen thousand physicians and dentists for more than nine years) found that eating more dark chocolate was associated with a reduced risk for developing diabetes, so something about dark chocolate helps with blood sugar and insulin regulation as well.

A tablespoon of dark, unprocessed cocoa powder has only twelve calories. Here are a few ways I get my daily chocolate brain boost. I recommend **one or two ounces of dark chocolate or two tablespoons of dark, unprocessed cocoa powder per day.**

- Add 1 tablespoon of cocoa powder to each of two cups of coffee each morning. This is my version of a mocha for breakfast.
- Add 1 tablespoon of cocoa powder to a smoothie. Frozen cherries, almond milk, kefir, protein powder, and cocoa powder are awesome in a smoothie and terrific for your brain, too. (See the basic smoothie recipe on page 255.)
- Consume 1–2 ounces of dark chocolate after dinner.
- Melt and drizzle dark chocolate over berries, pear slices, or other fruit and nuts, allow to cool, and enjoy. (See recipe on page 309.)

To achieve the benefits, noted in studies on cognitive function, from eating dark chocolate instead of cocoa, you would need to eat at least one or two ounces of dark chocolate, about half a typical dark chocolate bar. But if you like dark chocolate, it's not so bad, right?

8. Caffeine Sources (Coffee and Green Tea)

Over the last decade researchers have concluded that caffeine consumption from coffee and tea is harmless at levels of 200 mg in one sitting (around two and a half cups of coffee) or 400 mg daily (around four or five cups of coffee during the course of the day). Note: Throughout this section, I refer to eight-ounce cups of coffee or tea—not to smaller cups or to a double espresso from the local coffee bar.

Caffeine sources (tea and coffee, as well as caffeine tablets) have several positive actions on the brain in healthy people. Caffeine increases information processing, alertness, and concentration, and in some people it enhances mood and limits depression. It also enhances the effect of drugs used to treat migraines. Lifelong coffee/caffeine consumption has been associated with lower rates of cognitive decline and reduced risk of developing Parkinson's and Alzheimer's diseases. However, for people with mild cognitive impairment, adding caffeine in tablet form has almost no benefit, meaning the benefits of caffeine may not apply to people with established early memory loss. Long-term consumption appears to be protective, and benefits may take time to have an impact.

Coffee

Although most studies have shown that coffee is good for your brain, there has been some debate about the ideal intake, and about whether the benefit is from caffeine itself or from the flavonoid pigments in the coffee. When researchers analyzed several studies, with a total of more than 34,000 participants, comparing coffee intake with cognitive disorders (mild cognitive impairment, Alzheimer's disease, and dementia), they noticed a J-shaped-curve relationship between coffee consumption and the risk of developing memory loss. On the J-shaped curve, the lowest risk was in people who drank one or two cups per day, which was better than those who drank no coffee, or those who drank more. And in Japan, a study with over 23,000 adults older than age sixty-five showed a 20 to 30 percent reduction in advanced dementia in those who consumed two to four cups of coffee daily.

Several studies have shown that women display less cognitive decline than men as a result of consuming coffee. (Even decaf coffee has been shown to improve cognitive function and mood in men and women, so that cup of decaf can have some benefits, too.) If you like drinking coffee, enjoy it—**about two cups per day is the right amount.**

If you're also a tea drinker, don't exceed more than two cups of coffee and two cups of tea per day, unless the additional beverages are decaf. (If you're concerned about caffeine jitters and wondering why coffee-drinking affects people differently, see the box "That Caffeine Buzz—Is It Good for You?")

Tea

As promising as the science is linking coffee and brain benefits, tea looks even better. Tea provides flavonoids, caffeine, and L-theanine, an amino acid that helps cognition. Over decades, tea drinkers consistently show less cognitive decline than non-tea consumers, and as with coffee, women appear to benefit more than men.

In particular, the L-theanine in tea has special cognitive benefits. Supplied in capsule form, it has been shown to improve mental function and help achieve a state of calm, without the jitteriness that some people experience with caffeine. For millennia, monks have consumed tea while meditating for greater focus and clarity. In one study, researchers combined 97 mg of L-theanine and 40 mg of caffeine in a single tablet for one group of subjects and gave a placebo to another group. Those who took the combo showed a significant improvement in cognitive accuracy during task switching, an improvement in alertness, and less self-reported fatigue.

Getting this amount of caffeine should be easy, as a typical cup of tea has 25–35 mg and a cup of coffee has 60 mg. The challenge might be in getting this amount (close to 100 mg) of L-theanine without a supplement. **Two cups of matcha green tea** will do it, as matcha has 46 mg of L-theanine per cup. You would need to drink nearly **four cups of black tea** (which has 25 mg per cup) to get the right amount. With **regular green tea**, it would be hard to achieve—it has only 8 mg of L-theanine per cup, so you'd need more than twelve cups to get L-theanine's benefits. The challenge with green tea is that when a cup from a tea bag is brewed, most of the antioxidant capacity and L-theanine don't get into the tea; they are discarded with the solids in the tea bag. Not only is matcha green traditionally grown in the shade, which increases the leaves' L-theanine production, but matcha is stone-ground into powder, allowing the antioxidants and L-theanine to dissolve into the tea liquid far more effectively.

If you are going to choose green tea over coffee, choose matcha to get 500 percent more antioxidant and L-theanine benefits. Matcha has a similar amount of caffeine as other teas, but only about 25–30 mg, which is half that found in a standard cup of coffee.

If you happen to avoid caffeine altogether, you will still benefit from consuming decaf tea (which has L-theanine) and decaf coffee (which has flavonoid pigments), as their benefit is only partly related to the caffeine. Unfortunately, if you are an herbal tea drinker, any benefits relating to cognitive function or the prevention of memory loss are unknown. However, many herbal teas have antioxidant and/or anti-inflammatory properties, and drinking them will likely help lower the risk for all forms of neurodegenerative conditions, including Alzheimer's disease.

That Caffeine Buzz—Is It Good for You?

Do you need to drink at least two cups of coffee before you're firing on all cylinders, or are you wired after just one? People metabolize caffeine differently. About half the population are "fast" caffeine metabolizers, meaning their caffeine blood levels naturally decrease promptly after consuming their coffee or tea. The other half are "slow" metabolizers—their caffeine blood levels jump and stay high longer after consumption. How you break down caffeine is a genetic trait and can be measured with genetic testing—or you may know simply based on how coffee or tea impacts you. (I like drinking coffee and feel lucky to be a fast metabolizer.)

When scientists studied the impact of caffeine consumption on heart disease risk, they noticed that in the whole population, consuming zero to three cups of coffee daily had no cardiac risk, but consuming four cups or more increased the risk by 30 percent. Yet when they controlled the analysis for caffeine metabolism, the results looked very different. Fast metabolizers who consume one or two cups per day have less heart disease risk than those who consume no coffee. (Those flavonoid pigments in coffee are good for you.) They had to consume more than four cups daily to show even a small risk. Fast metabolizers who consumed two to four cups of coffee per day also had better blood pressure and blood sugar control than non-coffee drinkers.

The slow caffeine metabolizers' results are eye-opening, as spikes in blood caffeine levels that persist are a concern. Slow metabolizers who consume four or more cups of coffee daily have a 400 percent greater risk for a cardiovascular event. Slow metabolizers do fine with one or two cups per day, but clearly they should not exceed a second cup. Not only do they show an increased risk for cardiovascular events, but the extra coffee increases their blood pressure and blood sugar levels as well.

Caffeinated beverages may disturb sleep and cause insomnia, especially for slow caffeine metabolizers. It may also raise anxiety in highly sensitive people. If caffeine impacts your sleep or anxiety, avoid it. Caffeine does not seem to lead to classic dependence, although some people experience withdrawal headaches for a few days when they suddenly stop caffeine intake, which feel much like an intense migraine. If you drink coffee or tea regularly and want to assess how you would feel without it, I suggest you wean slowly and stop your intake over a couple of weeks, not all at once.

If you are not sensitive to caffeine, then a daily coffee and/ or tea intake can be part of a healthy diet for adults of all ages. If you feel better avoiding all sources of caffeine, you might consider taking an L-theanine supplement, as it has known cognitive benefits without any established significant side effects.

The greatest benefit derives from consuming one or two cups of coffee or three or four cups of tea per day, and not more. If you currently exceed this amount, either cut back, or be safe and ask your doctor to check your caffeine metabolism status, which is a measure of your CYP1A2 activity (the liver enzyme that metabolizes caffeine). Most likely your health insurance won't cover this type of testing.

I enjoy drinking **a couple cups of coffee in the morning,** and I drink **a cup of matcha in the early afternoon.** The evidence suggests that I'm making a smart choice for my brain and my heart. I have to limit myself to two or three cups of caffeine per day, because if I drink more, even as a fast metabolizer, I won't sleep well at night. I also look for organic brands, to avoid the pesticides used by large coffee and tea growers.

9. Red Wine

Moderate alcohol intake has complex biochemical neuroprotective and anti-inflammatory properties, and worldwide, multiple studies consistently show that those who consume alcohol in moderation experience less cognitive decline than those who have no alcohol intake. Red wine, a classic complement to the Mediterranean diet, has the most beneficial effect. *Moderate* consumption is described differently in various studies, but generally it is one to three servings per day for women and two to four servings per day for men. (A serving is 5 ounces of wine.) If you are wondering why men get larger servings, it's because generally men are bigger, distributing the alcohol over a greater body size; in addition, due to the effects of estrogen and progesterone, women metabolize alcohol more slowly. Even if a woman and a man of the same size drink the same amount, the woman will experience a higher blood alcohol level over a longer period of time.)

One serving of beer is 12 ounces, and one serving of distilled spirits is 1.5 ounces. Sorry, beer and hard liquor lovers—most studies that show cognitive benefits from alcohol reveal most of the benefit comes from wine, especially red wine. I think four drinks a day for most people is a considerable amount of alcohol (likely excessive), and more than that—particularly with beer and hard liquor—is associated with an increased cancer risk, so use your discretion. Overindulging in any form of alcohol will undo its benefits.

In one study, New York City residents older than sixty-five who drank wine (but not beer or liquor) had larger brain volumes, indicating less brain shrinkage, than those who didn't drink. (Women had one serving per day and men had one or two servings.) Whether they had the Alzheimer's-related ApoE4 gene or not, they showed the same benefit.

In Australia, researchers studied people age sixty-five to eighty-three who had a Mini-Mental State Examination score of less than 23 out of 30 (indicating mild cognitive impairment). Those who had two to four drinks a day over six years had less cognitive decline than those who were abstainers or used alcohol infrequently.

A study in the Netherlands tracked people age forty-three to seventy over five years. Those who drank two or three servings of red wine per day showed less cognitive loss than those who abstained or who drank *more* than three servings per day.

In France, researchers assessed alcohol intake in 3,088 middle-aged adults and measured their cognitive function thirteen years later. Women who consumed one or two servings of wine and men who had two to three servings had better cognitive function than those who had none or who had it infrequently. Again, heavy drinking showed worse cognitive function.

The consensus from multiple studies shows that even after controlling for other health factors (weight, diet, education, and various health issues), those who drink moderately, especially red wine, have less cognitive decline than those who don't drink at all and those who drink too much.

Red wine seems to be key. Though several studies showed some benefit from all alcohol intake, they showed substantial and additional benefits from red wine compared to beer or spirits (and wine, beer, and liquor contain varying percentages of alcohol). Something in red wine, apart from alcohol, benefits the brain—likely the red grape pigments, the polyphenols, and the nutrient resveratrol, found in the skins of dark grapes. Multiple studies with red grape juice have not found these benefits as consistently, likely because the sugar in grape juice offsets the benefits noted in red wine.

Red wine has not only brain benefits but other benefits as well—better digestion, decreased arterial plaque formation, decreased inflammation, and better blood sugar control and insulin sensitivity. For all these reasons, I recommend daily consumption of **one or two servings of red wine with dinner.**

Although the benefits seem clear, some people have good reason to avoid all alcohol. Not everyone likes it; nor can everyone enjoy a glass or two of wine and simply stop. For some, a few drinks leads to excess, and excessive alcohol is bad not only for your health but for families and job performance as well. If you do not wish to drink, for whatever reason, don't start. Instead, consume other red-purple plant pigments (red grapes, blueberries, cherries, and other berries) and consider taking a resveratrol supplement daily, discussed in Chapter 5.

10. Herbs and Spices

Seasoning your food with herbs and spices elevates it to another level—not only because of their great taste but because of their extraordinary health benefits. Fresh or dried, herbs and spices can add a kick of flavor plus a blast of antioxidant and anti-inflammatory properties. If you want to slow aging, protect your brain, and have fewer aches and pains, simply eat more of these wonderful plants.

The best-known mainstays of a Mediterranean diet are olive oil, heaps of vegetables and fruits, and even red wine—yet the diet's distinct spices and herbs likely have just as many benefits. Italian herbs and fine herbs—**rosemary, thyme, oregano, sage, basil, marjoram, tarragon, chervil, chives,** and **parsley**—are used throughout Mediterranean cuisine. They are loaded with medicinal properties, and eating them lowers inflammation, reduces oxidation, and slows aging. They also taste fantastic when combined with food.

Rosemary has been called a brain-boosting herb. Animal studies in mice and rats have shown that it slows cognitive decline and helps maintain memory. In Italy's southern regions, some locals eat rosemary-infused foods at nearly every meal. In one area near Naples, researchers have noted a very high rate of people who live into their nineties, with surprisingly low rates of dementia. I consider rosemary a terrific culinary herb; I grow it in my garden and cook with it several times a week.

Don't limit your palate to Mediterranean cuisine when you're searching out healthful, fabulous flavors. In southern India, where curry spices are used in abundance, you will find one of the lowest rates of Alzheimer's on the planet. Curry spices have amazing anti-inflammatory power. Eating them decreases joint pain, lowers cancer risk, and helps prevent memory loss. A typical **blend of curry spices** would include **coriander, turmeric, cumin,** and **fenugreek** and may also include **chili pepper, ginger, garlic, fennel seed, caraway, cinnamon, clove, mustard seed, cardamom, nutmeg,** and **black pepper.** The potential varieties are nearly endless, and they don't have to be spicy hot.

Curry powder is a spice mix of varying ingredients based on South Asian cuisine. Curry powder and the very word *curry* are Western inventions and do not reflect any specific South Asian food, though a similar mixture of spices used in India is called garam masala. The word *curry* is derived from the Tamil word *kari* meaning "sauce, relish for rice," although most people think of it as the essence of South Indian food. Curry-like mixtures have been used in South India for almost four thousand years. (Chili pepper spices, now essential to any curry powder, are relatively recent additions to the mix as chili peppers were brought to South Asia from the Americas in the sixteenth century.)

The best-known individual curry spice with brain benefits is **turmeric,** a yellow, ginger-like plant. Turmeric plays an essential role in curry spice blends. A variety of studies using turmeric have suggested that it slows cognitive decline and benefits cognitive function. The challenge is that it is generally poorly absorbed, and the quantities needed to show a benefit are *big:* you'd have to eat about three heaping tablespoons of turmeric every day. When I lived and worked as a volunteer in various hospitals in India, including a leprosarium near Calcutta, I likely ate this amount daily. I ate curry-flavored meals for breakfast, lunch, and dinner. But that was then, and this is now. I once tried to add a tablespoon of turmeric to yogurt and eat that three times per day, thinking, *Okay, this is good for me,* but I confess I didn't get past the first serving, let alone three per day.

Fortunately, the benefits of turmeric are also available as a supplement, called curcumin (discussed in Chapter 5). The brain benefits of turmeric can be replicated by taking one curcumin capsule daily, without any meaningful side effects, apart from occasional stomach distress noted with higher dosages.

Garlic and **ginger** have additional anti-inflammatory benefits. **Chili pepper spices,** derived from any number of chilies containing the ingredient capsaicin, help rev up your metabolism. **Cinnamon** improves blood sugar control and improves insulin sensitivity.

My challenge is to use more spices and herbs every day, and I encourage you to do the same, at least two teaspoons of dried spices or two to three tablespoons of fresh herbs daily.

David's Better Brain (and Body) Story: Adding the Right Foods

David was fifty years old and felt awful. Obese, struggling with type 2 diabetes, and depressed, he couldn't think straight. As an accountant, he was having more and more trouble focusing on tasks at work, and felt like his brain was beginning to fail him, just as his body had. His doctor recommended bariatric surgery and a slew of medications to take beforehand—for high blood sugar, cholesterol, and high blood pressure. Disheartened and unenthusiastic about the prospect of surgery and reliance on medications, he got motivated . . . and it started in the kitchen, at the grocery store, and on his plate.

David isn't one of my patients, but he did show up at my clinic months after his doctor suggested the surgery, wearing two pairs of jeans—at the same time. He wore a size 34 pair, and over that he had on his old jeans, size 48. This happy, smiling stranger had shown up to thank me.

It turns out that after rejecting surgery, David knew he had to do something to reduce his dangerous weight, repair his brain, and save his life. He went online and found my books—*Ten Years Younger* and *The 30-Day Heart Tune-Up*. His wife agreed to cook recipes from the books, and he took the leftovers to work for lunch, cutting out the junk and focusing on the core foods I recommended. While those books focused on foods for their anti-aging properties and their cardiac benefits, they are similar to the ones I recommend here for better brain health—foods like clean protein, fiber, red wine, nuts, and dark chocolate.

Within a month, David told me, he knew he didn't need the surgery. Instead, he added many of the same dozen foods featured in this book, and he cut out cereal, bread, crackers, and all beverages with sugar. He also started going for a walk twice a day, before and after work.

During the first month, he noticed that he had much more energy and slept better, and his wife noted a big improvement in his romantic performance. He enjoyed the foods he was eating and felt satisfied with his new meals and snacks. The biggest change was that he felt mentally sharper all day long. He was not just getting his work done on time but feeling like he could do more. His boss noticed his improved job performance as well, and he was promoted.

David kept losing about fifteen pounds per month. Uncomfortable with the physician who had thought drug therapy and weight-loss surgery were the only answers, he found a new doctor, who was almost as happy as he was with the results: David's blood sugar, cholesterol, and blood pressure were all back to normal. David had simply added the right foods and avoided the bad ones. What you choose to eat, and what you leave out of your diet, truly has a dramatic impact on your mind and body.

11. Beans

Beans are a tremendous source of nutrients, as they are likely the best source of fiber you can achieve from one serving of food. They are loaded with vitamins and minerals, such as mixed folates, magnesium, B vitamins, and potassium. They have the highest oxidation-blocking score of any food ever tested, meaning that they effectively fight destructive oxidation in cells—think of it as internal rusting—that can lead to accelerated aging and disease, including memory loss.

Best of all, eating a half-cup serving of beans improves blood sugar control and decreases insulin secretion, as the carbs in beans are absorbed slowly. We have known for decades that eating legumes can even improve blood sugar control and insulin production when consumed with other carbohydrates, such as rice and bread. Legume intake also helps with weight control.

Yet some people don't tolerate beans. Beans contain lectins, a compound that about 10 percent of the population cannot break down and digest. The result isn't merely gas—it's intestinal pain and discomfort, enough to turn you off from this otherwise amazing food. But there is a work-around. You can remove lectins from uncooked beans by soaking them in water a couple of times (commonly called sprouting, although you don't need to wait until sprouts actually appear). Simply soak beans overnight in water, drain and rinse in the morning, soak again for up to eight hours, and rinse one last time before cooking. This will markedly shorten the cooking time (a boon on a weeknight), and the beans will absorb and remove most of the lectins during this initial sprouting process. It will also decrease the common gassy effect from eating beans, too.

Canned beans are convenient and nutritious (though you can't remove lectins if that's an issue for you), and most supermarkets carry a terrific variety. Choose pintos, chickpeas (garbanzos), cannellini (white) beans, butter beans, lentils, or any bean or legume you enjoy; if you buy canned beans, be sure to purchase BPA-free cans. Soaking dried beans and cooking them from scratch is economical and easy, although it takes time. **Aim to eat at least one-quarter to one-half cup daily.**

12. Fermented Foods

A tsunami of research now connects the gut microbiome—the complex community of trillions of microorganisms that live in the digestive tract—to the brain. Have you noticed that when you know something isn't right, you get that "gut feeling"? That you develop "butterflies in your stomach" before a first date or a big interview? And how about "stomach rumbling" when you are stressed out? All these are everyday examples of the extraordinary gut-brain connection, a relationship that impacts your cognitive function.

Several books have explored this link, including *The Mind-Gut Connection* by Emeran Mayer, M.D., and *Brain Maker* by David Perlmutter, M.D. (the best-selling author of *Grain Brain*). Interviewing both of these internationally renowned physicians for this book made me even more aware that the gut communicates with the brain like no other part of the body.

Most of us have always had an inkling of the gut-mind connection (those butterflies!), but scientists have been slow to focus on it. Yet there are more microbes in our gut than there are cells in our entire body. The connection between the mind and the gut is bidirectional: the gut talks to the brain and the brain talks to the gut every minute of our lives, and the microbes living in our gut have a major influence over the quality of this exchange. When our gut-brain communication is off balance—due to diet, antibiotic use (which kills off valuable bacteria and other microbes), stress, or lifestyle—we experience physical and mental health issues, including depression, anxiety, fatigue, weight gain, and digestive problems. Recent studies have shown that a diverse, healthy biome improves cognitive function and decreases risk for depression, anxiety, and cognitive decline.

In 2015 I co-chaired the American College of Nutrition's symposium

"Translational Nutrition: Optimizing Brain Health," attended by scientists and clinicians from around the world. I was amazed how much research connects a healthy gut microbiome to brain function, and how an abnormal gut microbiome balance is associated with an increased risk for neurological problems, including Alzheimer's disease, Parkinson's disease, attention deficit disorder (ADD), and autism.

The needless use of antibiotics has harmed our gut microbiome (see the box "Antibiotics and Gut Health"), but so have acid-blocking agents (heartburn medications); it turns out that stomach acid is essential to a healthy microbiome. Some people may have a serious medical problem requiring the use of an acid-blocking drug (to name a few: Prilosec, Nexium, Omeprazole, Ranitidine, Zantac, and Lansoprazole). But in my clinical experience, far too often people overuse these microbiome-disrupting medications because they smoke tobacco or overindulge in coffee and alcohol, causing avoidable heartburn. If you are currently taking this type of medication, talk to your doctor about how you could safely avoid this drug class altogether.

We need a strong, balanced gut microbiome to detoxify chemicals, metabolize our own hormones, and control inflammation. A healthy gut microbiome depends on two primary factors:

- Fiber. Gut-healthy microbes eat primarily fiber—so you need to **eat fiber from vegetables, fruits, beans, and nuts** to keep your microbiome well fed and alive.
- Bacteria. If you haven't always eaten an abundance of fiber, you likely need to restore some healthy bacteria to rebuild your microbiome. The best way to do that is to **eat a diet rich in fermented foods,** which naturally are packed with multiple strains of valuable gut-healthy bacteria.

Fermented foods include, among others, sauerkraut, pickles, kimchi, kombucha, miso, tempeh, yogurt, and kefir. (You'll find the last two items in the Mediterranean-style diet, where fermented foods come from the dairy category.) If you aren't likely going to eat fermented foods daily, then taking a **probiotic supplement** would be another good option, which I'll expand upon in Chapter 5. Feed your gut—to fuel your brain!

Antibiotics and Gut Health

Even a short course of antibiotics can wreak havoc on your gut microbiome, killing billions of healthy bacteria and leading to an overgrowth of potentially toxic microbes. I am not suggesting that you avoid antibiotics for, say, pneumonia or an infected wound. Yet far too often antibiotics are prescribed for colds or minor infections when they are absolutely not needed. A single course of antibiotics can disrupt your gut microbiome for more than one year and, by changing the balance of gut microbes, cause you to gain substantial weight. Before you accept a prescription for an antibiotic treatment, clarify with your physician if you could safely do without it, even if it requires a follow-up visit.

Foods That Can Harm Your Body and Brain: Four Foods to Avoid

Adding the 12 Smart Foods to your daily diet will help you think more sharply and save your brain from decline, at the same time giving you satisfying, flavorful options to indulge in when you choose your meals and snacks. There are, however, some foods you should eat in moderation or avoid entirely, as they have the potential to hurt you in many ways. Some are obvious (nobody will recommend that you eat more partially hydrogenated fat), but others will be surprising, especially with regard to brain health.

1. Partially Hydrogenated and Hydrogenated Fats (Trans Fats)

Let's begin with the least controversial and most toxic substitute to avoid—any form of *trans fat,* also called *partially hydrogenated* or *hydrogenated fat.* For nearly twenty years, I have referred to these dangerous fats as "embalming fluid," an apt term because consuming them essentially embalms your insides—that's as bad as it sounds. The food industry creates trans fats in much the same way chemists create plastic. Manufacturers heat oil, such as vegetable oil, add noxious chemicals such as nickel, and pump in hydrogen gas to stiffen it. When you eat hydrogenated fat, you are in turn hardening your tissues, including your arteries and your brain. It's like being injected with liquid plastic.

Partially hydrogenated fats are almost fully saturated with hydrogen, a process that destroys most of the healthful chemical bonds that make fats delicate and flexible. Don't let the word *partially* fool you into thinking that's somehow better than all-out hydrogenated. Fully hydrogenated fats have no healthy double-bonded structures left within them; the hydrogenation process obliterates them. *Partially hydrogenated* means they are nearly 100 percent hydrogenated.

Why would the food industry do this? The answer is pretty simple—profits. Foods prepared with partially hydrogenated fats last for decades on the shelf, so they almost never go bad, and you can sell them forever. Because of hydrogenated oils, cookies and crackers, frozen pizza, and boxed rice pilaf won't go rancid. On the other hand, healthy fats have a far more limited shelf life (not the multiple years–plus of many hydrogenated fats), and products containing them must be thrown away after their sell-by date. Some locations have banned food with trans fats (restaurants in a number of states can no longer use them), and recently passed federal legislation will, I hope, eventually phase them out of our food supply. It's way overdue. Still, be aware that many baked goods, foods that come in boxes and cans, and numerous highly processed foods still contain these nasty compounds.

Avoiding them is fairly simple: read the ingredient list. If you see the words *hydrogenated* or *partially hydrogenated* (even if the nutrition label indicates zero grams of trans fat), return that item to the shelf and buy something else. Dining out is trickier, but you can ask what type of fat a restaurant cooks with. If you hear the words *partially hydrogenated* or mention of a restaurant-grade oil called *phase vegetable oil,* ask them to use another oil, such as virgin olive oil, or you should go somewhere else.

Another way to avoid hydrogenated fats is to avoid fried food, especially when you are eating out (and especially in fast-food restaurants). Many fats may start out healthy or harmless, flexible and clean, but when they sit in a fryer all day and then are heated to high temperatures, they become damaged and dangerous. As we saw on pages 65–66, even many healthy fats—including olive oil—can be destroyed and transformed into hydrogenated fat when heated for a prolonged time and above their smoke points. If you must fry a food, then at least use a healthy fat, like high-heat-tolerant avocado oil. Cook quickly at high heat, and don't reuse the oil.

2. Toxic Fats

Toxic fats originate in feedlots, among animals who are typically fed grains sprayed with pesticides and the chemical glyphosate (the active ingredient in the weedkiller Roundup), or given up to six different growth hormones to fatten them up before they are slaughtered for market. Over time, chemicals and hormones are concentrated in the animal fat. Eat a cut of meat or poultry from a feedlot-raised animal, or an egg from a factory-farmed chicken, and you eat a load of toxins. Something similar occurs with dairy products when cows and sheep are fed toxic grains and injected with hormones to increase milk production. The milk fat used to make cheese, butter, yogurt, or other dairy foods, as well as the milk itself, may be loaded with residual pesticides, chemicals, and hormones.

I've had a few colleagues challenge me with statements like "But those toxins only cause cancer, not dementia or heart disease." To which I say, isn't cancer bad enough? As it turns out, many of the harmful chemicals in toxic fats block insulin sensitivity, leading to diabetes and elevated blood sugar, thereby upping the risk for heart disease and dementia.

The solution is straightforward. If you buy animal protein and dairy, buy "mostly" products that are clean, as in grass-fed, or only organic-fed, and from animals that are not given hormones. Look for terms like *pasture-raised* and *wild,* as well as *grass-fed* and *organic,* and try to purchase products that come from smaller farms and producers as opposed to the food giants. Unfortunately, such marketing isn't a 100 percent guarantee that your food is clean, but at least it is a very good start. As for dairy, if you cannot find grass-fed and pasture-raised, at the minimum opt for organic.

3. Sugar and Refined Carbohydrates

Since elevated blood sugar is the #1 cause of dementia and heart disease, avoid sugar—especially added sugar—and refined carbs if you want to improve blood sugar and insulin control. How high your blood sugar rises after a meal is fairly predictable (and is explained more thoroughly in Chapter 4), particularly if you know whether you've consumed actual sugar—but that's where it gets a bit murky. Here is a partial list of alternative names for plain old sugar: *organic cane juice, syrup, glucose, fructose, high-fructose corn syrup, cornstarch, cane products, fruit juice, sucrose,* and *dextrose*—it's all just added sugar. And the more of these names you see in the ingredients list, the worse that item is for you (even if it's organic).

Don't be fooled by agave, either. Agave is often marketed as a "health food" because consuming it doesn't raise blood sugar levels, but agave is nearly pure fructose, which is stored in your liver as fat, basically turning your liver into pâté. Fatty liver is one of the causes of insulin resistance, which leads to disabling memory loss. Skip the agave.

4. Sweeteners (Sugar Substitutes)

Chemical sweeteners give you a sweet taste without any calories, but they have little upside beyond that. Some of these sweeteners kill off the healthy microbes living in your intestinal tract, disrupting the gut microbiome and causing a variety of serious health problems, ranging from weight gain to neurological injury to elevated blood sugar. Sucralose (found in Splenda) is really chlorinated sugar. Consider that we use chlorine to kill bacteria in public water supplies. In lab animal studies, aspartame (what NutraSweet and Equal are made from) has been reported to increase the risk for certain cancers, in particular leukemia and lymphoma. Furthermore, a natural calorie-free sweetener (even the plant-derived stevia, or the alcohol-based xylitol) will likely stimulate your appetite and cravings, causing you to eat more later and gain back some of the calories you were trying to avoid.

To make this message sweet and short: avoid most sweeteners, including the blue, yellow, and pink packets—aspartame (NutraSweet and Equal), sucralose (Splenda), and saccharin—as they all have the potential to harm your gut microbiome and/or raise your risk for other health problems. If you feel you must use a sweetener, consider natural options that don't adversely impact your gut, like stevia, erythritol, and xylitol, but don't overdo it. Erythritol and xylitol in excess can cause an unexpected reaction—diarrhea—and as mentioned above, even these natural sweeteners can spike your appetite and cause you to overeat.

Some Foods to Moderate

For many of us, celebratory foods are an important part of our family culture and ethnic heritage. We share them with others as we mark holidays, birthdays, weddings, anniversaries, and other major milestones. My goal is to keep you in good enough health so that you can enjoy life and have decades ahead filled with those special moments—the occasional high points in life that may call for a splurge at the table. That is why the most realistic and important focus with regard to food should be on the everyday: what you eat for breakfast, lunch, and dinner, including workdays, when you want to be mentally sharp.

With that in mind, let's look at a few food categories that fall into the "in moderation" category (including foods that often show up on those special occasions) and practical ways to navigate them.

Sweet Stuff

From my perspective, Americans as a nation take "treats" for granted, particularly when it comes to sweets, but sweets have taken a quantifiable toll when you look at rates of diabetes, heart disease, and dementia. We're swimming—and drowning—in a sea of sugar.

Our love of sweets started out naturally enough. It's a taste humans have enjoyed for eons. Breast milk, the first food for many infants, naturally contains the milk sugar lactose—humans are exposed to sweet before they taste savory. Early humans would get some honey from a beehive, for instance, or lick sugary sap from a rare tree, or chew a sweet-tasting plant. It wasn't often, and it was nice when we found it. Eventually we figured out how to manufacture sugar from sugar beets and sugar cane, though for centuries sweets were still a rarity reserved for the rich. That changed, of course, but it's unlikely anyone would have predicted today's astronomical levels of sugar consumption. The average American consumes twenty teaspoons of sugar every day and nearly sixty-six pounds per year. We're pouring it into our food supply, and it's damaging our bodies, hearts, and brains.

If your blood sugar and insulin levels are elevated, then avoid all forms of added sugar for at least thirty days. Often that will bring your insulin and blood sugar back into control.

If they are well controlled (fasting glucose less than 95 mg/dL and insulin less than 5 µIU/mL), then I think it's fine for you to have the occasional treat. Just use common sense—and remember the definition of *treat*. If you have it regularly, it's not one.

Given what we know about chemical sweeteners and their impact on the microbiome, I'd use a natural agent rather than a chemical one, so on occasion, if you have normal blood sugar control, then a bit of maple syrup in your oatmeal, honey in your tea, or a sweetener like xylitol, stevia, or erythritol is okay. Unless you are a long-distance athlete and you can tolerate much more sweet intake than most of us, just keep it to an occasional use, as in a few times per week. If that seems unrealistic, and you are going to take something sweet daily, then pick honey, and limit it to a teaspoon per serving, and not more than a couple of teaspoons per day. Honey acts as a probiotic with up to ten to fifteen gut-healthy bacterial species, and if you eat local honey it can help you with pollen allergies. Therefore, if you have well-controlled blood sugar and you want to use an occasional sweet in your food or beverages, make honey your top choice.

Most people report that gradually reducing their sugar intake is much easier than trying to do it all at once. And from a health perspective, if it is a choice between sugar or organic half-and-half in your coffee, choose the organic half-and-half.

What About Saturated Fat?

The topic of saturated fat is one of the most controversial in this book, especially when we are talking about brain health. If you ask ten doctors about the risks and benefits of consuming foods high in saturated fats, you will likely get ten different answers. From a heart perspective, the evidence is pretty clear. Eating clean saturated fat from animal protein and dairy isn't bad for your heart—but I can't say it's good for you, either. The evidence from multiple randomized clinical trials says it is neutral, meaning that clean meat and dairy won't improve your heart health, but they won't necessarily hurt you. If you want to avoid heart disease, it is vastly more important to focus on cutting your sugar intake than to worry about clean saturated fat.

During expert interviews for this book, I asked my colleagues, neurologist and author Dr. David Perlmutter and Dr. Daniel Amen, the brain health expert, psychiatrist, and author, about saturated fat and the brain. Neither was concerned about cognitive decline with saturated fat intake, because they both focus on eating the *right* saturated fats, in the right way.

The challenge is that the more saturated fat average Americans eat, the higher their risk for Alzheimer's disease. To appreciate why this might be, you have to consider the type of saturated fat that people are eating and what else they eat with it. The issues that link saturated fat intake with dementia and brain diseases are revealed with these questions:

1. Do you consume excess saturated fat when you have insulin resistance?
2. Is the saturated fat clean or loaded with toxins?
3. Do you consume saturated fat by itself or with sugar and/or flour?

First, as pointed out by Rush University professor Martha Clare Morris, Ph.D., epidemiological studies show that eating foods high in saturated fat likely increases the production of beta-amyloid in the brain, the protein associated with an elevated risk for Alzheimer's. Even worse, if someone is insulin resistant, then the enzyme that would normally remove beta-amyloid is busy removing excess insulin; thus especially for them, eating extra saturated fat may raise levels of beta-amyloid in the brain. This may be even more important for people with an ApoE4 genotype, as they already have trouble removing cholesterol from the bloodstream. For them, limiting extra saturated fat to a moderate intake might make good sense.

Because of this link, for the average person, Dr. Morris and most national organizations recommend following a Mediterranean-like diet and, as with the DASH plan, eating more vegetables and fruits and limiting the intake of saturated fat. With this approach, you don't have to give up saturated fat entirely; rather, just eat it in moderation.

Second, as discussed earlier, many sources of saturated fat have toxins and hormones that worsen blood sugar control, leading to insulin resistance, which damages brain cell function and triggers cognitive decline. Most saturated fat consumed in America today is dirty (the animals were fed pesticides or given hormones). There are no studies that compare clean saturated fat with dirty saturated fat and their respective impacts on memory loss (or even cancer), but based on what we do know, my position is this: if you eat animal protein, make it *clean*, not *mean* protein that hurts your brain and your health. I'm confident most of my medical colleagues would agree with that approach.

Third, as several studies show, when you combine saturated fat with refined carbs (such as sugar and flour), there is a much greater increase in inflammation than you get from eating either item alone. A study at the Veterans Affairs Medical Center studied twenty older adults with both normal cognitive function and early cognitive decline, comparing their diets and measuring beta-amyloid production in cerebrospinal fluid (the fluid that surrounds the brain). Those consuming a diet high in saturated fat and sugar had much more beta-amyloid production than those who ate a low-fat, low-sugar diet.

Americans typically eat saturated fat in the worst way possible for their brains: in cheese and crackers, butter and bread, steak and baked potato, burger on a bun, macaroni and cheese, frosted cupcakes, French fries (starch fried in fat), and of course, ice cream. You may be thinking, "Wait, cheese is fat, but crackers are salty," or, "The bun on the burger isn't sweet," but the white flour in both (whether it's gluten-free or not) as well as the starchy potato behave in your body the way table sugar does (as we'll see in Chapter 4).

A note on cheese: Cheese by itself, especially if eaten in moderation as in not more than one or two ounces per day, likely has a neutral impact on health. It is a decent source of calcium, and fermented cheeses act as a beneficial source of probiotics. To me, the issue with cheese is whether it is loaded with pesticides and hormones or is clean. If you eat cheese, choose minimally processed and organic varieties.

We simply don't have randomized clinical studies to answer the question, "Is there a healthy way to eat more saturated fat?" So we have to make the best guess as to what to do. When we lack evidence, my tendency as a physician who still sees patients most days of the week is to be cautious, not cavalier. So until we have studies that assure us that clean sources of saturated fat intake are safe for your brain, I'm going to advise this: Eat clean saturated fat in moderation, not to excess. And truly, that isn't so restrictive, as you could still have a couple of servings of foods with saturated fats each day.

Many health experts in my professional circle follow a Paleo eating plan (which aims to replicate how humans ate 20,000 to 70,000 years ago), and they will claim that you can eat all the extra saturated-fat-rich foods you like. But in truth, we don't come close to living like cavemen and -women anymore, and we live much longer, too. Sure—as long as Paleo followers have great blood sugar and insulin control, eat only clean animal protein, and don't combine saturated-fat-rich foods with carbs that raise blood sugar levels, then I'll admit that extra saturated fat may be just fine.

But until we know for sure, for the average American, especially for those with an ApoE4 gene, eating more saturated fat is associated not only with suffering from memory loss but also with dying younger and with a higher mortality rate. I'd rather be frank and share the latest information available, to help you make the best decision for yourself.

What About Salt?

Saltiness is one of the five types of taste, and our bodies require some amount of salt in our diet. For people who don't get iodine from eating seafood or from taking a multivitamin with iodine, iodized salt provides this essential mineral. The Better Brain Solution program provides salt in moderation to make your food taste delicious, but not enough to cause problems for those who are salt sensitive.

For years we have asked people to lower their salt intake, in particular those with high blood pressure, thinking that most people were sensitive to it. However, we now know that it is more effective to limit sugar than to cut back on salt for better blood pressure control. The average American consumes about 3,500 to 4,000 mg of salt daily. Many health organizations recommend that people limit their sodium intake to not more than 2,500 mg daily—there are 2,325 mg of sodium in one teaspoon of table salt.

Who needs to limit their salt intake?

Genetic testing shows that about 25 percent of people are sensitive to salt, almost 30 percent are minimally sensitive, and 45 percent are hardly impacted by salt intake at all. (Salt sensitivity means that increased salt intake increases blood pressure levels.) Being insulin resistant increases your salt sensitivity. The good news is that following The Better Brain Solution program will make you less salt sensitive so that you can enjoy a bit of salt without unhealthy consequences. People with high blood pressure, heart problems, and advanced osteoporosis may benefit from limiting their salt intake to 2,500 mg daily and should discuss it with their doctor. Recent studies have shown that people *without* bone loss or hypertension could enjoy a little extra salt without any harm.

For the rare person diagnosed with congestive heart failure or Ménière's disease (a disorder of the inner ear's balance center), limiting salt intake to not more than 1,500 to 2,000 mg daily is clearly a benefit. This may be about 2 to 4 percent of the population. For these individuals, I'd ask that they cut the salt content in my recipes by 30 to 50 percent, to ensure that they stay below 2,000 mg per day.

The goal for the recipes in *The Better Brain Solution* is to help people keep their salt intake moderate and consume close to the 2,500-mg-per-day limit. Adding extra herbs and spices to recipes provides an abundance of flavors, complementing the intended moderate food saltiness, to ensure you and your family love the meals you prepare.

What About Gluten?

Gluten is a protein found in wheat, rye, and barley. Every time you eat one of these three grains, you're consuming gluten. Wheat flour is by far the most prevalent source of gluten, used to make thousands of processed foods. It's a challenge to avoid gluten, but for gluten-sensitive individuals, it's essential.

Twenty percent of all Americans are gluten sensitive, meaning that if they consume this substance, they can initiate an autoimmune disease, including disabling and deadly ones like multiple sclerosis and inflammatory bowel disease.

An autoimmune disease means your body makes antibodies that attack and damage your own tissues. In the case of gluten sensitivity, your immune system "sees" the gluten protein and treats it like a foreign invader, making antibodies that attack the perceived enemy. Normally, the immune system's protective response is beneficial, but with an autoimmune disorder, many of these antibodies get confused and wreak havoc on your gut lining, joints, thyroid, sinuses, and even your brain.

When you have gluten sensitivity, you essentially have an autoimmune disease. Eating gluten even once has the potential to cause your immune system to attack your tissues for the next twenty to thirty days. You may eat gluten only once every two weeks, yet you may have symptoms all the time, because the antibody attack is relentless. The symptoms of gluten sensitivity include: gastrointestinal issues such as bloating, gas, and abdominal pain; brain fog; anxiety; depression; achy joints; sinus congestion; fatigue; weight gain or resistant weight loss; eczema and psoriasis rashes.

You could have all of these symptoms or merely one or two. I was surprised to discover that half of people with gluten sensitivity have no gastrointestinal issues but other systemic issues instead. At my clinic, anyone with any of these chronic, unexplained symptoms deserves laboratory testing or a gluten-free elimination diet trial for a minimum of three or four weeks. I wish it were simple, but the reality is that laboratory testing and going gluten-free are complicated; see the Resources section at www.DrMasley.com for details.

Gluten sensitivity is very serious. When you hear the term, don't confuse it with something annoying but not life-threatening like lactose intolerance. The good news is that the improvements in gluten-sensitive people who go gluten-free are really amazing.

Even people who are not gluten sensitive might benefit from giving up gluten. Absolutely no critical nutrients for your body are to be found in gluten products, most of which come in the form of bread, crackers, pretzels, and pancakes. The main thing you give up by not eating gluten is calories. Furthermore, the wheat grown on North American farms today is not the wheat that was grown fifty or a hundred years ago. It has been genetically modified and is more likely to cause gluten-related problems than before. People who are not truly gluten sensitive may nonetheless be intolerant of gluten and might feel better by avoiding it.

Mary's Better Brain Story: Gluten

Mary Beth was fifty-seven years old when she first came to see me, more than a decade after her diagnosis of multiple sclerosis (MS). Despite consulting several neurologists and trying a series of the latest available drugs, her symptoms were progressing. Her brain function seemed sluggish as she was increasingly forgetful, and she had tingling sensations down the left side of her body and some early signs of facial drooping. Her latest neurologist had ordered an MRI scan, confirming classic signs of MS. The medications were not working. When her neurologist indicated there wasn't much more he could do, she visited me.

In addition to her MS symptoms, she also had joint aches, marked fatigue, chronic sinus congestion, and bloating. That combination of symptoms made me think of gluten sensitivity, and I ordered a gluten antibody panel. Her tests were strongly positive for gluten antibodies, including transglutaminase-6 IgG, which is associated with brain antibodies and major neurological symptoms.

I asked Mary Beth to follow my program, add a dozen brain-protecting foods and extra nutrients (outlined in Chapter 5), and totally avoid all sources of gluten. Within a month, the tingling was disappearing, her memory and mental acuity were dramatically sharper, her energy greatly improved, and the joint aches had resolved. By five months, all her neurological symptoms had disappeared. At two years she has had no relapse of any neurological issues (totally symptom free), her energy and cognitive function are great, and as a bonus, she lost more than twenty-five pounds. I am convinced that if she had not started my Better Brain Solution, her symptoms would have progressed, and by now she would be disabled.

Putting It All Together: The Better Brain Way of Eating

One simple way to build meals around the 12 Smart Foods is to follow a Mediterranean-inspired diet. The heart-healthy benefits of the Mediterranean diet—famous for its generous use of olive oil, Mediterranean herbs and spices, and red wine, and for the longevity of its adherents—are well documented, but it offers impressive cognitive benefits as well. The overall diet is rich in plant foods and light on animal protein, and it is characterized by an abundance of bioactive phytonutrients, beneficial plant compounds, with antioxidant and anti-inflammatory properties.

This diet dates back to the early Greeks and Romans, but several decades ago nutrition scientists noted that people living along the Mediterranean basin had lower rates of cardiovascular disease and lived longer than other populations, including Americans. Today a typical daily Mediterranean diet includes five servings of vegetables, two or three servings of fruit, one or two servings of beans, five servings of fat (nuts, olive oil, seeds), one or two servings of fermented foods (like yogurt and raw milk cheese), an abundance of herbs and spices, and one or two servings of whole grains.

There is seafood three or four times per week, poultry two or three times per week, and red meat typically less than once per week. Its followers drink water, coffee, tea, and red wine. And in recent times, they have added cocoa and dark chocolate.

Many studies have linked the Mediterranean diet to overall longevity, but its impact on the brain is particularly striking. In one study of healthy elderly people (the average age was eighty, and they showed no signs of dementia), researchers analyzed diet and brain size. They discovered that individuals who ate more fish and less meat—consistent with the Mediterranean diet—had higher brain volume, a significant finding suggesting that memory loss and dementia are linked to brain shrinkage.

A hallmark of the traditional Mediterranean diet is a leisurely, pleasurable way of eating with friends and family, with fresh foods that are local and seasonal. Meals are heavily plant-based: animal protein is served in small portions or as a condiment, vegetarian dishes are drizzled with olive oil, and herbs play a major role at the table. The diet comes with an active lifestyle that is much more robust than that of most Americans. This was, after all, the diet of farmers, fishermen, olive growers, shepherds, laborers, and people who worked the land and sea.

The Japanese, famous for their longevity and low rates of Alzheimer's, also have a notably healthy diet that is worth mentioning here as it also features many of the 12 Smart Foods. At first glance, Japanese and Mediterranean cuisines may not appear to have much in common, but they are more similar than different: both have an abundance of vegetables and fruits, and more seafood than meat; both use herbs and spices in abundance, as well as legumes. The Japanese have fermented foods at most meals (miso soup, pickled vegetables, and natto), and although they eat less fat, they eat many smart fats such as nuts and fatty cold-water fish. Like a Mediterranean meal, a Japanese dinner is often a slow-paced, enjoyable affair that includes a moderate amount of alcohol. (The Japanese also walk much more than Americans do.)

The 12 Smart Foods show up consistently in the diets of healthy, long-lived people with sharp brains. Eat these foods more often— ideally, every day—to enhance your brain performance and fend off cognitive decline.

Now, let's move on to Step 2, for more ways to achieve optimal brain function and avoid the number one cause of memory loss.

Foods to Enjoy

These quantities are intended as a general guide, not to force you to measure and quantify everything you eat.

Green leafy veggies	≥ 1 cup per day
Other vegetables	≥ 2 cups per day
Fish (not fried)	≥ 2 serving per week, or supplement
Extra virgin olive oil	≥ 1 Tbsp. per day
Other cooking oils (heat-stable MUFA)	1–2 Tbsp. per day for cooking
Nuts	2 oz. per day
Other healthy fats (avocado, coconut)	1–2 servings per day
Berries	≥ ½ cup per day
Dark chocolate (or cocoa)	1–2 oz. (2 Tbsp.) per day
Caffeine sources	Optional, 2 cups coffee + 2 cups tea, or 4–6 cups tea
Wine	1–3 glasses per day (ideally red); if you don't use alcohol, eat more produce with blue, red, and purple pigments, and/or use a resveratrol supplement

Herbs and spices	≥ 1 Tbsp. mixed spices (dry), or ≥ 3 Tbsp. (fresh) (turmeric, garlic, ginger, Italian or fine herb blends, curry spices, chili) per day
Beans (including non-GMO soy)	½–1 cup per day
Fermented foods (plus 30 grams fiber)	1–2 servings per day, or supplement
Poultry (not fried)	Optional, 4–7 servings per week

Foods to Moderate

Whole grains*	Optional, up to 3 servings per day
Butter	Optional, grass-fed, 1–2 Tbsp. per day
Cheese	Optional, organic, 1–2 oz. per day
Red meat	Optional, grass-fed, 10–12 oz. per week
Natural sweets (honey, maple syrup)	Optional, 1–2 servings per week

Foods to Avoid

Partially hydrogenated fat (margarine)	Never
Fried fast food	< 1 time per week (if ever)
Refined sugar	Unless you are celebrating a special occasion, you shouldn't need cake, cookies, sodas, or sweetened drinks

---

Choose whole grains with a medium-to-low glycemic load (as explained in Chapter 4), and consider going gluten-free.

CHAPTER 4

More Ways to Feed Your Brain

Continue eating the 12 Smart Foods that are essential for better brain health, and avoiding foods that decrease cognitive performance. As soon as you are ready, for a truly sharper brain and even stronger protection against cognitive dysfunction and memory loss, take the next step.

Step 2: Eat Foods with a Low Glycemic Load

If we want to address the number one cause of cognitive dysfunction and memory loss—and abnormal blood sugar regulation—then we need to stop brain-killing insulin resistance. The easiest way to improve insulin sensitivity is to choose foods with a low sugar load, also known as a low glycemic load. A food's *glycemic load* refers to how high a person's blood sugar shoots up after eating a serving of it (*glyc* = sugar, and *emia* = blood level). Glycemic load is divided into three categories: low, medium, and high. (See pages 102–109 for lists of foods by glycemic load.)

Studies have shown that if you have insulin resistance, then eating even something as simple as breakfast can have a serious impact on your brain function. If you begin your morning with a high glycemic load meal (think pancakes, toast, cereal, bagels, pastries, orange juice), you will *immediately* decrease your cognitive function. It's not a great way to start your workday (or any day), right? But the reverse is true, too, and it's good news: eating low glycemic load foods and giving that breakfast a makeover (whole fruit with plain yogurt, eggs, or a protein- and fiber-rich smoothie) can improve your brain function, and your blood sugar control. A study of middle-aged, overweight women with insulin resistance found that eating a low glycemic load breakfast improved their cognitive function.

If you've been following dietary trends, no doubt you've encountered the term *glycemic index*—a numbered value that indicates how quickly and how high your blood sugar rises after eating a specific quantity of a specific carbohydrate, ranked as high, moderate, and low. After the glycemic index concept was introduced, it became quite popular in the dieting community, like calorie counting, since some saw it as a way to simplify and speed weight loss. The diet mantra was to avoid the "high GI" foods (because they were packed with sugar, the thinking went). People were encouraged to choose low GI, in the hope that the pounds would fall away. (Some food companies label products as "low GI" to attract diet watchers.)

Unfortunately, the glycemic index concept is not that simple. Though the index can be extremely useful when it is properly interpreted, it isn't the best decision-making tool, in part because it's quite impractical in the real world and easy to misuse. For example, the index rates pasta as a "moderate" GI food but carrots as "high." The average person might think that pasta, therefore, is a healthier (less "sugary") choice than carrots, but that's a gross misunderstanding of the data—and it leads people to false conclusions.

The index was largely developed as a research tool by Dr. Jennie Brand-Miller, a scientist at the University of Sydney in Australia, to help assess how foods impact blood sugar. Typically, researchers measure blood sugar levels after an individual consumes 50 grams of carbohydrates from a single food. That would be about 1 cup of cooked pasta, a portion that for most people would be pretty small. (You can easily eat twice that amount.) By contrast, to get 50 grams of carbs from carrots, you would have to eat nearly *nine large carrots* in one sitting, which most people couldn't do if you paid them.

Nutrient-dense carrots are good for you, and, like most vegetables, they have a very low impact on blood sugar. Avoiding them because they appear "high" on the glycemic index is a mistake, as carrots have a glycemic load of 4, which is low. As you'll discover in a moment, glycemic *load*—not glycemic *index*—is the gauge you should be using. Beets are another food with a high glycemic index but a low glycemic load. Their sugar impact per serving is low, so yes, eat your beets!

As it turns out, adding more fiber, especially from beans, is an effective way to improve glycemic control. The irony is that some people, including those who follow a Paleo diet, avoid beans because they are high on the glycemic index, but beans most definitely do not behave the way sugar does in the body!

I interviewed Dr. Brand-Miller, and we discussed the scientific merits of the glycemic index but also how it falls short in offering ordinary people usable information. To make the data more useful, she explained, researchers added another layer of information and started calculating a food's glycemic *load,* which estimates how quickly and how high your blood sugar rises after you consume a standard (real-world) portion of it. That makes it far easier to choose foods that will help you achieve blood sugar control. And that is why the glycemic load (GL) of a food has become my favorite tool for making blood sugar control easy. (I also refer to it as a food's "sugar load.")

A selection of low and medium glycemic load foods you can enjoy every day is found on pages 102–107, along with a chart of high glycemic load foods you should limit or avoid if you're trying to control blood sugar. For more extensive glycemic index and glycemic load lists, visit the University of Sydney website www.glycemicindex.com.

Here are some other factors to consider as you make your food choices.

Activity Levels (and what kind of shape you're in now) Count

The more active and fit you are, the trimmer you are; and the more fiber you eat, the more glycemic load you can tolerate without causing a rise in blood sugar or insulin. However, the proof is in the testing. If your fasting blood glucose level is less than 95 mg/dL, and your insulin level is less than 5 µIU/mL, then your food choices and active lifestyle are working well for you.

At the other end of the spectrum, most people with metabolic syndrome and poor blood sugar control will need to avoid all foods with a glycemic load of more than 10 (as indicated in the charts; 10 to 19 is considered a "medium" load food) to restore normal blood sugar and insulin regulation. If you fall into that category now or if you're sliding down that slope, you can do something about it now, and as you get healthier and increase your fitness through better eating and regular physical activity, you will be able to manage occasional indulgences.

Your activity level also influences your response to glycemic load, meaning that the more active you are, the less your blood sugar will rise after you eat a specific amount of carbs. As an example, an athlete exercising twenty or more hours per week can eat a great deal more pasta and maintain normal blood sugar than a person sitting at their desk all day who struggles to exercise even two or three hours each week. If you enjoy eating pasta and need to improve your blood sugar control, then spaghetti becomes a great incentive to exercise!

As a general guide:

- If you exercise less than 7 hours per week, then choose mostly foods from the low glycemic load list.
- If you are highly active (more than 7 hours of aerobic activity per week), you likely will tolerate 1–2 servings of medium glycemic load foods daily.

Everyone Is Different

Scientists debate how accurate the glycemic load tables are for users, and a recent study showed that people's blood sugar responses can vary by 20 to 30 percent. While scientists might quibble over a few points, generally the glycemic load tables are still useful if they can predict your response within 70 to 80 percent. Of interest, the two biggest factors that create variability in glycemic load response are blood sugar control and levels of inflammation, factors that this book will help you to improve, which will also make your use of these tables more reliable.

Sally's Better Brain Story: Low Sugar Load Foods

When I first met Sally, a new patient, she looked older than her age, which was sixty. But more than anything, she looked worried.

She'd been struggling with her weight—she'd tried at least a dozen diets as well as exercise programs, but the number on the scale seemed stuck. What worried her more than her weight, however, was that she felt she was losing her memory. She forgot details from meetings at the marketing firm where she worked. She had trouble remembering names of new clients. She was constantly misplacing her glasses and cell phone. Her brain felt sluggish. And what really scared her was that her mom, who had been diagnosed with Alzheimer's disease several years ago, had been transferred to a nursing facility the previous year. Would she wind up the same way?

We went over Sally's test results—including fitness and nutrition evaluations, as well as cognitive function scores—to come up with a plan. Her cognitive scores put her in the lower half for her age group, making her job responsibilities a real challenge. She also had elevated blood sugar and insulin levels, and from reviewing her eating plan, I could see why. She had been following a low-fat, high-carb eating plan, with lots of whole grains: whole-grain cereal for breakfast with nonfat milk, a sandwich for lunch, a granola bar for a midafternoon snack, and some protein with brown rice or whole-grain pasta for dinner, followed by a fat-free cookie for dessert. Sally thought her choices were in keeping with a healthy diet and would lead to weight loss, but she was actually sabotaging those efforts and compromising her brain health as well.

To help transform her brain function, Sally needed to pick foods with a low sugar load. I asked her to avoid eating any foods for the next month that had a glycemic load of more than 10. She didn't have to diet, but she had to limit her sugar load at each and every meal, and she also had to eat more healthy fats. She was to take a good-quality supplement as well (discussed in Chapter 5). And I wanted her to go for a walk, either in the morning or after work, for at least twenty to thirty minutes five days per week for the first month.

"That's it?" she said, with some surprise. "I already work harder than that every day." But as I told her, what she was doing wasn't working, so she agreed to give my plan a chance.

At the end of thirty days, she had lost five pounds. She looked more youthful, and her fasting blood sugar and insulin levels were totally normal. We repeated her cognitive function test, and she was now in the top twenty-fifth percentile for executive function, a 50 percent improvement. All those "healthy" whole grains and low-fat foods she had been eating had sent a large glycemic load into her bloodstream, causing her insulin levels to surge and her tissues to stop responding, making her insulin resistant. That resistance had made her brain cells unable to use the overly abundant glucose in her bloodstream. Choosing to avoid foods with a high glycemic load was the key that unlocked her from mental prison. With those accomplishments in place, we talked about ways she could step up her fitness, and additional supplements that she should consider to protect her brain over the long term—all part of the Better Brain Solution. Now almost ten years later, Sally looks and feels younger and is as mentally sharp as ever.

The Better Brain Glycemic Load Tables: Low, Medium, and High

What the numbers mean:
    0–9.9 = a low glycemic load food
    10–19.9 = a medium glycemic load food
    20+ = a high glycemic load food
    (You may find some slight variation on numbers in other sources.)

Table 1: Low Glycemic Load Foods (GL <10)

• *Enjoy Them Every Day*
Most of the vegetables and fruits, and all the nuts and clean protein sources, are low in glycemic load. Beans have a low glycemic load, and eating legumes actually offsets a jump in blood sugar caused by other

foods, such as bread or pasta. It provides a gradual release in blood sugar over hours—exactly what you'd like from eating food.

For nearly two decades, the mantra I have shared with my patients is for them to eat more clean protein, healthy fat, vegetables, fruits, beans, and nuts—with extra spice and herbs for flavor. The glycemic load tables will help you clarify which foods to enjoy more often.

Food Source	Serving Size	Glycemic Load
BEVERAGES		
Tea and coffee, unsweetened	1 cup	0
Milk, almond	1 cup	0
Milk, skim	1 cup	9
Milk, whole	1 cup	9
Milk, soy	1 cup	9
Wine, red or white	5 oz.	0
Beer	12 oz.	3
CEREALS		
Oatmeal, cooked, steel-cut	1 cup	9
SNACKS		
Chocolate, dark (70–85% cocoa)	1 oz.	4
Guacamole	¼ cup	0
Hummus (chickpea salad dip)	1 oz. (30 g)	0
FRUIT		
Apple	1 medium	6
Apricots	1 cup	6
Blueberries, wild*	1 cup	1
Blueberries, commercially raised*	1 cup	4

*The glycemic load discrepancy between blueberry varieties is because wild are small and tart, but commercially raised are modified to be larger, juicier, and sweeter.

Food Source	Serving Size	Glycemic Load
Cherries	1 cup	4
Grapefruit	1 small	3
Grapes	1 cup	5
Mango	1 cup (120 g)	8
Orange	1 medium	4
Peach	1 large	5
Pear	1 medium	5
Pineapple	1 cup	7
Plum	1 cup	5
Strawberries	1 cup	3
Watermelon	1 cup	4
LEGUMES (BEANS)		
Beans, black	½ cup	7
Beans, kidney	½ cup	7
Beans, white	½ cup	9
Chickpeas	½ cup	8
Lentils	½ cup	6
Soybeans (edamame)	½ cup	3
NUTS		
Almonds	1 oz.	0
Cashews, salted	1 oz.	3
Hazelnuts	1 oz.	0
Macadamias	1 oz.	0
Peanuts (actually a legume)	1 oz.	0
Pecans	1 oz.	0
Pistachios	1 oz.	0
Walnuts	1 oz.	0
VEGETABLES		
Asparagus	1 cup	3
Avocado (Florida or California)	½ fruit	0
Beet	1 cup	6

Food Source	Serving Size	Glycemic Load
Bell pepper, green	1 cup	2
Bell pepper, red or yellow	1 cup	3
Bok choy	1 cup	0
Broccoli	1 cup	0
Cabbage	1 cup	0
Carrot	1 cup	2
Cauliflower	1 cup	0
Celery	1 cup	0
Mixed greens, lettuce, and raw spinach	1 cup	0
Peas, frozen or fresh	1 cup	5
PROTEIN SOURCES		
Eggs, steak, chicken, salmon, pork	6 oz.	0
SMART FATS		
Olive, avocado, almond, and coconut oils	1 Tbsp.	0
Avocado (Florida or California)	½ fruit	0

Table 2: Medium Glycemic Load Foods (GL 10 to <20)

• *The More Active You Are, the More Glycemic Load You Can Handle*

For these foods, generally limit your portions to not more than one or two servings per day. You should notice that two commonly eaten foods, potatoes and bananas, are in this medium glycemic load group.

Food Source	Serving Size	Glycemic Load
BEANS		
Beans, baked	½ cup	10
VEGETABLES		
Potato, boiled white and purple	1 cup	14
Potato, instant mashed	1 cup	17
Sweet potato	1 medium (½ cup)	10
FRUITS		
Apricots, dried	¼ cup	10
Banana, regular yellow (without spots)	1 medium	10
Banana, yellow (ripe)	1 medium	15
Dates, dried	¼ cup	14
Papaya	1 cup	10
Raisins	¼ cup	18
GRAINS		
Barley, pearled, cooked (has gluten)	1 cup	11
Bread, pumpernickel	2 slices	13
Cereal, All-Bran (Kellogg's)	1 cup	16
Cereal, Cheerios	1 cup	13
Cereal, Grape-Nuts	1 cup	16
Cereal, Kashi GoLean Crunch	1 cup	17
Grits, cooked	1 cup	14
Hamburger bun	2 slices (1 bun)	18
Muesli (oats, nuts, dried fruit)	1 cup	16
Oatmeal, instant	1 cup	16
Oatmeal, rolled	1 cup	13
Quinoa, cooked	1 cup	18
Spaghetti, whole-meal, boiled	1 cup	15

Food Source	Serving Size	Glycemic Load
Tortilla, flour	50 g (1 tortilla)	15
Wild rice, cooked	1 cup	16
BEVERAGES		
Gatorade	1 cup	12
Juice, apple (unsweetened)	1 cup	12
Juice, fruit	1 cup	12
Juice, orange (unsweetened)	1 cup	12
SNACKS		
Cookies, oatmeal	1.5 oz.	18
Cookies, Vanilla Wafer	6 cookies (1 oz.)	14
Granola bar	2-oz. bar	18
Popcorn, popped	2 cups	12
Rice cakes	1 oz.	18
Tortilla, corn	50 g (2 tortillas)	12
DAIRY		
Yogurt, plain low-fat Greek	245 g (~1 cup)	10

Table 3: High Glycemic Load Foods (GL ≥20)

• *What Are You Celebrating?*

These foods are fine for your birthday but not every day. You should avoid them most of the time. You likely won't be astonished to learn from this chart that a doughnut or a candy bar is high, but you may notice a few surprises, too: whole-wheat bread and white bread have the same high glycemic load (20), a bagel is even higher (34), and "healthy" granola cereal is nearly (literally) off the charts (36). Also notice that none of the proteins, vegetables, fruits, beans, and nuts have a high glycemic load. You won't miss much avoiding high glycemic load foods.

Food Source	Serving Size	Glycemic Load
GRAINS		
Bagel, white	3.5-in.-diameter	34
Bread, whole-wheat	2 slices	20
Bread, Wonder	2 slices (2 oz.)	20
Spaghetti, white, boiled 10 min	1 cup	22
SNACKS AND DESSERTS		
Cake, chocolate, with icing	⅙th cake, 84 g	25
Candy bar, Mars	2 oz.	27
Cookies, Ginger Snap	1.5 oz.	24
Doughnut, glazed	One 4-in.-diameter	22
Ice cream, regular	1 cup	24
Pretzels, oven-baked	2-oz. bag	33
BEVERAGES		
Juice, cranberry cocktail (Ocean Spray)	1 cup	24
Coca-Cola	12-oz. can	25
Fanta (orange soda)	12-oz. can	35
Cereal, Coco Puffs	1 cup	20
Cereal, Corn flakes	1 cup	24
Cereal, Raisin Bran (Kellogg's)	1 cup	26
Cereal, granola (Kashi)	1 cup	37
Corn, sweet	1 cup	22
Couscous, boiled 5 min.	1 cup	30
Macaroni (elbow), cooked	1 cup	23
Macaroni and cheese (Kraft)	1 cup	32
Potato, russet, baked	1 medium (5 oz.)	26
Rice, brown, medium-grain, cooked	1 cup	22

Food Source	Serving Size	Glycemic Load
Rice, white, long-grain, cooked	1 cup	27
Rice, white basmati, quick-cooking	1 cup	28
Chips, potato	4-oz. bag	30
Nacho chips, tortilla chips, salted	3-oz. bag	35

Step 3: Consider Partial Intermittent Fasting

There is one more step you can take to improve insulin sensitivity and cognitive performance, and that is fasting—avoiding calorie intake for a prolonged period of time.

When we fast, we divert energy from digestion to higher purposes and accomplishments that are often attributed to greater mental clarity. Many historical figures and spiritual leaders, from the ancient Greeks to biblical figures to Gandhi, embraced the practice of fasting for a wide variety of reasons, and its use as a form of political protest continues to this day. Fasting has long played a major role in most of the world's religions (Christianity, Judaism, Islam, Buddhism, Hinduism, and more) and is incorporated into many holidays and rituals.

The traditional fast entails avoiding all food and sources of calories for anywhere from twenty-four hours to several days. Hydration with liquids including herbal infusions, tea, and broth, as well as water, is essential during a fast. To end the fast, start with water or broth, then progress to a broth or soup with vegetables. Gradually return to eating normally, with foods that are easy to digest. After a fast, most people report feeling more mindful and connected to the foods they consume. Fasting will not only improve some aspects of cognitive function but help us appreciate food and eating as well.

Partial intermittent fasting is a bit different from the traditional model, but it shows promise for improving blood sugar control as well as cognitive performance, especially for those who may be dealing with cognitive impairment.

How Fasting Impacts Brain Health

One of the benefits of prolonged fasting is that without calorie intake, you eventually exhaust your blood sugar supplies and start burning fat to make energy for cells, which forms molecular compounds called ketones. Many of your tissues can use ketones very effectively, especially your brain.

The challenge is that the longer you have to fast, the harder it is to follow, but for some individuals it's worth doing. "Partial intermittent fasting" is one of the more recent twists on this dietary practice (and is the basis of a number of popular weight-loss diets). Instead of the traditional twenty-four-hours-or-more fast, partial intermittent fasting can have many variations—for example, a fifteen-to-eighteen-hour calorie fast done two or three days per week, or for up to twenty-one to twenty-eight days. And it works for more than weight control.

Recent studies have shown that partial intermittent fasting can be as effective—and sometimes more effective—in improving cognitive performance than traditional fasting; plus it also improves blood sugar control. Avoiding calories (especially carbohydrates) for at least fifteen to eighteen hours will initiate ketone formation and shift fuel usage from glucose (sugar) to ketones (a molecular by-product of fat-burning). The brain's energy-producing factory, the mitochondria, then uses those ketones for fuel. Simply put, in ketosis, cells convert fat rather than sugar into energy, and the brain seems to like that.

At least in studies of mice, extending the time between feedings (without overall calorie restriction) to induce ketosis has shown several brain benefits. Researchers have noted that such intermittent fasting in mice stimulates the ability to handle brain oxidative stress, enhances the ability to memorize new information (neural plasticity), and induces actual brain growth through increased brain-derived neurotrophic factors and heightened brain cell mitochondrial function.

A second form of partial intermittent fasting is to limit calorie intake for one day to 500–800 very-low-carb calories, get into ketosis, then eat as much as you want the next day. During a three-week period, this method of alternating fasting (25 percent of calories) and feasting (175 percent of calories) every other day has been shown to improve insulin resistance and decrease markers of oxidative stress. The limitation was that the improvements in insulin resistance were about as equally effective as interval exercise training for twenty minutes three times per week. You'd have to decide for yourself, but to get the same results, I would find it much easier to add sixty minutes per week of interval exercise than to fast with only 25 percent of my normal calories every other day.

Yet another form of intermittent fasting is to follow an intense and extremely low carb diet for four or five days every month, basically changing the cellular fuel from glucose to ketones for several days in a row each month. During the four-to-five-day fast, carbs make up less than 10 percent of all food sources, with a modest amount of protein, and nearly 70 to 80 percent of calories during the fast are from pure fat. During this high-fat, ultra-low-carb eating plan, typical meals would include:

- Shakes with coconut milk, green leafy vegetables (like kale), and protein powder, and without any fruit or sugar
- Animal protein stir-fry with green leafy vegetables, like spinach, with ample cooking fat
- Liver, bacon, pâté, and other animal protein sources
- Nuts and seeds, avocados, coconut
- Avoiding all fruits, potatoes, grains, beans, and products with sugar
- Adding extra oil to everything you cook

Since the 1920s, and especially with recent protocols at all major epilepsy treatment centers, many people with difficult-to-control epilepsy have shown a marked improvement in seizure control by shifting their brain fuel from glucose to ketones. However, for epilepsy control, they follow this type of very-low-carb, moderate-protein, very-high-fat diet *all* the time, not intermittently. In particular, the brain is able to use ketones, which include the molecular compounds beta-hydroxybutyrate, acetoacetate, and, to a lesser degree, acetone. Based on the benefits shown for people with epilepsy, researchers have tried these same protocols for people with mild cognitive impairment and dementia.

In a small study, twenty-three older adults with mild cognitive impairment were randomly chosen for either a very-low-carb or a high-carb diet for six weeks. Those on the very-low-carb diet who showed signs of ketone formation (as evidenced by ketones being present in the urine and blood) showed improvements in not only their memory scores but also in their waistline and in their fasting insulin and glucose levels. This strategy appears to be effective for those with established cognitive decline, and it seems related to improving blood sugar and insulin control, but it was limited to those willing to follow this restrictive regimen. And we don't know yet whether this type of change yields long-term or only short-term gains.

While a person with epilepsy might be highly motivated to avoid a devastating seizure, a healthier person won't be inclined to adopt this restrictive fasting regimen long-term—it's tough to do. The difficulty in following this plan is a big reason why I have designated partial intermittent fasting as a Step 3 option, not Step 1 or 2. Another reason is that the long-term benefits aren't confirmed. They appear promising but are still being studied.

A Better Way for Women to Fast

One of my friends and medical colleagues, Dr. Anna Cabeca, an obstetrician/gynecologist from Emory University, has been studying the impact of partial fasting regimens for women to address menopause symptoms. Her clinical experience has been that women have much more trouble tolerating fasting with higher meat and fat intake, when they become physiologically acidotic (a state of increased acidity in the blood that may occur with ketosis). Typically, eating animal proteins, eggs, dairy, and grains makes us "acidic," meaning that we're forcing the body to eliminate acid in the urine to keep the blood acidity balanced; eating vegetables, beans, and nuts has the opposite effect. With prolonged acidosis, people lose bone mass and muscle mass and may initially report fatigue and brain fog.

There may be a gender difference in how we respond to fasting. After 100,000 years of history, men may adapt better to an eating plan focused on animal protein intake mixed with fasting, while women may do better with far more plant foods mixed between fasting states. Vegetables, fruits, nuts, and beans make us alkaline. Loading up on vegetables and beans the night before fasting ensures an alkaline fasting state, and Dr. Cabeca has found that having her menopausal patients do a vegetable feast before an overnight prolonged fast improves many aspects of their quality of life and makes fasting far more tolerable.

Fasting Options: Coffee with Milk, or with Fat?

When I talk to my clinic patients about fasting, we review the partial intermittent fasting options:

1. Fasting overnight for 15–18 hours (basically skipping breakfast) 2–3 days per week
2. Very-low-carb fasting every other day
3. Very-low-carb fasting 4–5 days per month

Thus far, in these short-term studies, all three approaches seem similarly effective. However, the vast majority of my patients say the first option—to skip breakfast (fast for fifteen to eighteen hours) two or three days per week—is the easiest to follow, and I predict that this approach would probably be the easiest for you, as well.

With the fifteen-hour overnight fast, there are two options. Option one is hydration (water, tea, herbal infusions, or broth), but no meaningful calories. A friend and colleague, Dr. Kellyann Petrucci, M.S., N.D., made this very popular with her Bone Broth Diet, as she has people limit their calorie intake to only bone broth for eighteen-plus hours two days per week.

Another, even easier-to-follow variation of fifteen-to-eighteen-hour fasting was developed by another colleague, Dave Asprey, who created the Bulletproof Diet. He asks people to eliminate all carbs and protein for fifteen to eighteen hours most days, just having coffee and fat for breakfast (see "Bulletproof Coffee" box, page 115). The advantage of adding fat to your coffee is that because you are adding 300 to 400 calories, you don't get hungry, but without carbs or protein, you go into ketosis as if you didn't consume any calories at all, minus the hunger.

To get the most benefit from adding fat to your coffee, you don't dump in half-and-half or cream and stir well. Instead, you use a medium-chain triglyceride (MCT) oil and clarified butter (ghee) and mix the fats with the coffee in a blender. MCTs, typically derived from coconut oil or palm oil, are a special form of saturated fat that has shorter chains than the saturated fats that come from meat, eggs, and palm oil. MCT oil breaks down pretty quickly into ketones and provides a very effective fuel source not only for people with epilepsy but also for competitive athletes who participate in long-distance sports and don't want to run out of fuel. While a person typically runs out of glycogen (sugar stored in chains in muscle cells) within 90 to 120 minutes with exercise, nearly all of us have enough fat stores to be used as fuel all day long, giving a big advantage to using fat as fuel for long-distance sports.

Because MCT oils break down into ketones, they are also being used as supplements for people with mild cognitive impairment and dementia. In 2009 Samuel Henderson (vice president of research and development for the biotech company Accera) and his research team evaluated 152 subjects with mild to moderate Alzheimer's disease in a ninety-day randomized study—in other words, nobody knew who was getting what. Instead of having the participants fast to create ketones, researchers gave them an MCT oil supplement or a look-alike placebo, initially ten grams of MCT oil per day during week one, then twenty grams per day for the remaining ninety days. Those getting MCT oil had a clear increase in ketone levels (especially beta-hydroxybutyrate, which is used readily by the brain as fuel), and their cognitive function improved compared to the placebo-treated group.

The biggest downside was that at the dosage of twenty grams daily, 25 percent of the MCT-treated subjects had diarrhea, more than four watery stools per day, sometimes with urgency and crampiness. This discomfort might be worth it for someone with established memory loss (a scary if compelling diagnosis) if they got a boost in brain function, but it's far harder to tolerate if you are looking for a bit of cognitive edge in your daily, healthy life. You'd have to decide for yourself if you'd prefer to generate ketones through fasting, or tolerate the gastrointestinal issues by adding a hefty dosage of MCT oil, about 1.5 tablespoons every day.

The other major concern with this study is that while there were some benefits for people with the ApoE2 and ApoE3 genotypes, 20 percent of the population with at least one ApoE4 gene showed no benefit. Those are precisely the individuals who have a 300 percent greater risk for developing Alzheimer's disease, and that's an unfortunate and frustrating finding because they are the group most desperately in need of a solution like this.

I personally know of one exception—and it's a striking one. In researching this book, I spoke to Dr. Mary Newport, a physician from Florida who was famous in a way that she would have preferred not to be: her husband was diagnosed more than a decade ago with premature Alzheimer's disease, and she was researching treatment options. All the medications available had failed him, and Mary was looking for additional options. Though he carried an ApoE4 gene, she tried him on a series of products, including coconut oil, later MCT oil, and finally beta-hydroxybutyrate (the primary ketone in MCT oil), finding moderate improvement with *all* of these treatments. Mary has spoken at a variety of physician meetings during the last decade and published articles related to her trials. Her husband's initial success clearly shows that although he had the ApoE4 gene, some individuals are still able to benefit from this type of plan, at least in the short term.

For some reason not yet known, the majority of people with memory loss and the ApoE4 gene are not able to use ketones effectively as brain fuel. Thus, if you have an ApoE4 genotype, it is much more important to prevent cognitive decline and maintain excellent blood sugar and insulin regulation. As noted in the study above, consuming MCT oil does not appear to be highly effective once memory loss has occurred, although partial intermittent fasting may still have other benefits for this high-risk population. For people with an ApoE4 gene, see additional tips to prevent cognitive decline in Chapter 10.

Bulletproof Coffee

Dave Asprey suggests how to make Bulletproof Coffee with MCT oil; he started the trend toward mixing organic, super-clean, mold-free coffee with butter and MCT oil. Always use a blender. If you pour MCT oil into hot coffee, the fat will float to the top and you may burn your tongue trying to drink it.

Start with 8 ounces of hot coffee, 2 teaspoons of MCT oil, and 1–2 tablespoons of butter or organic ghee. Ghee is essentially dairy free (no dairy protein), so people with dairy intolerance are able to use it without side effects.

First, pour hot water into the blender to warm the container; once that is done, pour the water out. Next, add the hot coffee and MCT oil and blend carefully (taking precautions so it doesn't splatter). Add a bit of butter (or ghee, organic clarified butter) to the mixture, making a nice, creamy suspension. MCT oil by itself is a bit bland, so blending in ghee adds flavor and richness. The minute amount of dairy protein in regular butter provides lasting foam formation when you blend the coffee, creating a cappuccino effect, so if you truly want foam, you need to use real butter. You can gradually increase the MCT oil to 20 grams daily over time.

A much simpler way to fast and not go hungry (and avoid putting coffee in a blender) is to add organic heavy cream to coffee. Two tablespoons provide 103 calories and less than 1 gram of carbs. If you are otherwise fasting, have one or two cups of coffee with fat, and you'll reach ketosis—start burning fat and making ketones. Using MCT oil as a fat offers a big boost in ketone levels and especially for people with MCI, might make preparing their coffee in a blender worth it.

Coffee Fat Chart

Note: This chart compares 20 grams of MCT oil to 20 grams of butter, half-and-half, or heavy cream per one 8-ounce cup of coffee; in relevant studies of MCT oil, the amount specified is 20 grams of fat. I've also included 30-gram listings for half-and-half and heavy cream, which is a standard prepackaged single-serving size. Aim to keep carbohydrate grams to less than 1 if you are trying to get into ketosis.

	Calories	Fat Grams	Protein Grams	Carbohy- drate Grams
MCT oil (20 g, 1½ Tbsp.)	164	20	0	0
Butter (20 g, 1½ Tbsp.)	143	16.2	0.2	0.01
Half-and- half (20 g, 1⅓ Tbsp.)	26	2.3	0.6	0.87
Heavy cream (20 g, 1⅓ Tbsp.)	67	6.7	0	0.5
Half-and- half (30 g = 2 Tbsp.)	39	3.5	0.9	1.3
Heavy cream (30 g = 2 Tbsp.)	103	11	0.6	0.8
MCT oil and butter	307	36.2	0.2	0.01

Another Way to Boost Ketones

If you don't want to add fat to your coffee, another alternative to taking MCT oil is to drink an elixir loaded with the ketone compound beta-hydroxybutyrate. Whereas MCT oil is converted into ketones, there are now products available that provide the ketones themselves. Popular with athletes and often sold in a powdered form (users compare the taste to Tang), these drinks are fairly expensive, at around four dollars per serving. These products have just started to be studied, however, and there is a concern that the initial ketone elixirs may be contaminated with other products that might cause harm. If you want to test this type of elixir, ensure that the product is pure beta-hydroxybutyrate, without acetone or formaldehyde by-products.

What About Coconut Products?

Coconut products (such as coconut milk and the meat of the coconut) and oil are different from MCT oil. "MCT oil" and "coconut oil" are *not* interchangeable terms, as coconut oil has only about one-fourth to one-eighth the concentration of medium-chain triglycerides compared to pure MCT oil. MCT oil is usually concentrated from coconut oil or palm oil. The MCT oil used in Dr. Henderson's study was more than 95 percent caprylic acid and caproic acid, which are shorter versions of medium-chain triglycerides. For those of you into biochemistry (or if you just want to understand the significance of molecular chain-length in this context): medium-chain triglycerides include caprylic acid with 8 carbon chains, caproic acid with 6, capric acid with 10, and lauric acid with 12. Here's the key fact: the shorter chains—in this case, caprylic and caproic acids—are better at forming ketones.

Coconut oil has only about 25 percent of these shorter MCT forms and is more than 50 percent lauric acid. It also has a wide variety of other fatty acids, including 223 mg (0.223 grams) per tablespoon of omega-6 fatty acids—part of the reason it has such a low smoke point for cooking, meaning it tolerates only cooking temperatures below 350°F. (It's a myth that you can safely cook at high heat with coconut oil, because it can convert to a damaged fat at temperatures above 350°F.)

If the goal is to produce ketones to be used as brain fuel, then MCT oil appears to be a better choice than coconut oil, as it has anywhere from four to eight times the potency of coconut oil. Yet consuming coconut oil is associated with several health benefits:

- The primary oil component in coconut oil is lauric acid, which, once digested, is very effective at killing microbes and fighting infections. It is often used by natural health practitioners to help remove GI pathogens.
- Coconut oil boosts metabolism (calorie burning) in highly active people, as the medium-chain fats are great for athletes to use as fuel, especially for prolonged exercise sessions, which is why athletes often combine coconut milk with their workout protein shakes.
- Coconut oil generally appears to be beneficial for cognitive

function and for people with neurological disease, as the medium-chain triglycerides will help to form ketones—less than pure MCT oil does, but far more than other oils.

Despite these benefits, coconut oil is still controversial because eating more coconut products increases cholesterol levels. Coconut oil and coconut products are made of 90 percent saturated fat, much more than is found in butter (64 percent) or beef fat (40 percent). Consuming coconut products daily raises LDL and total cholesterol by 40 to 70 points. That said, it increases healthy HDL levels as well and may even improve the healthy total cholesterol/HDL ratio. Another cholesterol benefit of consuming coconut products is that they increase LDL particle size (considered good); thus, although a conventional physician might be concerned by the shift in your cholesterol profile, the net change on cholesterol profiles may be more beneficial than problematic.

My concern, however, is we do not have any clinical outcome studies that show eating coconut is either neutral or beneficial, and at least one clinical study using coconut products showed that they decreased artery function and worsened HDL inflammation. For those reasons, I don't recommend coconut oil to my patients with established heart disease.

Skip the Coconut Water

I'm hesitant to suggest coconut oil for people with heart issues but I'm even more concerned about the highly popular coconut water—for anyone. A typical 11-ounce serving of coconut water has 12.5 grams of sugar, nearly 1 tablespoon, without any meaningful fiber. This is akin to drinking apple juice instead of eating an apple, which is far more sugar than I'd recommend for anyone. When some of my patients with diabetes started using coconut water as a sports drink during their regular workout activities, such as during a tennis match, they almost immediately went from well-controlled blood sugar to poorly controlled—and the only change was a few servings of coconut water daily. Plain water is a much better choice. If you can find unsweetened coconut water (without sugar), then it's fine to enjoy it.

My recommendation is that if you are in good health, or if you have neurological issues like memory loss, and especially if you are trying to follow a ketogenic diet, then it is likely smart to eat more coconut products. However, if you have established heart disease or are being treated by your doctor for abnormal cholesterol problems, I'd recommend that you consult with your doctor, avoid coconut oil in general, and enjoy the many other heart- and brain-friendly fats. Other fats to consider beyond coconut oil would be avocado and avocado oil, nuts and nut oils, dark chocolate, wild cold-water fish, and of course olives and olive oil.

If instead of pure coconut oil you are using coconut products, use coconut milk as well as coconut flour and meat, as they also provide fiber, flavonoids, and other vitamins and minerals. I remain enthusiastic that someday coconut products will be shown to have clinical benefits, which is why despite the lack of proven benefit, you'll notice that I use coconut flour and coconut milk in several of my recipes (see Chapter 10).

What Is the Best Form of Partial Fasting?

An overnight fast with nothing to eat after seven or eight p.m. a couple of days per week seems the easiest type of partial intermittent fasting to try first, allowing you some form of fat, in particular with your coffee or tea for breakfast, to suppress hunger. The evening before your partial fast, eat a big salad, extra vegetables, or bean-vegetable soup to help induce a more alkaline state. Don't eat anything else until noon.

Despite the potential health benefits of partial intermittent fasting, I have designated it as Step 3 of my food plan for several reasons. It is harder to follow than adding foods that are proven to enhance brain function (things like dark chocolate, berries, greens, coffee/tea, and red wine), as in Step 1, and more difficult than choosing foods that have a low sugar load, as in Step 2. Second, the limitations are that we don't know if this type of fasting intervention will work over the long term (as in years), or for just the thirty to ninety days they have been studied to date. Furthermore, we don't know which type of intermittent fasting is the most effective, although the initial data suggest that they all work.

Finally, although partial intermittent fasting and adding MCT oil to generate an elevation in ketones has been shown to help people with dementia and mild cognitive impairment over the short term, we simply don't know if they help people who are relatively healthy with normal brain function—those of you trying to optimize your current brain function and prevent future memory loss.

If you want to try Step 3, I leave it up to you to decide if following one of these fasting regimens matches your lifestyle. Certainly, doing Steps 1 and 2 will take you a long way toward achieving better brain health. Step 3 has the potential to take you even further.

The recipes starting on page 255 feature the brain-boosting foods at the heart of Steps 1 and 2. Weigh the fasting options in Step 3 as well as the use of MCT oil—all of which will improve your blood sugar and insulin control. You can start on those recipes now, and perhaps they will inspire you to try some of your own brain-boosting food combinations.

Now, to the second pillar of the program: key nutrients for brain health.

CHAPTER 5

Key Nutrients for Brain Health

At least 85 percent of all Americans have major nutrient deficiencies that adversely impact their health in a variety of ways, including accelerated cognitive decline. This seems shocking in a country where nutritious food is plentiful, but the problem is SAD—the Standard American Diet—that most men, women, and children are consuming.

Everyone needs a personalized plan to meet their key nutrient needs, and ideally they would do it with food. But in reality, and certainly after seeing thousands of patients over thirty years as a physician, I have yet to meet a person who eats well all the time. Furthermore, nutrient content in food has decreased substantially over the last several decades, as processed food has crowded out real food. Even whole foods—fruits, vegetables, and whole grains—have been diminished nutritionally through industrialized farming, the use of pesticides, and other practices, compounded by the amount of processing done by big food manufacturers. Considering all the toxins in our environment today, we need extra nutrients, certainly not fewer, to detoxify and remove these chemicals from our tissues.

Adding vitamins, minerals, and other valuable nutrient therapies can only enhance a healthy eating plan—they can't replace it. Supplements will never make up for eating junk food, skipping a workout, being stressed out, or getting poisoned by toxins like pesticides or hydrogenated fats. Eating well—especially choosing brain-boosting foods and reducing your sugar load—should be a priority if you want to correct any deficiencies.

It's important to note the limitations of looking at the effect of one nutrient or a single compound at a time on cognition; that isn't how Mother Nature works. Typically, dozens or hundreds of nutrients and compounds interact to enhance physiological function. One agent on its own often will not work as well as several compounds used together.

That is why many supplement compounds sold with claims to support brain function use anywhere from five to twenty ingredients at the same time, though most studies evaluate these compounds one at a time. (The reality is that those combinations are rarely, if ever, tested together.) Their manufacturers can't claim that a multi-ingredient compound will prevent memory loss or improve cognitive function, because such a claim would have to be substantiated with research, in complex and sophisticated studies that would cost millions of dollars. Instead, manufacturers typically rely upon a vague statement that doesn't require research, like "this product supports healthy brain function." (For an example of a product that has crossed the line in terms of claims and research, see the box "The Problem with Prevagen" on pages 144–145.)

With this limitation in mind, here are key nutrients—not compounds with a multitude of agents—that we know, without a doubt, are essential for preventing memory loss.

Step 1: Get the Essentials

These nutrients are necessary for optimal cognitive function, and strong evidence supports their use. Some of these nutrients can be found in food, but if that isn't realistic (because of the amount of that food you'd have to eat in a day), there are supplement options as well.

- Vitamin D
- Vitamin B12
- Mixed folates (also known as vitamin B9)
- Chromium
- Long-chain omega-3 fats (fish oil)
- Probiotic source
- Magnesium

Vitamin D

Vitamin D is a fat-soluble vitamin, but once it has been converted to its active form, it functions like a hormone. Nearly every cell in your body has a vitamin D receptor, and vitamin D modifies how your cells function.

For the last 100,000 years, humans have obtained vitamin D from sunlight. (The sun stimulates vitamin D production when a form of ultraviolet light reacts with a cholesterol molecule in the blood.) Early humans, their skin exposed with limited clothing, spent twelve to sixteen hours daily hunting and gathering in direct sunlight.

Today, of course, most people wear clothing and are indoors most of the time. And for six months of the year (late fall–winter and early spring), people living north of Santa Barbara, Dallas, and Atlanta don't make any significant vitamin D. And when we are in the sun, wearing sunscreen, which is essential for guarding against skin cancer, blocks the skin from making vitamin D.

While a twenty-year-old should be able to make enough vitamin D from twenty minutes of sun exposure, he or she would have to be on a beach or by a pool in a skimpy bathing suit (lots of skin showing and no sunscreen, for maximum sun absorption) between ten a.m. and two p.m. with peak sun. In contrast, the skin of someone fifty or older isn't nearly as efficient at using sunlight to convert cholesterol into vitamin D. That person may require sixty minutes to make the same amount of D, with similar attire and time of day. Spending an hour in the midday sun—without sunscreen—is a tall order for most of us. Even living in Florida, the Sunshine State, 90 percent of my patients are vitamin D deficient unless they take a supplement, and the majority of them need to take at least 2,000 IU daily to achieve an optimal level, above 40 ng/mL (nanograms per milliliter, as measured in the blood).

Experts argue about what constitutes a normal vitamin D level, but most would agree that a level less than 30 ng/mL is deficient; that greater than 30 is acceptable; and that 40–70 is optimal. More than 100 ng/mL is associated with significant (negative) side effects. Vitamin D supplementation is extremely safe, and dosing up to 3,000 IU daily has never been associated with any side effects or toxicity.

Without vitamin D supplements, most Americans become deficient and show bone loss and elevated risk for fracture, heart disease, diabetes, and weight gain. Randomized clinical studies have shown that giving vitamin D decreases the risk for cancer by up to 40 percent and also reduces the risk for autoimmune diseases. It also plays a major role in brain health.

Vitamin D crosses the blood-brain barrier, the protective cellular barrier that lets certain nutrients into the brain and keeps other substances out. Once vitamin D passes through, it diffuses easily into the cerebrospinal fluid. Several studies have shown that low vitamin D levels are associated with a higher risk for cognitive decline and dementia. Vitamin D deficiency increases your risk for multiple sclerosis as well. People with higher vitamin D levels appear to have larger brains than people with low vitamin D levels. The active form of vitamin D, called 1,25-dihydroxyvitamin D, stimulates brain cell growth, including in the hippocampus—the memory center—and activates numerous neurotransmitters in the brain.

Studies using vitamin D to slow existing cognitive decline are still needed. In a small pilot study in India with eighty subjects, randomized to receive either a placebo or a vitamin D supplement, those who received the vitamin D showed greater improvements in cognitive function based on their performance on the Mini-Mental State Examination (MMSE). More research is needed.

- *Vitamin D Better Brain Action:*
  Take 2,000 IU Daily

At some point, after you have been taking vitamin D consistently for at least three months, you should have your blood levels of vitamin D checked. A measurement of 25-OH would indicate that this dosage gives you a normal blood level of vitamin D. Some people may have poor absorption and require higher dosing, although 2,000 IU daily will be adequate for most adults. Gluten sensitivity can limit nutrient absorption. If you take a vegetarian form of vitamin D (such as vitamin D2), it is extra important to check your level, as most of us absorb vitamin D2 differently.

Key Ingredients in a Multivitamin

Before we discuss the Better Brain nutrients, such as B12, folates, and chromium, that are generally found in multivitamins, it's important to note a few facts about multivitamins, including how to locate quality supplements.

Most multivitamin supplements on the shelves of chain drugstores are low in quality and won't deliver the potent levels of nutrients your brain and body need. Consumer advocate groups, such as Consumer-Lab.com, which monitors the supplement industry, regularly conduct independent testing and point out that what is printed on the label isn't necessarily what is in the bottle. (A rock-bottom price, for starters, should always give you pause, especially if you're buying online and can't examine the packaging for ingredients and expiration dates. Good supplements are not inexpensive.)

For one thing, it's impossible to get all the vitamins you need in one small pill—all these nutrients cannot be combined and compressed to fit into a compact pill, due to their molecular structure. A quality multivitamin is most likely to be at least two pills, not one. My clinic offers four brands that I trust for quality: Designs for Health, Thorne Research, Metagenics, and ProThera. You can purchase their products online or through a health-care provider, including a licensed nutritionist or a physician.

If you want the best quality, here is a look at what should be in a multivitamin and what should not.

- **Folacin or 5-MTHF (mixed folates)**—*not only folic acid*
- **Mixed carotenoids**—*not solely beta-carotene*
- **Mixed tocopherols**—*not only alpha tocopherol (manufacturers are required to label alpha tocopherol content by itself, but it should contain mixed tocopherols as well)*
- **Protein-bound minerals (malates, glycinates)**—*not oxides (like magnesium oxide)*
- **Zinc-to-copper ratio of 20 or more**
- **Organic copper (copper glycinate)**—*not inorganic copper* (copper sulfate or copper carbonate), which is potentially toxic; see Chapter 8.

- **Chromium**—*at least 400 mcg*
- **Vitamin B12 (cobalamin)**—*at least 100 mcg*

Vitamin B12

Vitamin B12 is an essential nutrient used by cells to convert glucose into energy. Brain cells are particularly sensitive to an inadequate B12 supply. When vitamin B12 levels decrease to dangerously low levels, brain cells die. You can have permanent, irreversible nerve damage and develop dementia from vitamin B12 deficiency, which, alarmingly, is becoming common.

For the last 100,000 years, we consumed some of our vitamin B12 from eating animal protein, but a surprising, indirect source was also crucial—dirt! When we eat dirt, we consume bacteria, and these dirt-laden bacteria ultimately produce vitamin B12. Our ancestors ate dirty plant foods, including roots and leaves, and dirty meat. Even up until the last century, dirt was still making its way into our food supply, providing a guaranteed source of vitamin B12. Today our foods are washed, sometimes irradiated, and coated in plastic. There isn't much dirt left, and gone too are the helpful bacteria that triggered the production of a vital nutrient.

Certain groups of people are at high risk for vitamin B12 deficiency. First are vegetarians and vegans (not because they are eating dirt-free plant foods, but because they do not consume animal protein). If you are following a healthy vegetarian or vegan eating plan, you're likely well aware of this concern, and you know the remedy is simple: take a vitamin B12 supplement (50–1,000 mcg daily depending upon your health issues).

The much larger group at risk for B12 deficiency are people who lack stomach acid, as stomach acid is essential to absorb nutrients, especially vitamin B12. As we age normally, we lose stomach acid—and with it the ability to absorb vitamin B12. Sometimes this condition is mild, but it can be severe. Though there are symptoms (see list on page 128), the only way to know for sure is to have your vitamin B12 levels measured through bloodwork.

Over-the-counter and prescription heartburn medications, however, are a bigger issue than acid reductions caused by normal aging. Millions of people now take heartburn medications that decrease the absorption of vitamin B12 as well as other nutrients such as calcium. Acid-blocking medications negatively impact the microbiome. (Many such medications now carry a "black box" warning to signal their stomach acid– and nutrient-blocking side effects.) The most powerful acid blockers are the proton pump inhibitors, including Nexium, Prilosec, Omeprazole, Lansoprazole, Protonix, Aciphex, Dexilent, and Prevacid. These medications are effective treatments for those with serious gastric reflux issues, but they can also cause extensive nutrient deficiencies. If you are using these types of acid blockers, a high-quality supplement regimen is therefore very important. Other antacids that block nutrient absorption include Ranitidine, Zantac, Tagamet, Cimetidine, Tums, Rolaids, and Mylanta. If you use any of them regularly, be sure to check for the signs listed below.

Here are symptoms and signs suggesting vitamin B12 deficiency:

- Tingling, numbness, and burning in your extremities (neuropathy)
- Memory problems
- Poor balance, especially standing with your eyes closed (ataxia)
- Decreased vibratory sense
- Elevated homocysteine
- Anemia
- Elevated MCV (mean corpuscular volume) on a complete blood count (CBC) lab test

Don't miss these signs, as over time they can cause permanent neurological injury.

Testing for vitamin B12 deficiency is simple, although your doctor will need to order it as a blood test, and low-to-normal levels may require additional testing. Most labs consider a B12 level below 250–300 pg/mL (picogram/milliliter) to be low, and low-to-normal to be 300–500 pg/mL. Above 500 pg/mL is desirable.

If you have borderline low levels, and also the signs or symptoms noted above, then additional testing may be warranted. On occasion, a blood level could be above 250–300 pg/mL in the low-to-normal 300–500 pg/mL range, but such a result might not reflect the fact that intracellular levels are actually low. The result could be permanent neurological damage. A test to clarify borderline low B12 levels assesses vitamin B12 function, namely a methylmalonic acid level. Vitamin B12 should lower methylmalonic acid, so if this level is high, that is a functional sign of B12 deficiency.

In the past, we treated people with vitamin B12 shots and intravenous treatments, but fortunately those are not needed with the updated dosing that many physicians and other health-care practitioners now follow. The current recommended daily allowance (RDA) for vitamin B12, however, does create some confusion: it varies from 2 to 3 mcg daily, which is enough to meet the needs of a teenager without any intestinal problems but insufficient for many others. Many multivitamins provide 10 mcg of B12 to meet this RDA need, but for adults with stomach irritation and limited stomach acid production, including that caused by normal aging, this will leave too many of them vitamin B12 deficient.

That's why I typically recommend a daily multivitamin with at least 100 mcg, and the multivitamins I carry typically have 500 mcg of vitamin B12 to ensure it meets the needs of 99 percent of my patients. (Rarely, I'll meet a patient with gastrointestinal issues who requires 1,000–2,000 mcg daily.) Back when we were limiting our therapy to 10 mcg daily, B12 shots were pretty common, but now that we have dosing at the 1,000–2,000 mcg levels, that just seems like added expense and bother. Sublingual levels are also available with lower dosages, but they cost more than regular oral pills with 1,000–2,000 mcg dosing.

A variety of studies have tried treating adults with vitamin B12 to help prevent cognitive decline and improve cognitive performance. Thus far these studies have been pretty disappointing. Therapies with B12 have not slowed cognitive decline. They will work only for those who are vitamin B12 deficient. However, allowing yourself to become deficient in B12 will likely harm your brain. You can avoid deficiency with a good-quality multivitamin supplement.

- *Vitamin B12 Better Brain Action:*
  Take at Least 100 mcg Daily, and More If Needed

I recommend that you take a multivitamin with at least 100 mcg of vitamin B12 daily. If you have any of the symptoms noted on page 128, have your vitamin B12 level checked. If you use medications to treat heartburn or dyspepsia, you may need at least 500 mcg of vitamin B12 daily. In my clinic, I offer a multivitamin with 500 mcg of vitamin B12. Some people absorb vitamin B12 very poorly and need up to 2,000 mcg daily.

High intakes of vitamin B12 are not harmful, unless an individual has a deficiency in folate, a related nutrient. Because it is harder to diagnose folate deficiency when someone is taking extra vitamin B12, let's talk about folate deficiency next.

Mixed Folates (also known as Vitamin B9)

Folates, which are a group of B9 vitamins, are required for methylation, a process that repairs cellular DNA and removes toxins. People with folate deficiency are at elevated risk for depression, heart disease, cognitive decline, and dementia. Rich food sources of naturally occurring folates include leafy green vegetables, beans, and whole grains.

Most people can convert folic acid, the synthetic version of folate found in supplements, into active folates. (Folic acid is also added to foods such as flour and cereal.) Two examples of active folates that play a big role in brain health include folacin and methylenetetrahydrofolate (a tongue-twister of a name abbreviated as 5-MTHF). However, up to 40 percent of people are not able to effectively convert folic acid to these active forms, and most inexpensive supplements rely upon the assumption that you can do so. If you're in that group, then the five-dollar bottle of "folic acid" you bought at your drugstore isn't doing you much good; nor are those fortified foods.

Folate deficiency, like vitamin B12 deficiency, is associated with a metabolic problem: high levels of the toxic compound homocysteine. High homocysteine levels are strongly associated with increased risk for dementia, depression, and heart disease. Yet short-term studies tracking people with high homocysteine levels found that treatment with high dosages of folic acid and vitamin B12 did not prevent cognitive decline. The role of homocysteine remains a complicated topic, hotly disputed in the nutrition science community, but most likely homocysteine is a sign of a metabolic problem, not the true cause of the injury—in this case, dementia, depression, and heart disease.

We do know that both folate deficiency and vitamin B12 deficiency can result in cognitive decline and dementia, as well as depression.

Treatment with adequate dosing will help to prevent this. However, unlike vitamin B12, where excess dosages seem harmless, excess dosages with active folate can cause problems. Because folates help DNA repair itself (methylation), extra folates seem to repair cancer DNA as well, increasing the risk for colon cancer and colon polyp growth. Therefore, you don't want to take more folate than you need.

- *Folates Better Brain Action:*
  Take at Least 400 mcg Daily

Most people need at least 400 mcg of active folates, such as folacin and methylenetetrahydrofolate (5-MTHF), to prevent a deficiency state. But taking more than 1,000 mcg daily can lead to problems. People who eat plenty of beans, leafy green veggies, and whole grains can easily get 400 mcg of active folates daily. Adding at least 400 mcg of active folates in a daily multivitamin, and enjoying the healthy foods noted, will give you enough, but not too much, active folate, with a total supplement-plus-food dosage of 400–800 mcg daily. In some unusual situations, your doctor may recommend higher dosing, but this is a discussion I'll leave to you and your personal physician.

A multivitamin with cheap, inferior ingredients, such as only folic acid, puts up to 40 percent of the population at risk for folate deficiency. That is why your multivitamin should specify mixed folates, including folacin and 5-MTHF. Genetic testing related to this issue is discussed in Chapter 2.

Chromium

Chromium is a mineral that is essential for insulin sensitivity. I don't know of any studies that show an association between chromium and cognitive decline, yet people with low chromium levels are more likely to be insulin resistant, and insulin resistance is the most important reversible cause of dementia. Giving a chromium supplement in randomized trials has not improved blood sugar levels, as studies didn't target people with a chromium deficiency. However, in people with documented chromium deficiency, the supplement does improve blood sugar control.

Foods rich in chromium include meats, whole-grain products, high-bran cereals, green beans, broccoli, nuts, and egg yolks. Eating simple sugars increases chromium excretion—another reason to avoid added sugar. Ironically, people with diabetes are more likely to suffer from chromium deficiency, as chromium is lost with excess urination, worsening their already compromised blood sugar control.

- *Chromium Better Brain Action:*
  Take 400–800 mcg Daily

The solution is really simple. Ensure you take a good-quality multivitamin with at least 400–800 mcg of chromium daily.

You can get adequate vitamin B12, folate, and chromium from a good-quality multivitamin. (See pages 126–132 for recommended quantities.)

Next, let's focus on what you won't find in a multivitamin (besides adequate vitamin D): long-chain omega-3s, a probiotic source, and magnesium.

Long-Chain Omega-3 Fats (commonly called fish oil)

You read about the benefits of adding omega-3-rich seafood to your diet in Chapter 3. As a reminder, to reap the brain benefits of cold-water fish (such as wild salmon, sardines, or herring), I recommend you eat them at least two or three times every week. The least expensive way to get your long-chain omega-3 fats would be from eating wild canned salmon.

Yet at least 30 percent of my patients don't like those varieties of fish, and for them it isn't realistic for me to recommend it so frequently. I know from experience, as a physician and as someone who loves to cook and feed others, that if I ask an adult to eat something he or she truly dislikes, even if it's beneficial, chances are they will not stick with it for the long term, unless their palates change. For those who do not care for the taste of cold-water fish, therefore, a supplement is a good alternative. Still (one more plug for one of my favorite foods), the benefits of eating fish are well established and far less controversial than taking fish oil supplements.

If you take long-chain omega-3 supplements, there are a few major concerns you should know about. The first involves dosing. Some companies sell fish oil products that contain inadequate ratios of beneficial DHA and EPA components and diluted omega-3 components. The result is a less effective, watered-down supplement.

A number of manufacturers have developed modified ratios, with extra EPA, but most of them guessed wrong when they made these modifications. Recent research has shown that DHA appears to be more effective than EPA. DHA is better at improving lipid profiles, decreasing inflammation, and improving cognitive scores than EPA.

In 1,000 mg of most natural sources of fish oil, there are about 500 mg EPA, 400 mg DHA, and 100 mg of other mixed omega-3 fats. However, some forms are modified to have 70 to 80 percent EPA and only 10 to 20 percent DHA; I'd suggest avoiding those EPA-enriched formulas. Pure DHA would be excellent, but it is very hard to find and quite expensive, so considering the cost and value, a fish oil containing 600 mg EPA and 400 mg DHA is acceptable—just not less DHA to EPA than that ratio. Furthermore, whatever long-chain omega-3 supplement you choose should have at least 1,000 mg (combined) of DHA and EPA. You might find a 1,000 mg capsule of fish oil, but read the label. It could have 300 mg of EPA and 200 of DHA, and 500 mg of other mixed omega-3s. That is only a 500 mg dosage of EPA and DHA.

The second concern is contamination. Most fish oil sold in the United States would not be permitted to be sold in Europe because it is rancid. It has been cheaply extracted and/or improperly stored, and its molecular components have broken down. It tastes awful. Good-quality fish oil should not have a bad fish oil flavor. Rather, it should taste like fresh wild salmon, which is fishy but pleasantly so—not "yuck" fishy. (Unless you have no sense of smell, you're unlikely to miss the rank odor of bad fish. That's what you need to steer clear of.) The simplest way to test your fish oil is to taste it. When fish oil comes as a liquid in a glass bottle, that's easy, but when it comes in capsules, here is a tip—select one capsule from the bottle and stick a needle or pin into it, squeeze gently, and taste a drop. It should taste pleasant or return it.

High-quality fish oil with low levels of rancidity undergoes strict processing procedures, not something you'll find in most inexpensive fish oils. I'm not just trying to spare you the experience of getting a whiff of something rotten. Consuming rancid fish oil is quite bad for you because you are ingesting a big load of oxidized free radical fats that damage your cell membranes, including those in your brain. Find high-quality fish oil or skip it altogether.

A third concern surrounding the benefits from fish oil involves the ApoE4 genotype. In studies, if researchers don't control for the ApoE4 genotype (that is, identify and exclude it from trials), and everyone is given only 500 mg of EPA and DHA, then the entire group may not show any benefit. The results will be skewed if studies don't control for ApoE4. We know that people with the ApoE4 gene need bigger dosages to benefit, but they also benefit more than people without the ApoE4 gene. I recommend that people with the ApoE4 gene get 2,000 mg of EPA and DHA daily.

Long-Chain Omega-3 Fats Better Brain Action:
Eat Fish and Get 1,000 mg of EPA and DHA Daily

Ensure you are eating fatty cold-water fish two to three times per week (wild salmon, sardines, herring, sole), or multiple servings of seaweed weekly, or take 1,000 mg of EPA and DHA in a high-quality fish oil supplement.

Vegetarians can aim for 500 mg of DHA from a seaweed supplement daily. (Seaweed has DHA, not EPA.) Vegetarians probably don't need 1,000 mg. Animal protein consumption modestly raises inflammation levels. Vegetarians who eat well most likely have less inflammation than meat eaters, so 500 mg of DHA is likely sufficient.

The majority of people with an ApoE4 genotype should aim to consume 2,000 mg of EPA and DHA daily; check with your physician to confirm that this won't conflict with other medications you might be taking.

Probiotic Source

In the last few years, there has been an intense interest in the connection between the gut microbiome and the brain. Increasing the diversity of gut microbes is clearly associated with reducing the risk for many neurological conditions, including dementia. As part of Step 1 in the Better Brain food plan, you should be eating a variety of probiotic-rich fermented foods daily to increase the diversity and quantity of good microbes in your intestinal tract, such as sauerkraut, kimchi, miso, natto, plain unsweetened yogurt, and kefir. Also, to keep those healthy microbes well fed and alive, eat at least ten servings (30 grams) of fiber from vegetables, fruits, beans, and nuts daily. (See Chapter 3 for more on fermented foods.)

A depleted gut microbiome increases your risk for cognitive decline, depression, and dementia. In Chapter 3, I explained how chemical sweeteners can wipe out good bacteria, but antibiotic use perhaps does the greatest damage to the gut microbiome. You don't have much choice about taking an antibiotic if you have a severe infection (like meningitis or pneumonia), but you can safely cut your use of unnecessary antibiotics, such as those taken for a run-of-the-mill upper respiratory infection (the common cold). It will normally resolve with a bit of patience and time. If my own patients require antibiotics for infection, I recommend they add at least a two-month course of a probiotic supplement, and you should do the same.

- *Probiotic Source Better Brain Action:*
  Foods First, Then Supplement

If for years you have been consuming a cup of probiotic fermented foods and ten servings of fiber (30+ grams) daily, then I wouldn't fret over taking a probiotic supplement—you probably don't need one. But if you don't meet those criteria, add a supplement. Over the long term, I recommend that you consume at least 5 billion microbes daily, year round (along with adequate fiber); I typically suggest starting with at least 25 to 50 billion microbes daily for the first few months. If you've never purchased a probiotic supplement before, you may be thinking those "billions" sound extreme, but they aren't, when you consider that on average, a healthy gut is home to about 100 trillion microorganisms! Supplements with a variety of probiotic organisms are preferred, and better than one that provides only a few different microbes.

Magnesium

We know that magnesium improves blood sugar and blood pressure control, and that it is a strong predictor of shrinking—and not growing—arterial plaque. When I studied more than one hundred of my patients who shrank their arterial plaque load by at least 10 percent, I found that increasing magnesium intake was one of the most powerful predictors of improvement. And since arterial plaque growth, blood sugar, and blood pressure are all strong predictors of accelerated cognitive decline, I want to make sure you get your magnesium every day. Magnesium also helps reduce constipation, anxiety, migraine headaches, muscle cramps, and insomnia.

A challenge with magnesium supplements is quality. Inexpensive forms of magnesium come as salts, such as magnesium oxide, and can cause stomach upset and intestinal distress. Magnesium citrate is a bit better tolerated and is frequently chosen for its laxative activity. The best-tolerated form of magnesium with the highest absorption comes with protein-bound magnesium, such as magnesium glycinate and magnesium malate—magnesium chelated with protein. If taken in excess, all forms of magnesium can cause diarrhea.

Magnesium is also related to neuronal synaptic function. Synapses are the junctions between nerves, and neurotransmitters provide the biochemical connection between the synapses, impacting processing speed and function.

Magnesium appears essential for proper messaging to occur between brain cells. A recent small study with forty-four subjects randomized older adults with mild cognitive impairment to receive magnesium L-threonate or a placebo for twelve weeks. Multiple measures of cognitive function were obtained before and at the end of the study. In this small, short-term study, giving more than 1,000 mg of magnesium L-threonate daily improved cognitive ability and reduced cognitive impairment nearly to normal. The magnesium was divided into two dosages daily, likely to limit gastrointestinal side effects, which were equal in the two groups.

Good food sources of magnesium are seeds, nuts, beans, green leafy veggies, halibut, and bran, but 70 percent of people nationwide are deficient in this essential mineral, and in my clinic at least 50 percent won't get the minimum RDA recommendation of 400 mg from food alone. Most people need to eat the foods noted above, and also take a magnesium capsule with 150–200 mg at bedtime to help meet this critical need.

For people with mild cognitive impairment, speak with your physician about daily dosages of 2,000 mg of Magtein Magnesium L-threonate, including 144 mg of elemental magnesium, keeping in mind that some sources of magnesium penetrate from the blood into the brain more effectively than others. Magnesium L-threonate is the form used in the study of forty-four subjects noted above and has been shown to increase brain magnesium levels nicely.

- *Magnesium Better Brain Action:*
  Foods First, Then Supplement

Ensure that you get at least 400 mg of magnesium daily from food and supplement sources. For people with mild cognitive impairment, talk to your doctor about using higher dosages of magnesium L-threonate therapy.

MAGNESIUM CONTENT IN FOOD

Food and Portion Size	Magnesium (mg)
Pumpkin and squash seed kernels, roasted, 1 oz.	151
Brazil nuts, 1 oz. (1 handful)	107
Oat bran (100%), uncooked, 1 oz.	103
Halibut, cooked, 3 oz.	91
Quinoa, dry, ¼ cup	89
Spinach, frozen, ½ cup (or 3.5 cups raw)	81
Spinach, cooked from fresh, ½ cup	78
Almonds, 1 oz.	78
Halibut, 3 oz.	78
Swiss chard	76
Buckwheat flour, ¼ cup	75
Cashews, dry roasted, 1 oz.	74
Soybeans, mature, cooked, ½ cup	74
Pine nuts, dried, 1 oz.	71

Food and Portion Size	Magnesium (mg)
Mixed nuts, oil roasted, with peanuts, 1 oz.	67
White beans, canned, ½ cup	67
Pollock, walleye, cooked, 3 oz.	62
Black beans, cooked, ½ cup	60
Bulgur, dry, ¼ cup	57
Rolled oats, uncooked, ¼ cup	55
Soybeans, green, cooked, ½ cup	54
Artichoke hearts, cooked, ½ cup	50
Peanuts, dry roasted, 1 oz.	50
Lima beans, baby, cooked from frozen, ½ cup	50

At a minimum, make sure to meet your key nutrient needs for a better brain on a daily basis: Vitamin D, a good-quality multivitamin with adequate vitamin B12 and folates (vitamin B9), and chromium, plus long-chain omega-3 fats, probiotics, and magnesium. From there, it's not hard to make the jump to Step 2: adding other compounds to protect your brain from cognitive decline.

Peggy's Better Brain Story: Vitamin Power

Peggy was a careful eater. At age sixty-nine, she'd been a vegetarian for years, and local organic produce was a staple of her diet. She had once grown much of it herself in her backyard garden, but after she was widowed, she moved out of her house and into an apartment. She had recently been having burning in her feet and was growing forgetful. Her son, my regular patient, asked if I'd evaluate Peggy, after she set her kitchen on fire when she forgot about a pan on the stove.

Though she ate well, when I asked her about supplements, she said she didn't trust supplement companies and didn't bother with them. As it turns out, she was low in two key nutrients that have a major impact on memory and cognitive performance—vitamin B12 and DHA.

On examination, I noticed that she could not feel any vibration with a tuning fork. She could feel light touch, but her vibration sense was gone, clearly a sign of nerve damage—as was the burning in her feet. Her cognitive testing showed adequate processing speed, but her verbal and shape memory were both really poor, putting her below the tenth percentile for memory scores. From her diet, exam findings, and cognitive score, I could guess her lab results before they returned—sure enough, low B12 levels (less than 100 pg/mL, in contrast to a more desirable level of 500 pg/mL and above); and very low DHA levels.

I suspect that when Peggy gave up her garden, and her own organic-soil-raised vegetables, she lost an essential if unexpected nutrient—dirt as a source of bacteria that made vitamin B12. On top of that, she wasn't getting any long-chain omega-3s to support her brain. Now that she was buying her produce at the store, superwashed, sanitized, and packed in plastic, she wasn't getting the vitamin B12 she needed.

Once she saw her own results, and I assured her that some supplement companies could be trusted, I loaded her with 2,000 mcg daily of vitamin B12 for one month, then dropped the ongoing dosage to 500 mcg daily, plus 500 mg of vegetarian DHA from seaweed every day. By two months, the burning in her feet was completely resolved, and when we repeated her cognitive function, it had returned to normal. Prolonged vitamin B12 deficiency can cause permanent, irreversible memory loss and neuropathy. I had met Peggy just in time.

Step 2: Consider Some Additional Supplements

A handful of compounds come with compelling research and tremendous potential to prevent cognitive decline, but they are still being studied, and there isn't solid confirmation that they will work for everyone. And as their production is still fairly limited, they are also relatively expensive, especially when compared to sure bets like vitamins D and B12. However, especially if you have early cognitive decline, I would encourage you to discuss these supplements with your doctor and consider starting them now. If you have early memory loss, you may not want to wait for years while we keep studying them.

Curcumin

I'm putting curcumin at the top of the list of supplements to consider adding to your list of essentials in Step 1. That's in part because of its potential brain benefits but also because it has many other beneficial properties: decreasing inflammation, fighting oxidative stress, and helping symptoms of arthritis. It is also being studied for helping to prevent and treat cancer. Those are beneficial side effects I'd like to see with other treatments, too!

You can get curcumin from certain foods, as it is derived from the turmeric root—the yellow spice commonly blended with Indian curry dishes. Cultures that ingest large quantities of turmeric have some of the lowest rates of dementia and memory loss in the world. However, the challenge is the actual amount you would need to consume, as curcumin is poorly absorbed from the gastrointestinal tract into the bloodstream. You would likely need to eat at least three heaping tablespoons of turmeric spice daily to reach the same levels that can be achieved with a single 500-mg high-quality curcumin capsule. (By *high-quality*, I mean a form that has been studied to be well absorbed and is not contaminated with heavy metals, which are commonly found in turmeric from India.)

Because my parents had arthritis, and I have noted early signs myself, I concluded I should be taking this compound, too. Optimistically, since I like curry-flavored foods, one morning I spooned a heaping tablespoon into a half cup of plain yogurt and stirred, thinking, *I could easily get three tablespoons daily.* I took a brief taste—and was I ever disappointed by *that* experiment! It was awful! I was immediately motivated to find another way to get curcumin, and I set out to find the best absorbed form of clean curcumin in capsule form for myself and my patients. (See Appendix 2 for details.)

Beyond its anti-inflammatory, arthritis-relieving, antioxidant, and cancer-fighting properties, curcumin has been studied for its effects on cognitive decline. The challenge is that original forms were poorly absorbed, while larger doses (which might be the most effective for addressing cognitive decline) have caused significant gastrointestinal symptoms. Recently, improved curcumin formulations have been introduced, with much better rates of absorption and gastrointestinal tolerability. One study that used these newer forms of curcumin has shown improved cognitive function.

Dr. Katherine Cox and her Australian research team evaluated 60 healthy adults (without memory loss), age sixty to eighty-five. Subjects were randomized to receive 400 mg of a well-absorbed curcumin formulation and a placebo, and sophisticated measures were used to assess their cognitive function pre- and post-therapy. Even after only three hours, researchers noted improved cognitive function with curcumin, but none in the control group. After four weeks, those receiving curcumin showed better cognition, plus subjects reported more energy and less anxiety.

Additional studies in humans have shown that giving curcumin decreased blood levels of beta-amyloid (the brain protein associated with Alzheimer's disease); and in mice, giving curcumin enhanced hippocampal neurogenesis (regeneration of brain cells), helping to increase the size of the brain's memory center.

It's tempting to get excited by the potential of curcumin, but at least a couple of trials using less well-absorbed forms at higher dosages showed no benefit. One study showed no memory benefit to taking curcumin over forty-eight weeks, though this study did have some limitations. It was a small pilot study with only thirty-six subjects, and 21 percent of the curcumin treatment group dropped out due to gastrointestinal side effects. The dropout rate might have been related to the form of curcumin used, which had limited absorption. Another problem with the study was that researchers relied upon the Mini-Mental State Examination to assess for a change in cognition, which clearly might miss modest levels of improvement.

Although curcumin shows some clear promise, there is also uncertainty around it. Studies using it for arthritis, cancer, and cognition always find it to be highly safe, and there is ample reason to consider taking curcumin, even if in the end it isn't proven effective as a memory-enhancing therapy. In particular, its anti-inflammatory and antioxidant activity shows promise for high-risk individuals with ApoE4 genotypes, but that is yet to be proven. For now, I'm going to keep taking curcumin for my joints, with the hope it will protect my brain as well.

- *Curcumin Better Brain Action:*
  Take 500–1,000 mg Daily

Ask your doctor about taking a form of curcumin proven to be highly absorbable. This is crucial. I recommend taking 500–1,000 mg per day for arthritis symptoms or to support healthy brain performance. For information on curcumin products that have been documented to be highly absorbable, visit www.DrMasley.com/resources.

Resveratrol

Resveratrol is a compound, normally found in red grape skin and red wine, that has been found to have antioxidant and anti-inflammatory properties. It has also been shown to regulate physiological responses that are similar to those resulting from prolonged calorie restriction (as with fasting), such as a reduction in brain cell inflammation. Taking a resveratrol supplement, however, is much easier than dramatically restricting calorie intake.

A few studies focusing on the immediate impact of taking resveratrol have noted an increase in intracranial blood flow (in other words, more blood circulating throughout the brain—a sign of healthy cognitive function). But I can find only one small study where researchers specifically examined the impact of resveratrol on cognitive performance. In a German study, twenty-three subjects were unknowingly given 200 mg/day of resveratrol and matched with twenty-three who received a placebo. Neuroimaging, blood sugar regulation, and cognitive testing were performed before and after twenty-six weeks of therapy.

Those who received resveratrol showed an improvement in memory, blood sugar control, and functionality of the hippocampus as measured with functional MRI testing. The improvements in memory were highly correlated with better blood sugar control, as measured by testing HgbA1C, a long-term marker for blood sugar regulation. Obviously one small study doesn't mean we have found a major breakthrough in treating Alzheimer's disease, but it does give me hope that subsequent studies will continue to show promising results.

- *Resveratrol Better Brain Action:*
  Take 200–250 mg of Trans-resveratrol Daily

An important note on selecting resveratrol supplements: look for labels that say *trans*-resveratrol. This is the active form of resveratrol. A 250-mg capsule from a bottle labeled with wording such as "standardized to 10% of trans-resveratrol" is only giving you 10 percent of what you need.

MCT Oil (promising for some with memory loss, but not confirmed to work long term)

As discussed in Chapter 4, one study found that consuming twenty grams of MCT oil daily for ninety days improved cognitive function in people with mild cognitive impairment, though about a quarter of the study participants had gastrointestinal issues with the treatment. Unfortunately, this study showed no benefit for the 20 percent of people who have the ApoE4 gene. In healthy adults, the impact of MCT oil on cognitive function has not "yet" been studied, at least not with published long-term results. The gastrointestinal side effects with this therapy are not serious, just annoying for those who notice them.

I would certainly encourage anyone with any established cognitive impairment to discuss a trial of MCT oil with their own physician.

- *MCT Oil Better Brain Action:*
  Take 10 Grams Daily, to Start

After one to two weeks, gradually increase to 20 grams daily. If you have gastrointestinal symptoms at this dosage, decrease it to a level you can tolerate, and try to increase back to 20 grams daily in one month. If you suffer from cognitive decline, it would be very helpful if your doctor could order cognitive testing before and after twelve weeks of therapy, so that you can measure results.

The Problem with Prevagen

Perhaps the most widely marketed supplement on television, radio, and the Internet for preventing cognitive decline is Prevagen, "clinically tested" to improve memory, according to its advertising, often with a table showing a 20 percent improvement in memory. Its active ingredient is apoaequorin, a compound that binds calcium and occurs naturally in jellyfish. But despite its popularity, Prevagen is an example of a questionable supplement—a nutrient cocktail strongly marketed to its target audience but with few studies to back up its brain-boosting claims.

There is only one published study regarding this compound as it relates to protecting against cognitive decline, in the medical journal *Advances in Mind-Body Medicine*. The authors report a 15 to 20 percent improvement in cognitive function using Prevagen as directed for ninety days, although the benefit was only an extra 3 to 7 percent higher than that of a placebo. Furthermore, in the published article, the authors did not disclose their relationship to the product adequately: they all work for the company that manufactures Prevagen. In my opinion, the list of authors looks more like a corporate board than scientists studying a means to prevent cognitive decline.

Dr. Robert Speth, a noted professor of pharmaceutical sciences, wrote a critical summary about this publication on PubMed (a research tool for scientists), outlining a variety of valid concerns:

- A paid advertisement for Prevagen appeared in the same issue of *Advances in Mind-Body Medicine* that carried the study, without listing any financial conflict of interest in the article. (This lack of disclosure goes against the norm of most reputable journals and researchers.)
- In terms of how it works in the body and brain, it is unlikely this large a molecule would be absorbed from the

gut and less likely that it could penetrate the blood-brain barrier to impact the cerebral cortex. A separate study using apoaequorin in mice noted benefits in protecting against stroke damage only if it was *injected directly* into the brain itself—in other words, not taken in pill form like Prevagen.

- If apoaequorin was absorbed, Speth indicated, serious side effects might occur. But the authors did not elaborate on any side effects and suggested it was well tolerated.
- The statistical analyses were loaded with flaws and errors. Subjects in this small study went missing, and their absence was not explained; nor was an adequate description of the cognitive testing provided. In light of these anomalies, one would have to consider subjective bias in the conduct of the research and analyses, which was provided by the company selling the supplement.

Perhaps not surprisingly, after Dr. Speth reported his concerns, a class action suit was filed against Quincy Bioscience, the manufacturer of Prevagen. The Food and Drug Administration (FDA) has accused the company of not reporting adverse events, such as seizures, strokes, and worsening multiple sclerosis: more than one thousand incidents have been reported against the product. But to date the company has only followed up on two of these events. The product, as of this writing, is still available for purchase, and the ads continue.

Given all you know about the real causes of memory loss and dementia and how to prevent them, be aware of a questionably vetted product making a too-good-to-be-true claim—in this case, that a single pill or two will quickly deliver a "sharper mind" and "clearer thinking."

Step 3: Learn More About Supplements for High-Risk Individuals

If you or someone you know falls into a high-risk category for dementia and memory loss, or has signs of early cognitive impairment, it is worth learning more about additional supplements that might have benefits. However, I rate the following supplements as less promising than those in Step 2, until further research is available. Some items—like Prevagen (see box "The Problem with Prevagen")—are aggressively marketed for brain health, but do they really work? We don't have enough research to say. (In the case of Prevagen, the research seems to be highly flawed.)

Still, the following supplements—coenzyme Q10, phosphatidylserine, huperzine A, and alpha lipoic acid—stand out for their fascinating theoretical possibilities. You'll notice I don't include specific Better Brain action steps for these supplements, but still my suggestion is to learn as much as you can about them, discuss them with your physician, and decide if they're worth adding to your regimen.

Coenzyme Q10 (Ubiquinone) (potentially promising, not ready for prime time)

Coenzyme Q10 (CoQ10, also called ubiquinol or ubiquinone) is commonly recommended and marketed as a compound to help memory, yet I can find no solid evidence that it improves cognitive function. At high dosages, more than 200 mg per day, it is one of the only agents available that has been shown to slow the progression of Parkinson's disease. CoQ10 has also been helpful in reducing symptoms for people with congestive heart failure. With extensive study, it has been shown to be very safe and have few side effects.

Because memory loss is associated with decreased brain cell mitochondrial function, and CoQ10 has been shown to improve mitochondrial energy production, in theory it could help prevent memory loss.

In my clinic, the most common reason I recommend CoQ10 to my patients is if they are taking a statin medication for heart disease or cholesterol indications, since taking a statin decreases normal CoQ10 production.

You'll find a great deal of marketing hype comparing the two forms of CoQ10: the active reduced form, known as ubiquinol, and the oxidized form, which is ubiquinone (the form used in most supplements, and what most research is based on). They interconvert rapidly (meaning that ubiquinol turns into ubiquinone and vice versa), so I don't see a compelling reason to pick one form over the other, especially if you are asked to pay extra for the reduced form since ubiquinol is generally more expensive.

A major limitation with CoQ10 supplements is their absorption. Tablet forms typically only have 1 percent absorption—it won't do you much good if it can't get into your bloodstream. Oil-based capsules should have about 4 percent absorption, while some specially designed forms may achieve 8 percent absorption or more.

If you plan to use CoQ10, be sure to use a highly absorbable form and a high-quality brand. We know that cheap sources, particularly tablets, are not well absorbed, so it's a better investment to purchase a supplement that is. I'd recommend 50–100 mg daily. If you're in a high-risk category for dementia and memory loss, it's important at some point to confirm that you achieve a good level with this therapy, with an adequate dosage to achieve a blood level of >1.0 mcg/ml, or a more optimal level of 1.5–2.0 mcg/ml. Consult with your physician to identify your dosage and blood level.

Phosphatidylserine (potentially promising, not ready for prime time)

Phosphatidylserine is a normal component in brain cell membranes, accounting for 14 percent of the phospholipids, a type of fat molecule, in the human brain. It is required for healthy brain cell function. Like fish oil, phosphatidylserine intake nourishes the brain.

It was first isolated from cow brains back in the 1940s, and by the 1980s was used in supplements to support normal brain function. A mad cow disease outbreak (from consuming cow brain) put a stop to nearly all such supplements, and research shifted to synthesizing phosphatidylserine from soy products.

As popular as it has been as a brain support supplement for thirty years, evidence to show that phosphatidylserine improves cognitive function or prevents memory loss is still controversial.

A recent small study conducted in China with fifty-seven patients with established Alzheimer's disease were randomized to a placebo group or a group receiving 300 mg of phosphatidylserine (produced from a mixture of cow brain and soy products) for twenty weeks. Memory testing was performed before and after dosing. Those receiving phosphatidylserine showed a moderate improvement in memory compared to the control group. The same investigators also performed a similar study in rats, published in the same article, and found that those treated showed lower levels of inflammation in the hippocampus.

One of the limitations noted by the author was that it is unclear if this benefit would persist over the long term or would end after a limited period of improvement. To evaluate the safety of the product, a second pilot study treated thirty older subjects (age range fifty to ninety) with 300 mg per day of phosphatidylserine for twelve weeks. There was no placebo group for comparison. Four of the thirty people (13 percent) dropped out due to GI symptoms (similar to the MCT oil study). After treatment, memory and cognitive function improved, and although otherwise the phosphatidylserine was tolerated without any worrisome effects, we still don't know if these benefits would be achieved with long-term therapy.

The big controversy with phosphatidylserine as a treatment for memory loss involves its largest study. It compared 300 mg and 600 mg daily of soy-derived phosphatidylserine and placebo for six and twelve weeks of therapy, then used sophisticated measures of memory and cognitive function in 120 subjects with early cognitive decline. The results showed absolutely no benefit of any kind. There was some concern about the quality and shelf life of the phosphatidylserine product used, similar to that surrounding fish oil. (Rancidity may impact effectiveness—or even be harmful.)

Although phosphatidylserine seems safe in short-term studies, until further clinical investigations are performed that confirm its usefulness long term, its effectiveness remains uncertain. But as noted, people with cognitive impairment don't have the time to wait. If this treatment seems appealing, then check with your doctor to see if phosphatidylserine supplements might be appropriate for you.

Huperzine A

Huperzine A is a compound sourced from Chinese club moss (*Huperzia serrata*), an herb used in traditional Chinese medicine for centuries.

In China it's known for its cognition-supporting benefit and has been shown to be well tolerated in dozens of clinical trials. The limitation with this product, just like most of the other supplement agents discussed, is that none of the studies have yet to show long-term benefit in cognitive function or the ability to prevent memory loss long term.

Studies have shown that in rats, huperzine A inhibits the formation of beta-amyloid protein in the brain. A twelve-week randomized study of seventy-eight human patients with mild to moderate vascular dementia found that those sent to a vitamin C placebo group showed no cognitive improvement, while those receiving a daily dose of 0.2 mg of huperzine A had a modest improvement in Mini-Mental State Examination scores.

A review of twenty randomized clinical trials using huperzine A in a total of 1,823 subjects with dosages from 0.2 mg to 0.8 mg daily suggests that it provides modest improvements in cognitive function and activities of daily living for those with mild cognitive impairment and dementia. But the authors of this review conclude that the current studies are small, that many have flaws in their design or protocols, and that none have yet shown long-term benefits; thus further studies are warranted before they can recommend this promising compound.

It's worth noting that huperzine A acts just like four of the five drugs approved by the FDA to treat symptoms of cognitive decline. Four are cholinesterase inhibitors, which prevent the breakdown of acetylcholine, a compound that is involved in memory and cognitive function. And although these drugs provide some symptom relief, none of them have been shown to slow the progression of dementia or Alzheimer's disease. So a limitation is that huperzine A, like those drugs, may provide only short-term symptom relief without stopping long-term decline. (The side effects of these cholinesterase inhibitors are commonly nausea, vomiting, loss of appetite, and increased frequency of bowel movements.) As huperzine A appears to be safe, clarify with your doctor if it is a good choice for you.

Alpha Lipoic Acid as Support for Mitochondrial Function

Many supplements are designed to support healthy brain function with ingredients that are intended to enhance mitochondrial function. Mitochondria are microscopic organelles that produce the energy that keeps all your cells alive and functioning. Ingredients that enhance them would include items we've covered in Steps 1, 2, and 3 for key nutrients, such as fish oil (long-chain omega-3s), curcumin, resveratrol, and CoQ10. If you could boost mitochondrial function, especially in the brain, your brain cells would work better and be less likely to die.

One other agent that gets attention in this category is alpha lipoic acid, a natural compound synthesized in the mitochondria and also supplied in small quantities from the diet, primarily organ meats. Alpha lipoic acid is a powerful antioxidant, has anti-inflammatory properties, improves blood sugar control, and appears to enhance mitochondrial function.

Not surprisingly, many products designed to support brain health include alpha lipoic acid as an ingredient, although due to expense, they may not always provide an adequate dosage to be effective. Is alpha lipoic acid a key nutrient? For now, no studies show that it is effective in preventing cognitive decline, though as a proven antioxidant, it does offer other biochemical benefits. As far as offering brain benefits as part of a supplement, however, the right balance of multiple ingredients featuring this compound has likely yet to be created.

Another way, beyond the nutrients we've just discussed, to boost mitochondrial function, increase energy, and rev up cognitive function is exercise, the next pillar of the Better Brain Solution. Getting and staying active with regular exercise can lower your risk for dementia and memory loss.

CHAPTER 6

How to Move Your Body for a Better Brain

Regular exercise does everything from improving your sex life to decreasing your risk for cancer. When you are active, you have more energy, sleep better, manage stress more effectively, and have more regular bowel function. Exercise burns away fat, improves bone density, sweats away toxins, and lowers bad cholesterol and high blood pressure. It helps to prevent heart attack and stroke, as well as stop accelerated aging.

You may be familiar with all these reasons for getting and staying active—but more recently researchers have made an exciting connection between exercise and brain function: exercise plays a role in preventing memory loss. It targets the main causes of memory loss and dementia by reducing arterial plaque and improving blood sugar control and insulin sensitivity. (A mixture of aerobic and strength training is also one of the best ways to prevent or even reverse type 2 diabetes.)

Body and brain fitness are closely intertwined in a beneficial relationship, and the latest studies—including data from my own clinic—bear this out. In research I conducted on exercise and cognitive flexibility (a measure of executive function), I compared cognitive function in people who exercised less than once per week, three days per week, and five to six days per week. During a ten-week period, those who worked out three days (moderate exercise) had a 5 percent improvement in cognitive function; those who exercised five to six days, more vigorously, had a 25 percent improvement. Those who engaged in little to no exercise had no improvement. Separately, I have seen my own patients improve their executive function by up to 25 percent when they add aerobic activity to their regular routine, a significant improvement in mental sharpness! (See box "A Few More Push-ups Can Change Your Brain.")

My latest research, which has been accepted for publication by the *Journal of the American College of Nutrition,* has found that *fitness was the strongest predictor of overall cognitive function as well as executive function.* People with greater aerobic fitness and/or strength clearly have better brain performance.

While food and nutrients are a major foundation of the Better Brain Solution, compelling new research makes clear that daily activity—a brisk walk, a swim, or raking leaves in the yard—is one of the most important choices you can make, starting now, to decrease your risk for memory loss.

Whatever your current level of fitness—whether you haven't worked out in years and should start with Step 1 exercise basics, or you regularly run 10Ks and can jump ahead to Steps 2 and 3—physical activity will certainly boost your cognitive function.

Exercise is good for the heart, and it's great for the brain.

A Few More Push-ups Can Change Your Brain

To clarify the benefits of getting fitter: my clinic's most recent data analyses show that multiple measures of fitness predict greater cognitive performance and executive function. From hundreds of patients in my clinic, here's a quick glance at the numbers.

In patients who were able to:

- increase the number of push-ups they could perform by at least 10 percent, their overall cognitive score improved 18 percent
- increase the number of sit-ups they could perform by at least 10 percent, their overall cognitive score improved 17 percent
- improve their aerobic capacity by at least 10 percent, their overall cognitive function improved 19 percent

If you follow *The Better Brain Solution* and aim for a moderate enhancement in either strength or aerobic fitness, you can realistically anticipate a 16 to 19 percent increase in cognitive function. That is a huge improvement!

Bigger Muscles, Bigger Brains

Exercise gets your blood pumping, increasing blood flow to the brain; this additional blood flow protects and nourishes the brain by delivering more revitalizing oxygen, glucose, and nutrients to brain cells, as well as performing toxin removal and other life-supporting functions.

But working out regularly offers another brain benefit: preventing a loss in muscle mass over a lifetime helps prevent brain volume shrinkage. Even eighty-year-olds have been shown to increase the size of the brain's memory center, the hippocampus, by adding a regular exercise routine. And for people who already suffer from mild cognitive impairment, strength training by itself has been shown to increase executive function and memory.

The opposite of being fit is being inactive, which unfortunately describes the lifestyle of most Americans. "Inactivity," as defined by the U.S. Department of Health and Human Services, means doing less than thirty minutes of moderately aerobic activity daily. Now that you know that being physically active strengthens more than your heart and your muscles—that it can actually save your brain function—imagine what *no* exercise is doing to most of the population. It's easy to see why rates of diabetes, heart disease, dementia, and Alzheimer's keep rising. Being unfit not only keeps a person from reaching their true cognitive potential; it also can end life prematurely.

It doesn't take as much effort as you may think to go from inactivity to moderate activity and beyond. And even better (particularly for those of you who may balk at dedicating time to exercise), the fitter you get, the less time it takes to work out.

I recommend two modes of exercise that are effective in combination for both brain and body. (Note: If you're extremely fit and work out most days of the week, with a basic aerobic *and* strength-training routine, take a look at Steps 1 and 2 to confirm that you're beyond that level, particularly with regard to aerobic fitness and working at your maximum heart rate. You may be ready to go straight to Step 3.)

Aerobic Activity: Pedal a Bicycle, Power Your Mind

Aerobic activity is activity that speeds up your heart rate and maintains it for a minimum of twenty minutes; it's even more beneficial if you can maintain it for longer, at least thirty or forty minutes, most days of the week. A good aerobic workout revs up your metabolism so that you will burn calories for several hours afterward (even if you're sitting on the couch or working at your desk). It also strengthens your heart, improves brain speed and cognitive performance, and reduces stress levels. Any activity that significantly raises your heart rate is aerobic, like walking briskly, jogging, cycling, swimming, working out on an elliptical machine, or dancing. (If you have medical problems, especially related to heart disease or poor blood sugar, cholesterol, or blood pressure control, always check with your doctor before you start an exercise program.)

Strength training, which involves working with fixed or free weights or resistance bands, can be an excellent workout, but on its own it doesn't benefit the brain in quite the same way that aerobic activity does. In one study, after first establishing that both aerobic activity and strength training could improve memory in older adults, and that in young, healthy adults aerobic exercise increases hippocampal volume, a Canadian research team wanted to study how various forms of exercise might affect brain size. They selected eighty-six women with mild cognitive impairment and assigned them to balance training, strength training, or aerobic exercise, performing MRI brain imaging before and after six months. Those in the aerobic group showed a significant increase in brain size, in particular the hippocampus, compared to the balance and strength training groups, which both showed a decrease in brain size.

My own most recent database analyses from my clinic—of more than one hundred markers that influence cognitive function, apart from age itself—found that aerobic fitness was the most powerful predictor of overall better brain function, and that better strength improves overall cognition, too.

The simplest way to start an aerobic exercise routine—one that you will stick with over the long term—is to find an activity you *enjoy*, whatever it might be, and schedule yourself for twenty to thirty minutes, four to five days per week. Begin with a three- to four-minute warm-up, then pick up the intensity so you get a bit sweaty. You should be able to talk, but you should not be able to sing. (Save that for the shower afterward.)

If you haven't been active, this ease-into-it approach is ideal. (For those of you who are further along and are in search of better, faster results than what your current exercise plan may be yielding, I highly encourage fitness testing and a guided, personalized workout routine, discussed later in this chapter.)

Strength Training: Lift Weights for Mental Muscle

Strength training stresses your muscles through the use of weights and resistance, stimulating them to increase in mass. Most people lose at least 1 percent of their muscle mass every year after age thirty, and as a result they have more muscle and joint pain (in part because muscles become too weak to support joint movement and function). But there's more to it than those "everyday aches and pains." When muscle mass declines, insulin sensitivity decreases, growth hormone and testosterone levels drop, bone mass decreases, and our ability to burn calories plummets, setting us up for later-in-life weight gain.

Each pound of muscle in your body burns forty calories daily, even if you are sitting at your desk. As that mass decreases, so too does your ability to avoid gaining weight—unless you maintain muscle and guard against its loss. Gaining a pound or two over the course of a year may not seem alarming, but it's problematic if that pattern continues for several years.

Even more important, muscle mass is essential to blood sugar control and insulin sensitivity. The less muscle one has, the less capacity one has to store glucose as energy after a meal. Building muscle mass improves blood sugar control and insulin sensitivity. Strength training also decreases inflammation, improves blood pressure control, and makes a big difference in losing body fat and achieving a trim waistline.

Women in particular benefit from strength training, as they typically have less muscle mass to begin with than men. Strength training won't make women bulky and muscle-bound (unless it's done at extreme levels and combined with a protein-heavy diet designed for body build-ers), but it will help to create shapely, trim, and sexy curves.

Stronger muscles also help to create stronger brains. In a study in Australia, men and women fifty-five or older were randomly assigned into groups for cognitive training through a computer program, or doing a strength training routine two to three days per week. Those in the computer-based cognitive training group did show modest improvements in memory, but only those in the strength training group showed significant improvements in cognitive function and memory.

To begin a strength training program, identify eight to ten big muscle groups, as you get more benefit from working big muscles such as your biceps, glutes, and pectorals. (Generally, the big muscle groups include arms and legs, back, chest and core.) If you have never done strength training before, work out with an exercise physiologist the first few times; he or she can get you started properly and help you identify the muscles you want to work.

Choose a weight that you can lift at least eight to ten times. (If you are using resistance bands, the same guidelines will apply; instead of lifts, you will be pulling or pushing for the same feeling you'd get with weights.) The last few lifts should make your muscle feel fatigued; if you notice a little shakiness at the end, that's a good sign because you've worked the muscle to exhaustion, and now it will begin to recover and build back up again, increasing the muscle mass. Being able to lift a weight ten to twelve times and then noticing shakiness is a just-right feeling. If you can lift the weight fifteen times without shakiness, it is time to select a heavier weight. You want to be able to feel that you're "working it," and if you move up in weight choice, rather than simply adding more reps, you will build muscle more efficiently. If you only add reps, you increase your endurance but you aren't putting enough healthy stress on muscle fibers to build muscle mass. And adding more reps takes longer to do. If you want more muscle mass, you need to gradually increase the weight.

Using those guidelines, you should be able to quickly figure out how much weight to use, though be mindful of going too heavy with your selection. If you can't lift a weight for a minimum of eight repetitions, it may be too heavy, and you might get injured. *You should aim to exercise each major muscle group with a strength training routine one or two days per week.*

If you are inexperienced with strength training, work with an exercise physiologist; most well-staffed gyms offer this service. (An exercise physiologist has completed years of study for a bachelor's or a master's of science in exercise physiology, as opposed to a certified "personal trainer," who holds a certificate.) If your budget for help is limited, another option is to work out with a partner who can spot you while you lift (and you get to rest and spot them while they lift) and who will motivate you to keep up with your workouts. Studies show that people who exercise with a partner are more likely to exercise consistently and achieve better results.

Here is a list of a dozen highly effective strength moves:

- Abdominal crunches on an exercise ball
- Back extensions
- Chest presses or push-ups
- One-arm row
- Bicep curls
- Triceps extensions
- Overhead press
- Ball squats
- Lunges
- Hamstring bridge
- Calf press
- Rotator cuff lifts

For details on a dozen muscle groups to use and how to do the exercises, visit www.DrMasley.com/resources.

Aerobic exercise and strength training are the foundation of an effective Better Brian Solution workout.

- For those of you who are starting with little daily activity, begin with **Step 1: Get Moving.**
- If you already have a regular exercise routine, you are probably ready for **Step 2: Rev Up Your Heart Rate and Add Strength Training.**
- If you're *truly* fit (confirm you're hitting all the aerobic benchmarks in Step 2), you may be ready to jump ahead to **Step 3: Mix It Up for a Better Brain.**

Power Food

The guidelines on what to eat before or after a workout vary tremendously and should be personalized for your needs and level of exercise intensity. Still, there is one consistent recommendation that I can offer: a boost of protein intake after a strength training session. Strength training stresses your skeletal muscles, and they need amino acids (protein building blocks) to repair themselves. You will build muscle mass more effectively if you consume at least 20 grams of protein within thirty minutes of your workout session, delivering the amino acids your muscles need. It is more effective to drink your protein than to eat it, so liquid protein (like a protein shake) is better than eating edamame or chicken, although protein foods will still help you build muscle mass. And you will build muscle better if the protein you consume contains extra-branched-chain amino acids, such as leucine, valine, and isoleucine. A good food source for branched-chain amino acids is whey or soy protein.

Unlike strength training, regular aerobic training does not cause the kind of muscle stress that requires quick repair. For everyday training, you can eat before or after a workout, whichever makes you feel better, and you will want a balance of healthy protein, fat, and carbs, such as a protein shake with protein powder, fruit, greens, and either nut butter or MCT oil, or alternatively a vegetable omelet. If you are preparing for a stressful aerobic activity, then aim to eat a meal that balances protein, carbs, and fat at least sixty minutes beforehand to ensure fuel to sustain you.

Long-distance athletes, in particular those aiming for Ironman events, benefit from training in a state of ketosis. Athletes who aim to load up on carbs generally find that they run low on fuel after a few hours of exercise, as the glycogen stores in their muscle tissue are depleted. They "hit the wall" when their blood sugar levels drop; athletic performance plummets, and even confusion can occur. In contrast, the body has dramatically greater reserves of fuel stored as fat than we could ever store as carbohydrates. The challenge is that athletes need to shift their metabolism to using fat as fuel in advance of the event and preferably spend weeks training in this zone. With ketosis exercise training, nearly 70 percent of the diet is in the form of fat with 10 to 15 percent coming from protein and carbs. Coconut milk, avocado, nuts, and fatty, clean meats become the major source of calorie intake.

For my patients who are not athletes, I ask them to focus on eating a healthy, balanced meal before their workout (such as my protein shake; see the recipe on page 255), and to ensure they get at least 20 grams of protein in liquid form after a strength training session.

Step 1: Get Moving

Step 1 is for people who don't exercise at an aerobic level—those with no regular workout routine. If this is you, perhaps you get some form of light exercise like walking the dog or the occasional bike ride, but you never huff and puff, you don't break a sweat, your heart doesn't pick up the pace when you move, and you stroll instead of walk. In addition, any person with a heart rate recovery of less than 25 beats per minute during fitness testing should also start with Step 1. (See the box "Heart Rate Recovery: Why It Matters" on page 162 for more information on calculating your heart recovery rate.)

The Better Brain Solution exercise plan features increasingly intense phases of aerobic activity. Step 1, however, focuses solely on getting you moving and helping you increase your capacity for brain-boosting exercise. Here is your plan:

- Start by counting your daily steps. Get a high-tech fitness tracker or old-school pedometer (whatever you're more comfortable wearing and using), or just take a walk, if you have a regular route around home or work, and count miles walked. Your goal is to build up to 10,000 steps per day, which is the equivalent of walking four to five miles. If you are inactive, your baseline may be only 2,000 to 3,000 steps per day (about one mile), and it likely will take a few weeks to reach your daily 10,000. Try adding an extra 2,500 steps (an extra mile) each week until you are walking 10,000 steps per day. Or anticipate that you walked the equivalent of one mile while at home and work, and build up to taking a four-mile walk on your own. People who are active at home or work will likely find it much easier to count steps than miles.

- After you reach 10,000 steps per day consistently, it's time to "step" it up and move on to Step 2. If 10,000 seems like a staggeringly high number, keep this in mind: every step counts toward this goal, and you're probably already doing about a third of that amount—when you're walking down your sidewalk to pick up the newspaper . . . when you're going to the car . . . when you're shopping in the supermarket.

People who count steps tend to notice opportunities to reach their daily goals (and add on to their total): parking the car further from the entrance; taking the stairs instead of the elevator; walking down the hall to see a colleague rather than calling their extension; playing actively with a child or pet. The more you count steps, the more excuses you will find for walking. Most healthy people, including those who've been inactive for a while, should be able to easily build up to 10,000 steps every day.

Please note: If you struggle with major health problems, like uncontrolled high blood sugar, hypertension, diabetes, or heart disease, always check with your doctor before modifying your current activity, including beginning a step-counting program. The good news is if you are challenged with such health issues, exercise—even if you start small and build up—is one of the most potent and proven treatments available.

Getting aerobically fit can work magic on your heart and your brain. In research conducted by my clinic, we showed that people who were highly fit had far less arterial plaque, as measured with carotid IMT testing. Whether we measured heart rate recovery (see the box "Heart Rate Recovery: Why It Matters" on page 162) or MET levels achieved (see the box "Aerobic Fitness Testing: You Don't Have to Do It, But . . ." on page 166), or minutes that they could last on a progressively more difficult treadmill protocol, all measures of fitness showed that being fit helps predict having less arterial plaque—and your level of arterial plaque load is one of the strongest predictors of cognitive function. Just start step by step.

Step 2: Rev Up Your Heart Rate and Add Some Strength Training

For maximum brain benefits, the one-two punch of aerobic exercise and strength training is more powerful than either one of them alone. Two large national studies featuring more than five hundred subjects with type 2 diabetes focused on improving blood sugar control with exercise. Without a doubt, the key to controlling blood sugar was combining the two forms of exercise, as either aerobic activity or strength training by itself was clearly less effective.

I know from treating thousands of patients that everyone has a different fitness level; starting points and exercise intensity, once you're up and running (or walking, swimming, or biking), can vary greatly from person to person. Still, it's possible to create guidelines by breaking aerobic fitness goals into phases.

The Three Phases of Aerobics: Finding Your Level

You will get the most out of an exercise routine if you work out at just the right level. You don't want to overdo it so that you feel wiped out or, worse, get injured. You should feel energized after your exercise routine, not in pain or utterly drained. (Chances are, if you feel that bad, you're unlikely to keep at it.) Still, some healthy exhaustion is good—you don't want to underdo it and only achieve a minimum benefit.

Follow Your Heart—Heart Rate, That Is

It's important for you to determine what you are capable of doing aerobically. Perhaps the best option is to find your heart rate target—the cardiovascular sweet spot where exercise conditions your heart (like the muscle it is) and makes it stronger without overworking it.

You could use the heart rate charts you've seen at the gym, which are generally age-based, or the chart on page 317. The charts calculate 220 minus your age to arrive at your maximum heart rate, then suggest you work out at 60 to 80 percent of that maximum. For example, for a fifty-year-old woman, her calculation looks like this: 220–50 = 170 heartbeats per minute—her estimated maximum heart rate. The standard recommendation would be for her to exercise at 60 to 80 percent of 170 beats per minute, meaning a heart rate of 102 to 136 beats per minute. A drawback is that such heart rate charts are based on average levels of fitness, so for a third of the people who try to use them, they are simply too hard, and for another third, they are too easy.

It's much better to get an accurate heart rate calculation that reflects your personal aerobic capacity. To find that rate: when you've completed your running, walking, cycling, etc., and when you are at your maximum exertion level, measure your heart rate for 15 seconds and multiply it by four. This number is your real maximum heart rate.

If making these heart rate calculations sounds too complicated (honestly, it takes a bit of skill to measure your own heart rate while exercising), it is much easier to use a heart rate monitor to measure your heart rate accurately while you exercise, such as a wearable chest/wristband device or the pulse-monitoring hand grips on gym equipment such as treadmills. The ones that come with a chest strap work the best.

You can also pay for a onetime workout with an exercise physiologist. A trained, educated pro can help you personalize a safe and effective workout zone, and he or she will probably make the experience more fun, setting you up for success. Knowing your maximum heart rate is quite important if you want to get more benefits with less pain and in less time.

Heart Rate Recovery: Why It Matters

A powerful predictor of aerobic fitness is the drop in your heart rate after you stop exercising, also referred to as your heart rate recovery. At maximum exertion, your heart may race as high as 180 beats per minute. When you stop, the faster your heart rate drops, the faster you recover from stressing your heart. Published studies using treadmill testing at the Cleveland Clinic on tens of thousands of patients found that poor heart rate recovery was the strongest predictor of future heart attack and sudden death. Normally, after sixty seconds, your heart rate should drop by at least 25 beats. Some of my really fit patients have a 40-to-60-point drop. If yours drops less than 20 beats, that is concerning. If it drops less than 12, I call that alarming. However, if you happen to take medications that slow your heart rate, then these markers will likely not be reliable, so check with your doctor. To measure your one-minute heart rate recovery, first measure your maximum heart rate, immediately after stopping your exercise, walk slowly for 1 minute during your cooldown. After sixty seconds, measure your heart rate with a heart rate monitor, or measure your pulse for fifteen seconds and multiply that number by four. To calculate your one-minute heart rate recovery, subtract your one-minute recovery heart rate from your maximum heart rate. For example, at peak exercise Susan's maximum heart rate is 170 beats per minute. One minute after her cooldown, it is 145 beats per minute; 170–145 = 25. Her one-minute heart rate recovery is normal, with a 25-beat drop.

Here are three aerobic phases to choose from when deciding what level to start at for aerobic activity. For these guidelines, I will assume you work out by walking briskly or running, though the same benchmarks would apply for other aerobic exercise such as cycling or swimming. It is always a good idea to talk to your physician before you change your exercise routine. This is especially important if you have medical problems.

Aerobic Exercise Phase 1:
Target Heart Rate 60–70 Percent of Your Max

If you don't work out consistently, then start by working out with a heart rate that **is 60 to 70 percent of your calculated (or estimated by** age—see page 317) maximum heart rate. For example, if your maximum heart rate is 160, then 160 × 0.60 = 96, and 160 × 0.7 = 112, so your initial aerobic zone would be 96 to 112 beats per minute.

In Phase 1, aim for spending **twenty to thirty minutes, four or five days per week, in this aerobic zone.** Most people will be ready to shift to Phase 2 after one or two weeks. And if you feel uncomfortable for whatever reason making the shift, then the best step is always to consult your physician.

Aerobic Exercise Phase 2:
Target Heart Rate 70–80 Percent of Your Max

Once you're working out consistently (four or five times a week), you can kick it up to the next level of aerobic capacity. You're ready for Phase 2 if you:

- Can exercise at 60 to 80 percent of your maximum heart rate for 20 to 30 minutes and feel comfortable doing so.
- Have a heart rate recovery of at least 25 beats after one minute. To calculate that rate: When you've completed your running, walking, cycling, etc., begin your cooldown; after one minute, check your heart rate. If you aren't wearing a monitoring device, take your pulse and multiply by four. Your heart rate should drop by 25 beats (compared to your max rate); that indicates a good rate of recovery and fitness. (For more on the one-minute heart rate recovery, see the box "Heart Rate Recovery: Why It Matters" on pages 162–163.)

In Phase 2, you should be aiming for **an aerobic heart rate that is 70–80 percent of your maximum heart rate.** For example, if your maximum heart rate is 180, then 180 × 0.7 = 126, and 180 × 0.8 = 144, so with a max heart rate of 180, your Phase 2 aerobic zone would be 126 to 144 beats per minute. A good heart rate recovery would be more than 25 beats per minute. An optimum Phase 2 routine is to **exercise for at least thirty to forty minutes, four to six days per week, in this aerobic zone.**

Aerobic Exercise Phase 3:
Interval Training: Target Heart Rate 85–90 Percent
of Your Max

It typically takes two to four weeks to be ready to shift from Phase 2 to Phase 3. You can take your aerobic exercise routine to the next level if you

- Can work out for at least 30 minutes at a time, at the top of your Phase 2 aerobic zone (70 to 80 percent of your maximum heart rate).
- Have a heart rate recovery that is more than 25 beats per minute, which shows good exercise tolerance.

Phase 3 **combines a moderate Phase 2 aerobic workout two or three days per week and interval training (also called burst training) two or three days per week** for achieving optimal results.

Interval training consists of short bursts of intense exercise, typically for one or two minutes at a time. To begin, warm up in your normal aerobic zone for about ten minutes.

To shift to interval training, push yourself to 85 to 90 percent of your maximum heart rate for one minute. You will likely huff and puff. Then slow way down and walk or jog gently for another minute to recover. (Back in high school, my track coach had us do something similar: sprint for a minute, walk for a minute, sprint, then walk.)

Ideally your workout will consist of at least five or six high-intensity sessions, followed by five or six easy sessions, and with a warm-up and cooldown afterward; the whole session would take about twenty minutes. For maximum benefit, I suggest interval training two or three times per week, but not every day, as that would be overdoing it.

Several studies have shown that interval training improves blood sugar control and enhances insulin sensitivity. And in a major benefit for those concerned about taking time out for exercise, it takes less time than a traditional workout. A study in the United Kingdom assigned ninety inactive subjects to either daily moderate aerobic activity or interval training. Those in the interval training group exercised for twenty minutes three times per week (about one hour total per week).

Those in the moderate aerobic group worked out 125 minutes per week (more than two hours), spread across five days. The results showed both groups had the same reduction in insulin resistance.

With that in mind, would you rather work out

(a) 20 minutes per day, three days a week, or
(b) 25 minutes per day, five days a week, to get the same results?

Even though the exercise would be more intense, I would rather get the same results in less time. With interval training, you can get fit, healthy, and sexy—and keep your brain healthy—using a time-efficient workout that's easy to squeeze into any schedule.

Aerobic Fitness Testing: You Don't Have to Do It, But . . .

I've designed the Better Brain workouts in this chapter so that you don't need to seek out fitness testing. (But as mentioned, I do advise at least one workout with a professional who can help you with weight-training technique and aerobic zone calculations.)

Still, if you want to get the most brain, heart, and body benefits from exercise, having a fitness test will give you a big advantage. In an ideal world, everyone would be able to have a free fitness test; it would be the first step on the road to good health for so many people. In fact, the American Heart Association has finally suggested that cardiorespiratory measures, obtained through aerobic fitness testing, should be added to the standard list of vital signs gathered by clinicians, just like measuring blood pressure. It's about time. During the last fifteen years, I've made presentations at medical meetings to thirty thousand physicians, with my data showing that fitness is more important in predicting death rates, cognitive function, and cardiovascular risk than most of the things doctors measure.

In reality, a thorough fitness test—such as a stress test conducted by a physician, or a less elaborate fitness test done by a certified exercise physiologist—may not be free, but it's worth it over the long term as it's such a powerful predictor of health, including cognitive function. (If you choose to go without help from an exercise physiologist, get your doctor's permission before starting a serious exercise routine; he or she knows your medical history. Particularly if you have any cardiovascular issues or have been inactive for a while, it's important to do a test like this with someone who's aware of your background.) In my clinic, we offer detailed fitness testing to clarify a patient's current abilities and personalize a workout plan. If I could have you determine just two measures of fitness as we do at my clinic, they would be (1) your MET level, and (2) your one-minute heart rate recovery.

Let's look closer at METs. Shorthand for METabolic equivalency level, this is a measure of how much energy you burn while performing a particular activity. Physicians worldwide now use METs to assess cardiac function, and many exercise machines calculate activity in METs.

- 1 MET is the energy you expend lying quietly in bed.
- 2 METs is the energy you expend sitting at a desk, writing, or talking on the phone.
- 2.5–5 METs is the energy you expend walking at a moderate (not brisk) pace.
- 4–6 METs is the energy you expend gardening or doing housework.
- 5–10 METs is the energy you expend in brisk-to-vigorous walking or cycling.
- 10–18 METs is the energy you expend running on a treadmill.

Most healthy people should be able to "comfortably" work out at a level of 10 to 12 METs, and in my clinic I have eighty-year-olds who can still reach this level of exertion. Some of my more athletic patients reach 15 to 18 METs with no strain.

To measure your MET level on your own, you will need to exercise on a machine that can calculate your MET level. Many computerized treadmills and elliptical machines will do so. (Follow the directions for entering data like your age and weight, or gripping hand sensors when prompted.) Wear a heart rate monitor to check your heart rate as well. Start with a three-minute warm-up, then gradually push yourself, increasing your exertion level every two to three minutes, until you start to sweat, huff, and puff. When you reach a point where you can't speak more than one or two short sentences, stop. Don't push it to the point that you stumble and someone has to catch you. You are finished, but before you stop, note your MET level as displayed on the machine, and check your pulse with your heart rate monitor, too. (If you're working with a physician or exercise professional, they'll do this for you—far more accurately than the machine's computer program. For more details on METs and fitness testing, visit my website, www.DrMasley.com/resources.)

As you get fitter, every time you increase your maximum MET capacity by 1, you decrease your risk for a heart attack and stroke by 12.5 percent. Increase your fitness by 2 METs, and you decrease your cardiovascular risk by a whopping 25 percent.

You've decreased your risk for memory loss and dementia as well.

Step 2 Has a Second Step: Add Strength Training

In addition to aerobic activity, add one or two strength training workouts a week. You can do them on the same day as your aerobic workout, or you can do them on the off days.

I also want to emphasize the importance of moving on to heavier weights when you're ready. (See tips for strength training at www .DrMasley.com/resources.) Challenging your muscles seems to challenge your brain, with positive results. Dr. Teresa Liu-Ambrose started her Ph.D. work in Vancouver to help older adults prevent falls and debilitating fractures. For various reasons, many of her subjects seemed unable to benefit from aerobics, but they were able to make substantial gains with strength training. A key to their success was continued progression to heavier and heavier strength training; each time a person reached some level of improvement, Liu-Ambrose added 10 to 20 percent more weight to their routine. Not only did the subjects get stronger and have fewer falls, but they seemed mentally sharper as well. Her more recent research focuses on how strength training improves memory and attention in older adults.

Tracie's Better Brain Story: The Exercise Factor

Tracie, a successful forty-five-year-old hairstylist at a popular salon, was doing everything right, or so she thought. She ate well, took some appropriate supplements, and even meditated daily. Her home life was happy, with well-adjusted teenagers and a husband with a successful career. Yet she felt tired all the time, was unable to concentrate, and even struggled to interact with her clients. She had gained fifteen pounds over the last couple of years, and half of her clothes didn't fit. The weight gain, she complained to me, was bad enough, but her inability to think straight was really gnawing at her. When I asked her about physical activity, she looked at me like I was nuts. "Activity? I'm standing on my feet at work for six hours every day. Isn't that plenty of activity?"

When I tested Tracie's fitness level, she was shocked to learn that she was only at the twentieth percentile for her age—80 percent of women her age were more fit. Her one-minute heart rate recovery dropped by only 18 beats, showing that her level of aerobic fitness was cause for concern, reflecting an increased risk for serious heart problems. Her cognitive testing results showed that she had a good memory, but her processing speed and executive function were in the lower quartile for her age, confirming sluggish cognitive performance and explaining her inability to focus at work. When I suggested regular exercise, she said she was too tired and time-pressed to go to a gym for a workout, so I asked her to wear a pedometer to track her daily steps. Tracie was averaging between 3,000 and 4,000 steps every day, which to me is the definition of inactivity. I asked her to add an extra 2,000 steps every week until she reached 10,000 steps daily, taking a brief walk in the morning, at lunch, and after dinner with her husband.

In six weeks of 10,000 steps or more, Tracie lost eight pounds, her clothes fit better, she was sleeping well, and her exhaustion was melting away. Furthermore, her mental sharpness improved, and she no longer had trouble interacting with her clients. Then I had Tracie add some Phase 1 aerobic exercise four or five days per week, and strength training twice per week. Within another month, she felt fantastic. Her mind was clear and focused, all her clothes fit, she had energy, and she felt renewed. She was so grateful that she hugged my staff. I never fail to be amazed at how powerfully fitness impacts cognitive function.

To summarize all the research on exercise and cognitive function: we know that each form of exercise (aerobic, interval, and strength training) has brain benefits and multiple other health benefits as well. Once again, as we've seen with food and nutrients, and as is reflected in the whole Better Brain Solution philosophy, the maximum benefit will come from a combined approach to exercise, which leads us to the next level in brain and body fitness.

Step 3: Mix It Up for a Better Brain

Step 3 is intended to give you the greatest benefit for the time you spend improving your energy, drive, appearance, sexual function, and give you the maximum brain and heart improvements. To get these results:

- Include some moderate aerobic activity two or three days per week (Phase 2–like activity, such as brisk walking, cycling, swimming, dancing, or vigorous yardwork, or working out on an elliptical machine)

- Add interval training two or three days per week and strength training one or two days per week
- Do something for movement, core strength, and balance once or twice per week, such as Pilates, yoga, or tai chi (all discussed below)

These activities could be combined in the same day, such as an aerobic workout and strength training, or you could also take a yoga class and get credit for balance, stretching, core work, and strength training all at the same time.

At a minimum, you will work out at least four or five days per week. I usually encourage at least one rest day per week so your body has time to recover, but if you like being active every day, you could consider some low-impact activity, such as yoga or tai chi, on your off day.

Pilates

Pilates is a form of activity developed in early twentieth-century Germany by Joseph Pilates. His father was a gymnast, and his mother was a naturopathic physician. His exercises were intended to help build core strength, balance, and flexibility, especially useful for dancers and gymnasts. Over decades his work has been extended to many people wanting to enhance their strength and balance, and you can now find Pilates classes all over the country. In my clinic, I recommend Pilates to help those with neck and back pain. A Pilates session offers balance, strength training, and stretching, but you will still need some form of aerobic activity to complement it for maximum benefit.

Yoga

There are a variety of different types of yoga, but in general, it is an excellent form of exercise that includes strength training, stretching, balance, and breathing, often with a meditation component. Studies have shown that yoga helps improve blood pressure, insomnia, muscle mass, and balance; it deters falls, reduces chronic pain, and enhances cognitive performance.

Yoga is a collection of physical, mental, and spiritual practices that originated in ancient India nearly five thousand years ago. Yoga classes vary from easy to difficult, from beginner to advanced. If you are brand new to yoga, talk to the instructors beforehand to get placed at the correct class level.

Tai Chi

Tai chi is a noncompetitive martial art known for its slow and even movements and health benefits. This ancient Chinese tradition has evolved to alleviate modern stress and anxiety and build balance. Tai chi is a good option for those wanting to combine movement with meditation. (It has earned the nickname "meditation in motion.")

In studies, tai chi has been shown to decrease stress, anxiety, and depression, improve physical capacity, and enhance balance and flexibility.

Pilates, yoga, and tai chi aren't the only movement options for core strength, balance, and stretching, though they're the ones I recommend. Adult ballet classes (or other dance forms); bar exercise classes; tae kwon do, karate, and some of the other martial arts; stability classes that use an exercise ball; and many other options are available to you, at locations ranging from specialized schools and studios to your local Y, gym, or community center.

Exercise—particularly meditative movement like yoga and tai chi—can offer something else beyond cognitive and physical fitness and flexibility, and that is relief from stress. Effective stress management can offer vast brain benefits that we will explore in the next chapter.

CHAPTER 7

Calm Your Brain

S ome stress is good, like short-term stress that jump-starts your problem-solving abilities or motivates you to accomplish more, at work or at home, giving you a sense of purpose. When stress transforms into triumph—over a looming deadline at work, a physical challenge, or a complicated issue you want to resolve—the result is a pleasurable feeling of achievement and joy. Your body and your brain are challenged, in a positive way, and when you are successful, your self-worth and confidence levels skyrocket.

But lingering, ordinary stressors, in contrast to motivating ones, have the potential to overwhelm us in both mind and body. Everyday problems like family discord, dysfunctional relationships, workplace issues, and financial worries, particularly when they flare up in combination (as is often the case), can be difficult to untangle. As we struggle with them, these stressors can destroy personal time and deplete physical and mental energy, generating a type of chronic stress that ultimately impacts brain function.

Over time, uncontrolled stress can cause a 500 percent greater risk for heart attack or stroke, decrease bone density and muscle mass, reduce skin healing and growth, impair immune function (which can lead to more frequent infections and even cancer), elevate blood sugar levels, increase belly fat, drop DHEA levels (an important adrenal hormone that helps us cope with stress), and shorten telomeres (which speed destruction of our cellular DNA). In fact, studies suggest that high levels of unmanaged stress accelerate DNA aging by at least ten years.

In the short term, persistent stress can lead to poor self-care choices, ranging from unwise eating habits (featuring sugar and bad fat, the classic comfort foods) and inactivity, to lack of sleep and an overreliance on stimulants like caffeine or depressants like alcohol. If you are a normal person trying to cope with life's more challenging moments, taking the time to work out, rest, and relax, or to prepare a nourishing meal can easily fall to the bottom of your priorities list. (And if you are an ordinary person facing extraordinary circumstances, taking care of yourself may go out the window.)

The best way out of the maze of stress is to make time to manage it. You may not be able to control your environment or the people who populate it, but you can control your response to the stress they generate. And doing so is vital for healthy brain function.

The Hormonal Stress Spiral and How to Stop It

The negative impact of stress on the overall system is well known to researchers. What is particularly troubling is that stress has a physiological impact on brain structure. Chronic, high levels of stress can damage brain cells, decrease memory and learning, and even cause the hippocampus to shrink. The primary culprit here is the stress hormone cortisol, released by the adrenal glands. A sudden surge in cortisol, whether it stems from your reaction to a missed flight or an argument with a spouse, can cause a brain-damaging rise in blood sugar and, ultimately, a thickening waistline.

Cortisol, famously known as the fight-or-flight hormone, is responsible for making sure you have the energy to battle or escape from your "enemy"—it's energy in the form of glucose (blood sugar). When you are stressed, cortisol arms your system with high blood sugar, but it doesn't much care what happens to that extra glucose after you've dealt with the stress; once you've been rebooked on another flight, or the argument is over, excess glucose may eventually get converted and stored as hard-to-lose fat. Unmanaged stress can cause your cortisol levels to stay elevated, "on call" to deal with the constant need for fight-or-flight responses. Therefore, blood sugar levels will stay elevated as well, and over time that can accelerate the development of heart disease, dementia, and memory loss.

The adrenal glands may not be able to keep up with the constant and excessive demand for cortisol; should that happen, cortisol levels will drop and eventually crash. Now, without the fight-or-flight mechanism, we can't handle the extra stress, leading to exhaustion and depression. Chronic stress causes similar imbalances with DHEA (dehydroepiandrosterone), a beneficial hormone that helps the body recover from stress. DHEA, also produced by the adrenal glands, gives us drive, energy, and libido. If DHEA levels decrease, which they are likely to do when cortisol levels are too high, our ability to handle stress plummets even further. This hormonal imbalance feeds on itself, generating a downward physical and mental spiral that gets harder to halt with time—yet it can be done.

Reducing stress isn't easy. You can't swap your children, parents, or relatives. Switching jobs is hard to do, and opting for the simple life isn't realistic for most of us. But rather than trying to eliminate stressors, a much easier and more successful strategy is to adapt to the stress by proactively taking steps to manage it. Stress is not all about the situation we are in; it is also about how we respond to it. If we can't change our environment, we can change how we react to it. And that starts with a calm brain.

Your goal now is to achieve that state, to reverse the spiral of stress and find balance, which you can do with some basic lifestyle adjustments. One hormone that helps reduce stress is oxytocin. You can think of it as the "cuddling" hormone, as it enhances that warm feeling mothers experience when they are nursing their infants, and that lovers feel when they are caressing each other. Another group of brain chemicals that modulate stress is endorphins, which are released when you exercise and promote pain relief and relaxation. Both of these neurochemicals will ease your transition toward a greater sense of calm, and both are yours to create and control.

As you take steps to manage your stress and achieve hormonal balance, you will sleep better, eat more wisely, work out more, be mentally sharper, and feel better all the way around. With time, your cortisol, DHEA, and adrenaline levels will stabilize, and you will feel calmer. As your stress management improves, it will become easier for you to sleep, to maintain a healthy diet, and to work out regularly.

A calm brain is a better brain.

Step 1: Focus on What You Can Control—Your Lifestyle Choices

Add Daily Exercise to Release Tension

The first step toward managing your stress is to get a decent workout each day, and you can use the Better Brain exercise guidelines to do so. At the least, accomplish Step 1 of the exercise plan by moving every day; the sooner you move to Step 2, adding some aerobic activity and strength training, the sooner you will start feeling calm and relaxed. (If you're tracking your Better Brain progress and working through each of the four pillars, give yourself credit for taking two steps at a time— Step 1 of exercise and Step 1 of stress management.)

In addition to increasing your executive brain function, burning fat, and protecting your heart, daily exercise is likely the most powerful therapy for burning away stress. Tension tends to pour out of us like sweat during a good workout; no drug is as effective for reducing tension. Vigorous physical activity gives you a surge of endorphins. Many people don't sleep well unless they are physically tired, not just mentally fatigued. A daily workout is a must for optimal stress management.

Get a Good Night's Sleep

Every person needs a fresh start every day, but a good night's sleep is often elusive. Many people suffer from a combination of insufficient and poor-quality sleep, especially adults older than age seventy. Up to 25 percent of older adults have insomnia and have decreased cognitive function due to lack of sleep. A popular myth has it that as you age, you need less sleep. In terms of pure hours, babies, children, and young adults certainly do need more sleep than older people, but falling into a pattern of getting less than seven hours of sleep at a time can be harmful, physically and mentally, regardless of age.

Whether it happens frequently or is an occasional occurrence due to a late night, no one enjoys the morning-after feelings of physical sluggishness and nervous exhaustion resulting from lack of sleep. Trying to kick-start the system with caffeine (or a sugary snack) might "help" by providing a temporary burst of energy, but after the coffee and candy wear off and the body and brain crash, you will feel even worse. And of course it is particularly damaging if this is a regular way of life. It is well documented that poor sleep habits lead to decreased calorie-burning capacity (low basal metabolic rate), which can result in weight gain and the many health problems it can trigger. (If you are trying to lose weight or maintain weight loss, it is very difficult to do if your body doesn't get the sleep it needs.)

As far as brain health goes, sleep deprivation at any age results in poor cognitive performance. Research with college students has shown that those who sleep seven to eight hours nightly have better memory retention than those sleeping less than seven hours, even if they spend the extra waking time studying. Among older people, the results are the same—more sleep results in a better memory. The act of sleeping helps the brain store and protect memory. When we're awake and well rested, those memories are more functional, whether we are trying to remember the solution to a problem, a person's name, or the important task we must do that day. If we're sleep deprived, it doesn't mean our memory center has been erased, but it is very difficult for a tired brain to access and use those memories.

In my clinic, our patient data shows that the right amount of sleep is critical to overall cognition and especially problem solving and executive function. Those who consistently had seven or eight hours of sleep each night had the best brain performance. If they slept less than seven hours, their function dropped. However, those who slept more than eight hours consistently showed a drop in performance, too. Initially, I was surprised by that eight-plus-hours finding. But when I searched the literature, I noticed that studies outside my own clinic confirmed it: those who slept more than eight hours had lower function than those who slept seven or eight hours each night.

Studies have also shown that those who sleep five to six hours during the workweek and sleep nine or ten hours on their days off to catch up never really catch up. Yes, it is better than sleeping only five or six hours every night, but it takes at least a week of regular sleep to restore normal brain function. The majority of people would be more productive if they slept at least seven hours every night and stopped depriving themselves during the week.

What About Sleep in People Who Are Cognitively Impaired?

When my mom was caring for my stepdad after his procedure-induced stroke and subsequent acquired dementia, her biggest challenge as a caregiver was that he would roam the house 24/7. He lost his normal sleep-wake cycle when his brain was injured, and my mom ended up totally exhausted caring for him.

Studies show that people with moderate to advanced cognitive impairment have altered sleep, especially with their circadian rhythm, which provides a normal sleep-wake cycle. In adults with Alzheimer's disease, a classic example of this is "sundowning," in which they become agitated and confused as the sun sets and there's a shift from daytime to nighttime.

Whether sleep problems accelerate cognitive decline remains controversial. Studies suggest that people with insomnia are twice as likely to develop dementia over three years as adults with normal sleep patterns. But what isn't clear is whether the lack of sleep is directly causing the cognitive decline or if cognitive decline disrupts sleep and insomnia is just another sign of early cognitive impairment.

It is probably a bit of both. And either way, we need to take steps to help prevent and reverse insomnia in older adults and take steps to help people with cognitive impairment to sleep better. This should be done not only for the person suffering from cognitive impairment, but also for the caregiver of the person impaired.

The Better Brain Way to Optimize Sleep Quality

If you are already getting seven to eight hours of sleep nightly, protect and enhance your sleep with these tips.

- BE CONSISTENT: Aim to go to bed and wake up at the same time every night and every day. If you must go off-schedule, try to keep the variation to one hour (two hours max), even on weekends. Otherwise you're exhausting yourself. For instance, if you usually go to bed at eleven p.m. and rise by seven a.m., but you stay up extra late on Saturday night and sleep till ten a.m. on Sunday, you will feel the equivalent of jetlag on Monday, and you'll need a few days to get back on schedule. You've essentially altered your time zone.

- YOUR BEDROOM IS FOR BED: Sleep, rest, and be romantic in bed, and keep computers, TVs, smartphones, and all other screens out. (Pinging smartphones are especially encroaching on our bedtimes. Put cellphones "to sleep" at night, preferably in another room.) Books or magazines, if you want to read for fifteen to twenty minutes or so, are fine—but not office work. And if you're engrossed in your story, watch the clock—twenty minutes can turn into forty-five. If you're reading an article or news that irritates or disturbs you, consider if you'll have trouble sleeping as a result. Some people can hit their internal "off switch" when it comes to this; others can't.

- SCREEN OUT THE SCREEN LIGHT: If you like to read in bed on a device like an iPad, be aware that exposure to white or blue light from even the smallest screen will make it harder for you to fall asleep. Change the background to a dimmer sleep-friendly setting, or wear orange-tinted glasses for screening out artificial and bright light. Try to avoid white or blue light from screens for at least an hour (preferably two) before bed. This includes working on your computer—if you must, change the background from white/blue to red, which is more restful.

- GO DARK, GET QUIET: Bright light—from screens, from lamps, from the streetlight outside your window, or from the clock on your bedside table—is an impediment to sleep. Humans evolved to sleep when it was dark, and to wake with the light, and the production of the hormone melatonin helps this process along. Orange and red lights tell your brain to make melatonin and to get ready to sleep (just as those orange-red sunsets cued our cave-dwelling ancestors 100,000 years ago). But bright light (which tells the brain to wake) blocks the production of melatonin. Therefore, eliminating bright light is fundamental. Do an inventory in your bedroom and eliminate as many sources as possible. Try a sleep mask or blackout shades if necessary. Some people even outfit their bedside lamps with red bulbs

to help induce sleep. And don't forget the earplugs, if noise
is a problem—a quiet environment is as important as a
dark one.

- STAY COOL (BUT AVOID COLD FEET): Don't
  sleep in a warm room. At night, body temperature naturally
  drops, which helps us fall asleep. To help your body do
  what it wants to do, keep the air cool but your hands and
  feet warm. Unless it's really cold, you may not need all
  those blankets and flannel pajamas (but wear socks if you
  need to). Check the setting on your thermostat; 68 to 72
  degrees F is what many people prefer, but adjust as desired,
  and use a quiet fan if necessary. (Some people like the
  added bonus of a quiet fan's "white noise.")
- BED DOWN IN COMFORT: Much is made of
  "making your bedroom a sanctuary," but you don't
  need to go overboard with five-star hotel bedding to
  sleep comfortably. A decent mattress is important, but
  don't overlook the value of a high-quality pillow. That
  is something that you can afford to replace annually, if
  needed. An orthopedic-shaped pillow can help if you have
  neck problems. If you prefer down pillows, a fill-power of
  650 to 775 works well for most sleepers.

If You Can't Fall Asleep (you have insomnia) or You Sleep Poorly

- **Be selfish:** If you have a partner who tosses and turns,
  snores, reads in bright light, or otherwise is keeping you
  awake, speak up and figure out a solution. There is a
  lot at stake. (He or she may also be suffering from sleep
  deprivation, and it may be time to reboot your bedtime
  routines together.) And if a pet or a child is invading your
  space, gently send them to their own beds. They'll be
  grateful when you're no longer sleep deprived and seem
  happier, and when your brain and body are rested.
- **Limit caffeine.** If you drink coffee (or other sources of
  caffeine), limit it to one or two servings in the morning. An

afternoon (or late-day) caffeine serving may be contributing to poor sleep.

- **Limit alcohol.** Many people mistakenly think that alcohol will ensure sleep, given its association with relaxing effects. But alcohol can actually cause wakefulness—when you least desire it. If you drink wine with dinner or have other alcohol at night, be aware that when alcohol levels in the body drop, it can startle the body awake—usually at around two a.m. It can be very hard to fall back asleep once this happens. Don't drink more than two servings of alcohol at night, and avoid it entirely in the two hours before you go to bed.

- **Consider limiting fluids before bedtime.** If you wake up to urinate at night and you find it hard to fall back asleep, consider limiting fluids starting a couple of hours before your bedtime (particularly caffeine and alcohol, as they act as a diuretic, which stimulates urination). If you cut back on fluids and you're still waking nightly to urinate, particularly if you're getting up more than once or twice, discuss with your doctor, especially if you have bladder or prostate issues.

- **Try sleep-friendly food and drink.** Tryptophan-rich foods (like turkey, peanut butter, bananas, and skim milk) will help you sleep if you consume them sixty minutes before you go to bed. (However, if you suffer from heartburn, the heartburn may be worse than the benefit of eating tryptophan-rich food, so if this applies to you, avoid eating within two hours of bedtime.) In addition, some herbal infusions may help you fall asleep, in particular valerian.

- **Time your workouts.** Exercise daily for 30–60 minutes but not within two hours of your bedtime. The energizing effects of exercise will make it hard for you to fall asleep.

- **Nap smart.** If you're a daily napper, limit your rest to no more than half an hour, and don't nap after four p.m.

- **Shut down the stressors.** The two-hour period before your bedtime really is important. It sets you up for restful sleep, physically and mentally. (That's why so many of these recommendations specify "within two hours of going to bed.") Don't do work or engage in stressful activities within this two-hour period. Even a tense phone call or an argument can get in the way. Finding calm before sleep is crucial if you have insomnia or poor-quality sleep.

- **Fade to black.** In addition to following all the recommendations for optimizing your sleep quality (reducing light and noise), do something extra: dim the lights in your surroundings about half an hour before you head to bed. This will cue your brain that you're preparing to ease into sleep.

- **And when it's time to wake up:** If you have as much trouble waking up as you do falling and staying asleep, you may need bright light to help your sleep-wake cycle get into sync. Sunlight is ideal, but you can also purchase a full-spectrum bright light that activates with an alarm clock. Let yourself be in bright, increasing light for 5–30 minutes from the time you awake until you actually get out of bed. You'll feel more alert.

If you just can't stop tossing and turning, don't be a clock watcher and worry about your inability to sleep. Go ahead and get up and do something calming for ten to twenty minutes and then try again. Have an herbal infusion or a tryptophan snack, meditate or pray, write in your journal, or pick up a book that will soothe you. (Avoid content that will excite and absorb you, and do not turn on the TV or check your phone!)

If the problem persists, talk to your doctor. Sleeping supplements and medications can be helpful, but it's best to reserve them for occasional rather than regular (nightly) use. In particular, ask your physician about herbal supplements that have been shown to be effective in improving sleep quality, such as valerian and GABA. Over the long term, sleeping medications can become habit forming and actually disrupt the natural sleep cycle. Ideally, you want your body rhythms to dictate a healthy sleep cycle—not prescription drugs or supplements.

If you're in menopause, symptoms like night sweats may be disrupting your sleep. Ask your doctor about how to manage menopause-related sleep disorders. They can often be treated successfully with natural as well as bioidentical hormones. (Extracts of Siberian rhubarb root can be helpful for night sweats or other sleep-disrupting symptoms.)

Don't Overuse Stimulants and Alcohol, Especially If You're Stressed

Caffeine

The brain benefits of caffeine are discussed thoroughly in Chapter 3, but it is a stimulant, and everyone responds to caffeine differently. For those who are sensitive to its effects, it can backfire when it comes to stress management, particularly in its most commonly ingested form, coffee. Drinking one or two cups of coffee or tea will help some people focus and pay attention, while even one cup makes others feel wired. Data from my clinic shows that nearly everyone has a drop in cognitive function if they drink more than three cups per day. You may be wide awake but are not truly more functional when you have this much caffeine.

To manage your stress well and achieve a calm brain, you must put limits on stimulant use, including coffee and other caffeine-containing beverages and foods. Pay attention to how your body responds to caffeine, particularly when you are tired or feeling burned out. A hot, steaming mug of aromatic coffee might help you come alive in the morning, but if you're relying on it throughout the day, or if you're sensitive to its effects, you'll wind up feeling wired and tired at the same time. Your brain won't benefit, nor will your heart: excessive caffeine not only makes your heart race but can cause stiffening of the arteries and higher blood pressure. Considering all the data, as well as how you metabolize caffeine, it's best to limit yourself to two cups of coffee a day and definitely no more than three. If you feel wired after consuming caffeine, refer back to the box on caffeine metabolism, "That Caffeine Buzz—Is It Good For You?" on pages 72–73.

If you want to enjoy a stress-busting hot (or iced) drink to replace that extra coffee you're cutting out, try a few cups of tea with or without caffeine. Caffeine levels in most teas are dramatically lower than in coffee, and tea has calming effects as well as brain and heart benefits. Another option is a cup of magnesium-rich hot cocoa, with the added bonus of fiber and anti-aging compounds. (Cocoa also counts as a source of dark chocolate, which—like caffeine—is on the Better Brain list of 12 Smart Foods. While dark chocolate does contain some caffeine, it's only 5 mg—about what you'd find in decaffeinated tea or coffee.) Herbal infusions are yet another satisfying option, particularly in the evening when you want to wind down.

Tobacco

Tobacco is another stimulant, and despite the classic image of relaxing with a stress-busting cigarette, it does not have a calming effect on the brain. Data from cognitive testing in my clinic show that using tobacco increases attention span, but at the same time it decreases executive function and lowers overall brain performance. So although you might feel more alert, your brain function actually drops. Don't confuse that decrease in cognitive function with a decrease in stress. Tobacco also increases your risk for dementia and Alzheimer's disease, as well as cancer, heart attack, stroke, erectile dysfunction, emphysema, bone loss and fractures, gum disease, stomach ulcers, and heartburn, and it accelerates skin wrinkling and other outward signs of aging.

If you use tobacco, stop! It will be one of the most important things you ever do for your health.

Alcohol

Too much alcohol can be even worse than too many stimulants, particularly when you are trying to manage extra stress—because alcohol is a depressant, one that in excess can lead to major depression. Caffeine and tobacco, like alcohol, are too often mistakenly used as relaxants—the steaming cups of coffee, the reward of a cigarette, some drinks at the end of a long day to unwind. But alcohol, unlike caffeine and tobacco, is not a stimulant that will focus attention or cause a burst in energy, though as noted earlier, a late-night drink can startle a person into unwanted wakefulness a few hours into sleep.

Though one or two servings of red wine with dinner can benefit your brain function, blood sugar control, and cardiovascular risk, developing a reliance on alcohol—whether it is wine, hard liquor, or beer—and having more than three servings day after day is not healthy, physically or mentally.

Don't use alcohol to manage stress, particularly if you're facing a difficult time. It's like pouring gasoline on a fire. Drinking in excess might dull feelings of anxiety, tension, or pain, but that won't help you manage the problems that are causing your anxiety. In fact, alcohol has the opposite effect because it can disrupt and fray the personal and professional relationships that may be the source of your stress—or that may offer you a lifeline of support. You can't communicate effectively and honestly, and you will not be able to manage your reaction to stressors in a healthy way.

A numb brain is not a healthy brain.

To summarize, Step 1 for managing stress, boosting cognitive performance, and enhancing overall health focuses on stress-proofing your brain with smart lifestyle choices, including:

1. Get a workout each day, and sweat away tension.
2. Get enough sleep, seven or eight hours each night.
3. Don't overconsume stimulants or coffee. Don't use tobacco, and when stressed, don't exceed one or two servings of caffeine and/or alcohol daily.

Once you have incorporated these habits, you're ready to move to Step 2.

Sudden Stress: Stop the Spiral

In an instant, an unexpected event can unleash chaos into your life and send you into a stress spiral. Whether the new stressor is work-related or is triggered by a personal crisis, at times like these the default action is to set your normal routine aside and react to the urgent matter at hand. If you need to prioritize your time and postpone a social engagement or move an appointment, that's understandable, but a downward stress spiral is easy to fall into and hard to halt and emerge from *if you fail to adapt to the stress.* If all you are doing is reacting to the crisis, you begin to sleep less, eat

poorly, and skip your workout. You feel worse and worse—
and subsequently more stressed. The longer this cycle persists, the greater its impact on your health, including your
cognitive function.

If you are faced with a sudden jump in stress, you can take
steps to halt the spiral and better manage your circumstances.

- Don't turn to alcohol. It's okay to have a glass of wine with
  dinner, but don't rely upon alcohol to manage acute stress,
  and don't consume more than two servings per day.
- Do go for a workout and sweat. Exercise is fantastic
  for helping you manage stress. Many people use the "I
  don't have time *now*" excuse, but it is when you are most
  stressed that exercise is most effective and therapeutic.
- Eat well, and avoid skipping meals. Your brain and body
  need quality fuel, especially now. If you don't have time to
  cook, you can still make wise choices, particularly if you're
  following the Better Brain Solution.
- Carve out time for seven or eight hours of sleep. As with
  exercise, sleep needs are frequently ignored when stress is
  overloading all circuits. But don't burn the candle at both
  ends when you are stressed out. (And if it's job-related,
  don't pull an all-nighter—perhaps you managed that in
  college, but rarely will you produce your best work.) If
  you are too stressed to sleep, at least get some rest. If this
  persists over several days, consider a sleep supplement or
  talk to your physician.
- If you know how to meditate, schedule twenty minutes
  to do so once or twice per day. Don't set this beneficial
  practice aside when you most need it. It may not be
  a realistic coping technique if you are not a regular
  meditator, but at the very least, try the effective
  "Relaxation Response" breathing exercises on pages
  192–193.
- Make it a point to engage in a daily calming activity just
  for yourself, particularly if you are not a meditator. Do
  something that relaxes you, such as practicing a craft,

working a puzzle, reading, playing an instrument, taking a
hot, soothing bath, or getting a massage.

- Don't ignore personal relationships. You need friends and
loved ones during times of stress. Go out with people who
make you laugh and feel good, and do something two or
three times per week that brings you fun and joy. You are
not being selfish. You are being smart about adapting to
stress and, by doing so, stopping the spiral.

Step 2: Unplug, Recharge, and Reset

Schedule Some Peace and Calm Every Day

It may sound counterintuitive to "schedule" time to relax—schedules
are rigid and demanding, the opposite of relaxation. Yet, that is exactly
what my most successful (healthiest) patients do. They build time into
their days to find what I call peace and calm—some form of downtime
that will benefit the brain. Yes, you will sleep at night and rest your
mind and body then, but if you are trying to manage your daily stress
level more effectively to protect your brain, setting aside a specific time
to do so—scheduling it, the way you would any appointment—is the
best way. You can eat wisely, exercise, and improve your sleep quality,
but if you don't set aside time to regularly relax, everyday stress will find
its way into your life more easily.

Here are some favorite ways to incorporate peace and calm into your
life, which perhaps will inspire you to come up with your own ideas.
Some of these you can do on a daily basis—just aim for ten to twenty
minutes of brain-calming, soul-soothing activity—and some are more
occasional.

- Be in nature. If the weather is pleasant, take your morning
coffee or tea, or just yourself, outside and sit for a moment.
- Take a walk—this isn't aerobic, it's just a relaxing stroll.
(This might be best done solo. If you decide to bring your

energetic dog or meet a talkative friend, keep in mind that
your goal is to reduce your stress, not send it upward!)

- Enjoy soothing sounds and fragrances. Listen to pleasing
  music without interruption, or to any gentle sounds of
  your choice, like a bubbling fountain. If you like scented
  soaps and lotions, indulge yourself daily. For some, the act
  of cooking a meal and filling a kitchen with pleasurable
  aromas is the height of relaxation.
- Take time for deep prayer. Prayer time can provide peace
  and calm. If you are inclined, don't miss out on this
  opportunity. (If you prefer meditation, see the tips on pages
  191–194.)
- Make a monthly appointment for a soothing massage
  (or better yet, a weekly one). A good massage releases the
  neurotransmitter oxytocin, which naturally triggers a sense
  of calm and well-being.
- Try yoga. If "hot" yoga or power yoga classes are too
  strenuous (and if you're stressed out that you're doing it all
  wrong), go for something less athletic, with an emphasis
  on stretching; you may even be able to find a candlelight
  yoga class in your community. Gentle stretching classes, as
  well as movement classes such as tai chi, can also be very
  calming.
- Enjoy romance and sex with your partner at least two or
  three times per week; human contact releases oxytocin and
  lowers cortisol levels. If you don't have a partner, sharing
  hugs with friends offers some of the same healthful benefits.
- If you've gone through your whole day without a moment
  to spare, you can build in peace and calm at the end of your
  evening. Try a hot soak in a tub by candlelight (and with
  the door locked, kids in bed, and phone unplugged). If that
  doesn't appeal, then revisit your bedtime routine and build
  in at least 10–20 minutes of relaxation before you go to
  sleep. Keep a journal, meditate, or pray, or just breathe out
  the stress and breathe in the peace and calm.

Go on Vacation (even if you don't leave home)

Getting away from your regular routine with a regular vacation—even a short one—can restore your energy and help you get some perspective on stressful situations. But don't wait to get on a plane before you give your brain a break.

Cellphones. E-mails. Texts. Everyone you know is probably reachable twenty-four hours a day, every day. And if you live in the modern world, you are, too. You're just a dial or a "hit send" away from someone who wants to reach out and—potentially stress you. Technology was supposed to make our lives easier, but all too often it does just the opposite. Therefore, sometimes you have to make an extra effort to unplug so that you can recharge your own batteries and de-stress.

We often caution the young people in our lives to put their phones down or quit staring at whatever screen has captured their attention, but how often are we guilty of doing the same thing? It's very easy to be unaware of how much technology rules our lives, so the trick is to become self-aware. You may not want to go so far as to keep a log of how often you are on your computer or your phone (like a food diary), but if you do, you might be surprised at how often your attention is diverted by these devices—and that's not good for our brains. Research shows that the Internet is "rewiring" our brains, impacting our ability to focus and even retain memory.

Your brain can benefit from technology, but don't let it become another stressor. Unplug, and not just on vacation. Weekends are a great time to unplug and spend time with loved ones and nature.

This Is Your Brain on CNN

Whether their quality is high or low, the quantity of news stories is overwhelming these days. It can be hard to avoid the 24/7 deluge, whether it pours from your social media feed, talk radio, an old-fashioned newspaper, or a late-night talk show. While staying current is important for staying connected, when you are trying to reduce your stress and find peace, the media can act as a major stimulant, especially at bedtime. Taking in late-breaking news or details of a terrible crisis right before you try to fall asleep will generally rile you up (or depress you), rather than calm you down. Even if you don't yell back at the television, it's not unlike having a stressful, troubling conversation right before bedtime.

If you are a news junkie and take pleasure in following current events, make sure you have a thick enough skin to handle what is coming at you, and that your media consumption isn't contributing to your stress levels or poor sleep. If you are sensitive to what you see and hear in the news, it's best to take in the state of the world early in the day, after your brain has rested and recharged from a good night's sleep. (Some wellness experts even recommend a "media diet" from time to time—a self-imposed period of no news feeds, particularly during vacation.)

Of course, not all "news" comes from news outlets. In addition to their bounty of breaking news apps, our smartphones can be set to ping every time a boldfaced name tweets, a friend texts, a boss e-mails, or a store is having a sale. Cellphones are handy, but they are also pocket-size stressors, constantly asking for our attention. Be self-aware about your cellphone, iPad, and hand-held gadget use, and make sure you aren't overly attached to your device. When you are, it can be like carrying tension and anxiety around in your pocket. You can resist and control its impact on your brain (and your blood pressure) with a quick flick of the finger: mute, airplane mode, or power off.

Step 3: Go Deeper to Get Calmer

If you're ready for more challenging techniques that have real stress-management benefits but require some practice and commitment, move on to Step 3. Consider it a toolkit for reaching a deeper state of calm.

Meditation

Meditation is an ancient practice with modern benefits, including its ability to help us manage stress. People who meditate combine calm with a sense of focused and heightened awareness—two seemingly disparate states that are related. However, meditation does take training and practice.

Meditation can lower blood pressure and heart rate, relax muscles, lower cortisol levels, and improve sleep quality. (One of the first benefits new meditators often report is that their sleep improves dramatically.) It is also an excellent way to reverse the effects of stress within the brain itself.

During times of stress, blood flow is shunted from the frontal and temporal lobes of the brain—the forebrain area that is involved in problem solving and inhibiting impulsive behavior—to the "feed me now" midbrain. In other words, stress short-circuits normal and beneficial brain blood flow. However, during meditation (as noted in Chapter 7), blood flow to the frontal lobes is increased, which nourishes the calm and sensible forebrain. This is why meditation can be an ideal way to stay focused and control impulsive behavior, which can be especially helpful in stressful situations.

In most traditional meditation styles, meditators use a mantra (a personalized word or words, selected just for them by a teacher), a special sound or chant, or a meaningful phrase that gives them focus and comfort. Breathing is also an important component. (It doesn't need to be exaggerated to be effective. The idea is to become aware of one's breathing, which can become a focal point in itself.)

A comfortable sitting position is also important, but a ramrod-straight back is not required. In fact, sitting with the back comfortably supported (but not sliding into a semi-reclining position, which can cue the body for sleep) is best.

Meditation is fairly challenging. You are aiming to stay focused and relaxed for ten to twenty minutes at a time. It's also important to be consistent. Most teachers recommend daily seated practice—and some meditators will do ten to twenty minutes twice a day once they become hooked on its benefits.

You don't need to do it in pristine surroundings and sit like a yogi, but you will need to learn proper technique. While it is possible to learn some fundamentals of meditation from a book, the best meditation instruction is in person with a teacher, either in a group setting or one on one. Look for a meditation teacher—not a yoga instructor with some meditation training—as their guidance and instruction will help you reap the most from this experience. Numerous online courses offer guided meditations, and apps like Headspace offer step-by-step audio instruction. See www.DrMasley.com/resources for meditation details.

Whether you choose to pursue more formal instruction or not, these two simple options will help you develop some basic meditation skills, such as focused breathing, that can help you lower stress.

1. Simple Breathing Exercise: A One-Minute Meditation

Sit comfortably in a quiet spot. You can also do this when you're lying in bed, preparing to fall asleep.

- Breathe in 5 seconds, then breathe out 5 seconds. With each breath, recall a positive, joy-filled memory (a loved one, a vista from a treasured vacation) or something that fills you with gratitude and well-being.
- Repeat six times. As your mind becomes more peaceful and your body relaxes, your heart rate will slow, and you will feel calmer.

2. Prolonged Breathing-Meditation Exercise

This more involved exercise takes ten to twenty minutes. It can drop your blood pressure by 10 points, lower anxiety, and reduce chronic pain as it helps you manage stress. My suggestions are based, in part, on the techniques of Herbert Benson, M.D., who developed the famous "Relaxation Response" approach to meditation.

- Find a spot where you will not be disturbed. Make sure your phone is turned off (or better yet, in another room).
- Close your eyes, and sit upright but comfortably, letting your shoulders relax. Become aware of your breathing as you inhale and exhale rhythmically.

- You are now going to relax each muscle group in your body, beginning with your toes. Work your way up and focus on gradually releasing muscle tension from your toes, calves, thighs, buttocks, abdomen, back, chest, shoulders, neck, jaw, and scalp. Try to keep each muscle group relaxed as you progress to the next one.
- Focus on your breathing, which will help you avoid thinking of your to-do list. Repeating a meaningful sound or phrase, like a mantra, will also focus your process. Think or say your mantra out loud when you exhale. (Speaking it aloud will help you to exhale.)
- Don't fight the fleeting thoughts that will enter your brain. Just envision them passing through you. Use your breathing and your special sound or words to keep you focused.
- Continue for 10–20 minutes. You can open your eyes to check the clock.
- After the allotted time, don't rush to stand up. Just let yourself sit quietly. After a few minutes, open your eyes and gradually begin to move normally.
- You should feel considerably more relaxed after completing this longer exercise. If you like the feeling, try doing it daily. It gets easier and more fulfilling with each attempt.
- Repeating a mantra—any words that calm you, whether they have spiritual meaning for you or are simply a motivational reminder—can be useful in stressful situations. Whether you're about to have a difficult phone call or tough meeting at work, or are coping with insomnia, the ritualistic repetition can:
  - improve heart rate variability
  - decrease sympathetic tone, which is associated with rapid heart rates, which can sometimes be dangerous
  - synchronize respiratory and heart rate cycles
  - free your mind from daily thoughts and worries

If you like how you feel after doing these exercises, consider finding a full-blown meditation class. They are plentiful in most communities.

It does take skill and practice. (Many new meditators give up in part because they are self-taught and their errors are keeping them from enjoying the benefits of the practice.) If meditation reduces your stress and leads to a calmer brain, it's more than worth the time.

HeartMath

Many of my patients find meditation too difficult, but they are having success with the software program HeartMath, which provides biofeedback to help the brain find a state of peace and calm similar to that with meditation. The technique combines relaxation with positive feelings of gratitude, while monitoring heart rate variability. When you are in a relaxed state, your heart rate speeds up and slows down gradually and cyclically—it has nice variability. But when you are stressed out, it lacks this type of rhythmic variation.

People in the military, firefighters, and law enforcement officers suffering from post-traumatic stress disorder (PTSD) have had great results training with HeartMath. Hearing about its success with first responders, companies started offering this form of therapy to highly stressed corporate executives and saw signs of improved productivity. I first heard about it through my work with corporate wellness programs. Now this type of intervention has gone mainstream and is easily available to anyone.

You can install HeartMath on your computer or smartphone. The goal is to work with the program ten to twenty minutes every day. It focuses your mind as it guides you through controlling your physiological stress response through breathing; meanwhile you measure your heart rhythms with a special attachment as you concentrate on positive emotions. The hardware attachment measures your pulse and translates it into computer graphics. As you practice the protocol, the graphs change to reflect how your heart rate, mind, and emotions have become balanced and synchronized, leaving you in a much more peaceful and creative place.

The makers of HeartMath point to clinical studies showing that their program helps participants improve focus, sleep, and reduce anxiety. In my own practice, I have found it useful in patients who suffer from stress but who can't (or won't) meditate. For more information on HeartMath, see www.DrMasley.com/resources.

Finally, Have Fun

For most people, making time for fun is the hardest step of all when it comes to battling back the effects of stress and achieving a calmer, healthier brain.

During times of stress, it is challenging enough to do the most basic self-care. Having fun isn't just seen as a luxury—it's seen as unneeded. There are bills to be paid, work to do, children and elderly parents to care for. Fun? Love? Laughter? Forget it.

Yet the feeling of joy is a powerful tonic for the brain. It is what stimulates the brain to release powerful endorphins that promote relaxation, calm, pain relief, and happiness. Joy can come from cracking up at a silly joke, playing with a pet or a child, meeting a good friend for coffee, or simply smiling at something that makes you feel good.

Being connected—to your community, to your loved ones, to the wider world—also creates joy, as does having a sense of purpose, particularly as we wind down our work lives and our families become less dependent upon us for the day-to-day basics. For the good of your brain—and your overall health and well-being—schedule some fun for yourself, no matter how stressed you may be.

Look for activities and companions that lift you up—and be aware of those who bring you down. As discussed at the outset, while we can't control the circumstances that trigger brain-harming stress, we can control our responses to manage its physical and mental impact—and part of the way we can do that is by consciously choosing a beneficial, joy-filled environment.

Now that you have all four pillars of the Better Brain Solution (food, nutrients, fitness, and stress management), it's time to shift to another essential aspect of protecting your brain. You could eat great food, meet your nutrient needs, get truly fit, and manage your stress beautifully, but it would all be for naught if you poisoned yourself.

Let's clarify what those brain toxins are, and learn how to avoid them.

CHAPTER 8

Protecting Your Brain from Toxins

For 100,000 years, humans lived in a pristine environment. Our bodies didn't need to know how to detox because our planet was clean. But in our modern environment, we've changed that picture. Now it is far too easy to become loaded with toxins, even from birth, and our bodies haven't developed enough mechanisms to remove them.

Over the last century, chemistry has brought us an amazing array of "useful" products, from plastics to pesticides. The challenge is that most of us assumed that the chemicals included in these products were tested and proven to be safe for humans. But that has not been the case. There are around two hundred chemicals in the blood of newborns before they are even born, many of them harmful. In fact, only a small fraction of the thousands of chemicals in use in the United States have been tested for safety.

Take just one example, a brain toxin that has crept into our food chain with ease. Bisphenol A, or BPA, is commonly found in the lining of canned food containers—and until recently, in plastic baby bottles and the ubiquitous sippy cups used by toddlers and very young children. When a toxin like BPA is ingested, it can impact the body's ability to regulate blood sugar, the number one cause of cognitive decline. It is easier to accumulate BPA than you might think. Consuming two servings per week from cans and containers lined with BPA will, over the long term, increase blood and urine levels of BPA and block insulin receptors, and it may double your lifetime risk for developing diabetes. BPA has also been shown to spike an increase in blood pressure, after participants ingested a single serving of food from a BPA-containing can.

Compounds known as phthalates are used in the manufacturing of plastics, including plastic water bottles and other food packaging, as well as common household items like shower curtains and plastic flooring, furniture, children's toys, and electronic devices. Studies have shown that repeated exposure and ingestion of chemicals like BPA and phthalates may increase your risk for cancer and diabetes. Phthalate tissue levels are also associated with lower IQ scores in children.*

Fortunately, BPA is now banned in baby bottles, but children and adults still need to avoid toxins that make their way into everyday life. It's challenging, but not impossible. You can start by looking for BPA-free canned goods—it should say BPA-free on the can. To avoid phthalates, don't cook or microwave in plastic containers, and avoid drinking out of plastic bottles. The box "Getting Brain Toxins Off Your Plate" on pages 202–203 offers more suggestions.

It's much easier, however, to target major brain toxins that can be eliminated in a very straightforward way, through conscious choice and lifestyle changes.

Seven Brain Toxins You Can Start Avoiding Now

Though a healthy diet with proper nutrients, as well as exercise and stress management, will promote a better brain and protect it, each of these toxins is capable of undermining those valuable efforts and harming your health and memory. You will recognize many of the toxins on the list below as substances that are clearly harmful to humans. What is new and that you may not realize, however, is the extent of damage that these "everyday poisons" can do to your brain. If you are exposing yourself to any of the following, it's time to detox.

1. Tobacco

Using tobacco products raises your risk of developing early-onset dementia and Alzheimer's disease. Tobacco, of course, is also highly

---

*In 2012 the FDA officially prohibited the use of BPA in the manufacturing of baby bottles and cups, though this was after declaring it safe in 2008, and then reversing that decision in 2010, ultimately banning it two years later.

addictive, and quitting is very hard, even when the stakes are known. Unfortunately, because of the immense power of the global tobacco industry, one of the most damaging and deadly products in the world will likely remain legal to use.

Tobacco usage will increase your risk for heart attack and stroke, as well as more than a dozen fatal cancers, skin wrinkling, bone loss, and debilitating fractures. Smoking is the primary cause of emphysema. It gives you frequent respiratory and sinus infections, bad breath, and heartburn. It worsens sexual performance, especially for men, as tobacco is a leading cause of erectile dysfunction.

Its links to cancer and cardiovascular risk are well researched and documented, but many people don't realize the damaging impact that tobacco can have on the brain. One reason for this lack of consciousness may be that tobacco is a stimulant frequently associated with heightened awareness. Smokers will point out that using tobacco helps them pay attention. It's true that as with many stimulants, tobacco does wake you up and can help you focus. In fact, data from my own clinic reflects this—up to a point: Though patients who use tobacco do show an improvement in attention scores, more importantly they show decreased executive function (problem solving) and *decreased overall neurocognitive performance.* Over the long term, tobacco use worsens overall cognitive function.

If the other widely publicized risks of smoking and using tobacco aren't enough to motivate users to stop, perhaps the fact that brain health hangs in the balance will do so—the sooner the better. There are now dozens of sponsored programs to help you quit. (Check with your doctor.) Many of these programs are free, even if you don't have medical insurance.

Here is some information I share with my clinic patients to help them stop smoking. If you don't smoke but have loved ones who do, perhaps these guidelines will benefit them—and their brains.

Better Brain Action Steps to Quit Tobacco

1. *Pick a quit date.* Some people are motivated by selecting a birthday, anniversary, or a child's upcoming graduation or wedding as a quit date. Announce the date to friends and

family to prepare them as well—if you get a bit grumpy or tense, they'll be more forgiving if they know you are quitting an addictive habit. By going public with your intention and tying it to a specific date, you are enabling them to provide added support.

2. *Talk to your physician about using medications to help you quit.* Specific drugs, such as Chantix and Wellbutrin, increase your success at quitting. Talk to your doctor about whether they are a good option for you. They work by blocking the pleasure gained from using tobacco. If appropriate, start using the medication two weeks before your quit date.

3. *Before you quit, identify the three W's.* When do you smoke? Why are you smoking (what need is being met)? What else could you do to meet that need? Write down the answers on a notepad. It's easy enough to answer the first question (when), but dive deeper into the why and the what. Most people credit their tobacco products with helping them accomplish certain things: to relax, to take a break, to stop eating. In their minds, those are all good reasons. The challenge is to identify why and then make sure that need is met in another, more healthful way—for instance, by meditation, taking a bike ride, or eating a better diet.

4. *Plan to meet your needs.* One is the habit or the action, and the other is the addiction. One option for quitting is to first break the tobacco habit, then tackle the addiction. If you have identified why you smoke and what need it is meeting, develop a plan to match that need. If you require a five-minute break every hour, then take one without lighting up. If you like the hand-mouth movement, then switch to drinking tea, or chew gum with a harmless sweetener such as xylitol. Be prepared for this step. If you don't have a plan, you might be tempted to substitute food for cigarettes—particularly handfuls of junk food—and gain weight.

5. *Ask your physician if you are a good candidate for nicotine replacement.* Cigarette manufacturers have altered tobacco processing to make it easier to inhale and thus to absorb higher amounts of nicotine. In addition, they have

modified tobacco plants to increase nicotine content. The overall effect is to make tobacco more addictive today than it was fifty years ago. Likely, if you use more than half a pack of cigarettes per day (or the equivalent in other forms of tobacco), then you'll have to break a nicotine addiction. If your physician thinks nicotine replacement is a good idea for you, then the general rule is to use 1 mg of nicotine patch for every cigarette you use daily. If you smoke a pack a day (20 cigarettes), that means you need a 20 mg patch per day. (Conveniently, patches commonly come in 21 mg, 14 mg, and 7 mg daily patches.) For a pack-a-day smoker, start with a 21 mg patch daily for 2 weeks, then 14 mg daily for 2 weeks, and then 7 mg daily for two weeks. By six weeks, you will have found other ways to meet your needs and it will be much easier to break the nicotine addiction. When you do stop, celebrate, do something really fun, and thank the people who helped you succeed.

6. *To prevent weight gain, add an exercise routine.* People often gain weight when they quit smoking, typically ten to twenty pounds. Before you balk at the health implications, studies show that you would have to gain eighty pounds to do as much damage to your body as smoking a pack a day does. Exercise revs your metabolism and burns calories. It also reduces stress, which can trigger the urge to smoke. Following the Better Brain Solution eating plan will help you avoid gaining weight.

If you happen to restart the tobacco habit, just schedule another quit date, and repeat the steps above. Don't waste time feeling guilty. In some ways, it is like riding a bicycle—it's normal to fall several times before you get the hang of it. Just get back on and do it again. Research shows that the more times you try to stop, the more likely you will be to succeed in the end.

2. Excessive Alcohol

As we have seen, having one or two daily servings of alcohol, especially red wine, is good for your brain. (One serving is 4.5 ounces of wine, 12 ounces of beer, or 1.5 ounces of liquor.) But excessive amounts are not good for your health or that of your family, co-workers, or loved ones. If you can't keep your alcohol intake moderate, then don't use it at all.

Excess alcohol turns into sugar and promotes both weight gain and insulin resistance, which will damage your cognitive function; it basically pickles your liver, heart, brain, and tissues. Although wine has the least risk, alcohol also increases cancer risk, especially if you exceed three servings per day.

Toxins naturally build up in your bloodstream, such as extra chemicals in the food chain, excess nutrients, and even the naturally occurring by-products of food breakdown. Like clockwork, your liver provides the lifesaving "cleaning service" of eliminating these toxins. Alcohol, once it's in your bloodstream, acts like a VIP, jumping to the head of the liver detox line and blocking the removal of toxins. When you consume alcohol, your liver stops its everyday detoxing process until all the alcohol has been processed. In the meantime, other toxin levels build up, often to dangerous levels.

Because of excess alcohol's toxic impact on the brain, as well as the other damage it can do to mind and body, it's bad enough even a few days per week. It is especially harmful if it is happening every day.

Better Brain Action Step:
If You Drink Alcohol, Pay Attention to How Much
You Are Actually Drinking. Don't Consume More
than Two to Three Servings per Day.

3. Nitrosamines

Nitrosamines are preservative chemicals used in the production of most processed meats—such as sandwich meats, hot dogs, sausages, pepperoni, ham, and bacon—to extend their shelf life. Not only are they associated with greater risk for cancer and overall death, but studies performed on rodents show they are brain toxins.

Dr. Suzanne de la Monte, professor of pathology and laboratory medicine at Brown University, has shown that administering nitrosamines to rodents not only causes insulin resistance, diabetes, and fatty liver but leads to neurodegenerative injury and Alzheimer's disease. When she and her colleagues injected a nitrosamine-related compound (streptozotocin) into mice, they immediately acquired insulin resistance and showed signs of brain injury.

Tobacco also contains brain-damaging nitrosamines (another reason to quit using it). Dr. de la Monte and her colleagues have demonstrated that the harm associated with tobacco goes beyond cancer. Emerging data indicate that nitrosamines found in tobacco products—cigarettes and their smoke, chewing tobacco, and e-cigarettes—have harmful effects on the brain. These findings help to account for the increased rates of neurodegeneration and insulin resistance among smokers.

Better Brain Action Steps to Avoid Nitrosamines

1. Check labels. Don't buy foods that contain nitrosamines. Names for nitrosamines include: nitrosamine, nitrite + an amine, and other nitro- compounds, as in NDMA (nitrosodimethylamine) or NDEA (N-nitrosodiethylamine).
2. If you purchase deli meats, bacon, ham, sausage, hot dogs, or other cured meats, it is especially important to read the label as well as the ingredients list to confirm you aren't getting this toxin. Look for items that are organic, pasture-raised, and nitrosamine (nitrate) free. Many brands, such as Applegate, now make organic, nitrate-free meat products.
3. Quit tobacco, including cigarettes, chewing and dipping tobacco, and e-cigarettes. If you don't smoke, be aware that passive smoking can expose you to nitrosamines.

Getting Brain Toxins Off Your Plate

The most effective ways to reduce your exposure to BPA and phthalates are straightforward, but because many common convenience foods are sold in packaging that contains these toxins, it may require some adjustments to how you shop, prepare, and store food.

- Avoid or limit consuming food and beverages stored in plastic or in BPA-lined cans and cardboard cartons or boxes (including water bottled in plastic). Store your food in glass, not plastic, containers.
- Don't microwave food in plastic containers. Heating plastic increases the leaching of phthalates into food. Use glass for microwaving.

Choosing a more carefully packaged product is worth the extra money you may pay and the extra time you may take.

Some toxins that impact insulin sensitivity and the risk for type 2 diabetes have been in the environment for decades, even though their manufacturing has declined dramatically. Examples include:

- DDT (dichlorodiphenyltrichloroethane, the infamous pesticide used in the United States until 1972)
- Dioxins (released from fuel combustion and other industrial processes)
- PCBs (polychlorinated biphenyls, a compound widely deployed in coolant fluids, copy paper, and electric fluids that winds up in water)

These compounds linger in our environment for decades, waiting to be consumed and to accumulate in our tissues. DDT, banned in the United States more than fifty years ago and worldwide in 1986, still finds its way into our food chain. In one study, a DDT residue known as DDE was four times higher in elderly patients with Alzheimer's than in a control group of healthy elderly individuals.

People are commonly exposed to DDT and other pesticides, dioxins, and PCBs by eating animal products, particularly fatty meats and fatty dairy. One way to lower your exposure to toxins that impact blood sugar is to choose wild, cage-free, organic-fed, pasture-raised, and grass-fed products. If you avoid animal products that come from large-scale commercial feedlots, you will greatly reduce your exposure to pesticides and other brain poisons. When this isn't realistic, avoid fatty meat and dairy. (When animals consume contaminated feed or water, toxins are stored in their fatty tissues.)

4. Mercury

Mercury is a common metal that has been used in manufacturing and in scientific and medical applications for hundreds of years. Unfortunately, mercury is also a well-established brain toxin.

Even in otherwise healthy people, elevated mercury levels are common. Over the course of fifteen years, I have measured the mercury levels of nearly every patient in my clinic, and my data show that a full 25 percent of them have elevated mercury levels. Measuring serum (the liquid in blood itself) is not an effective way to measure for mercury, and whole blood samples are required. Most labs consider a normal level to be less than 11 µg/L (micrograms per liter). More than 14 percent of my patients have levels that are above 15 µg/L. At levels higher than that, my patients exhibit a drop in complex information processing, and when levels exceed 20 µg/L, the drop in function becomes substantial.

The single most common cause of elevated mercury levels is eating too much big-mouth fish, such as tuna or swordfish. Over the last thirty years, mercury levels have increased globally from burning mercury-laden coal, with the result that ocean and lake mercury levels have dramatically increased. Mercury is in the plankton in tiny levels, far less than 0.1 parts per million. But as we rise up the food chain from plankton to tiny copepods, to shrimp, to small fish, to bigger fish, and finally to large-mouth fish, mercury levels accumulate exponentially.

Fish with high mercury levels would be tuna, grouper, snapper, sea bass, kingfish, tilefish, swordfish, and shark. The larger and older the fish, the higher its mercury level will be. Wild salmon are a fairly big fish, but they have small mouths and eat mostly shrimp and herring, which are low on the food chain. That helps explain why wild salmon have very low mercury levels.

In 2012 my colleagues and I analyzed my clinic database to study the relationship between fish intake, mercury levels, and cognitive function in four hundred patients. We noted a clear improvement in cognitive function when people ate more fish and consumed more omega-3 fats, up to the point that their mercury levels reached 15 µg/L (15 parts per million). Levels greater than 15 showed a continued drop in their ability to process complex information. And a level more than 20 displayed an even greater drop in function.

An individual's ability to remove mercury after consuming it varies with the liver's ability to detoxify it, so detoxification varies greatly from person to person. Within a family whose members eat the same food, mercury levels fluctuate significantly among them. For example, my wife seems able to eat big-mouth fish weekly, and her levels have never been more than 5 µg/L. I have to be more careful, and if I eat even a couple of big-mouth-fish servings per month, my levels will be 15–20 µg/L or higher.

Our study published in *Integrative Medicine* in 2012 found that among people who ate big-mouth fish at least three or four times per month, 30 percent had an elevated mercury level that could harm their cognitive performance (a level more than 15). If you are eating more than two servings of big-mouth fish per month, have your doctor check your whole blood mercury level. Your level may well be normal (less than 11), but if it is higher, stop eating so much big-mouth fish. If it is more than 20, talk to your doctor about treatment options, and/or visit my resource center at www.DrMasley.com/resources.

Jeffrey's Better Brain Story: Removing the Toxins

Jeffrey, a highly successful CEO for a local company, came to see me as a patient because he was concerned he was losing his memory. For the previous few months, he couldn't remember names of staff he had known for years, nor a seven-digit phone number for long enough to dial it. He felt exhausted, dragging himself through the day, and he had ringing in his ears. We gave him the standard Mini-Mental Status Examination, and his result was completely normal, but he missed four out of ten questions on our clinic's Brain Symptom Score questionnaire. His computerized cognitive testing was clearly abnormal, with decreased memory and low executive function scores. His history revealed that he had changed his diet six months earlier to get healthier. His brother had had a heart attack the year prior, so he decided to give up eating meat and was eating five to ten servings of seafood each week, in particular ahi tuna. His examination was normal, as were all the laboratory studies noted above, except that his mercury level was 44 µg/L, extremely high.

I asked Jeffrey to eliminate all big-mouth fish from his diet. The only seafood he was to eat would be wild salmon, sardines, wild sole, cod, or shellfish. Because his levels were so high and he had neurological symptoms, we also started him on an oral chelation regimen with DMSA and supplemented him with ingredients that would double his liver's detoxification of heavy metals. (For information on chelation therapy, see www.DrMasley.com/resources.) Three months later his memory was better, the ear ringing had stopped, and his mercury level had dropped from 44 to 18. At six months, his mercury level was 10. (As a reminder, less than 11 µg/L is the normal reference range for the laboratory we use.) His symptoms resolved, and his computerized cognitive function was back to normal. The good news is that his condition was identified and treated fairly quickly. In a different clinical setting, this could very easily have been missed, and he would have likely suffered permanent memory loss.

My general recommendations are that if you eat big-mouth fish more than three times per month, or if you have concerns about your memory function, check your mercury level.

What About Other Sources of Mercury?

Many patients ask me about amalgam dental fillings and mercury levels. Most dental amalgams are at least 50 percent mercury. Mercury amalgams release about 1 microgram of mercury every day. They typically account for a 2–5 point rise in blood mercury levels. As the half-life for mercury removal is about two months, it can take substantial time for your body to remove this added mercury load. If you need a new dental filling, avoid amalgam fillings and opt for porcelain instead. (Some dental insurance may not cover the difference in cost, as amalgam fillings are less expensive.)

If you already have some fillings with amalgam in your teeth, talk to your dentist about a plan to gradually exchange the mercury fillings for porcelain fillings. You'll need to ensure that the dentist uses proper dams and venting for this type of procedure, as removing amalgam fillings can inadvertently increase mercury levels in the short term. In the dental world, dentists using proper techniques to remove dental amalgams are called ecological dentists. However, if you are concerned about your risk for high mercury levels, keep in mind that big-mouth fish intake is likely a more pressing issue.

Rare cases of mercury exposure don't relate to big-mouth fish or dental amalgam. You might recall as a child breaking a thermometer and playing with the slippery, magical-looking "quicksilver"—highly dangerous and toxic liquid mercury. Today, if we break a mercury thermometer in a medical office, we might call in an occupational health agency to handle the cleanup because we are now acutely aware of how poisonous this metal is in any form.

Though we are far more careful these days about handling mercury, other sources of mercury exposure include wood preservatives; fungicide sprays for lawns, shrubs, and landscaping; batteries; lab and industrial equipment; cosmetics; mercury-containing vaccines (though you can get mercury-free vaccines); and industrial polluted waters, especially those associated with mining.

Better Brain Action Steps to Avoid Mercury Toxicity

1. Don't eat more than two or three servings per month of big-mouth fish (grouper, tuna, snapper, sea bass, kingfish, shark, tilefish, or swordfish). If you do eat this much big-mouth fish and hope to continue doing so, then ask your physician to measure your whole blood mercury level.

2. If you enjoy eating seafood, select wild salmon, sardines, sole, flounder, cod, tilapia, and shellfish.

3. Avoid amalgam dental fillings. If you have them, have an ecological dentist remove the oldest, most worn-out fillings first, a few at a time.

4. Don't be exposed to fungicide sprays used in landscaping.

5. If you work in industrial manufacturing or mining, be aware of mercury-related compounds.

5. Lead

In Flint, Michigan, local government officials chose to save money on water service and collect acidic water from a local polluted river. The acidity corroded the city's old, outdated lead pipes, leaching lead into the local drinking water. People who consumed and bathed in the water became ill, developing digestive issues, skin conditions, hair loss, fatigue, and brain fog. Particularly for babies and children who ingested the poisoned water, the potential health issues are catastrophic, as lead poisoning can cause irreversible damage to a still-growing brain.

This issue isn't limited to Flint, as public water in many areas of the country has elevated lead. Even in minute quantities, lead is a brain toxin, potentially causing permanent harm to children and adults. If you live in a house or work in an office that was built prior to 1978, lead paint may have been used, which can contaminate the structure. Lead pipes used through the 1960s are another source of common lead exposure.

I recommend lead testing for all children and even adults who live in a home or work in an office built before 1978, especially if you have any symptoms of cognitive dysfunction. Don't hesitate to ask your physician to check your lead level—it should be zero. Children with lead levels of less than 5 mcg/dL have lower IQ scores than children with zero lead. If testing reveals that you have measurable lead levels, talk to your doctor about chelation therapy options to remove it.

6. Copper

Copper is an essential trace mineral that at low levels is critical for healthy blood cell formation, immune function, and nerve and bone health. However, at high levels it is toxic, especially when present as inorganic copper, one of the two forms we might ingest. (The other is organic copper.) The recommended daily allowance for copper is 0.9 mg (900 mcg) daily.

Organic copper comes from food sources and from supplements that are bound to amino acids (protein bound). Rich food sources of organic copper include nuts, seeds, beans, mushrooms, and green leafy vegetables. Healthy blood levels of copper can easily be achieved by eating these foods regularly.

Inorganic sources of copper come from plumbing (such as copper pipes in your home) and inorganic copper salts that are commonly included in many cheap vitamin supplements.

Only recently has copper emerged as a risk factor for Alzheimer's, and the data are startling. In animal studies, giving mice inorganic copper supplements (also called copper-2 or divalent copper), compared to giving a placebo, caused increased beta-amyloid production in the brain, plus an elevated rate of Alzheimer's disease. If you recall, beta-amyloid is the sticky protein that overaccumulates in the brains of those with Alzheimer's disease.

Researcher and physician George Brewer, M.D., MACN, has studied the relationship between inorganic copper intake and the dramatic recent increase in Alzheimer's rates. He draws a very strong relationship between copper pipes used in home plumbing and the rapid rise in Alzheimer's rates in the United States. His data demonstrate a correlation between levels of copper in public water supplies and Alzheimer's disease. Copper levels should be less than 0.01 parts per million, but Dr. Brewer's data suggests that two-thirds of all homes have copper levels in water that exceed this level.

In the past fifty years, Alzheimer's rates began to climb rapidly, perhaps not so coincidentally as Americans were first being exposed to inorganic copper. The use of copper piping in U.S. home construction was in full swing in the early 1960s, when we began to see a significant rise in dementia. By 1970 copper was the typical material of choice for water piping, and it is now estimated that more than 90 percent of all homes built after 1970 have copper pipes. Water with pH levels below 6.5 can corrode copper pipes. This breakdown of the pipes dramatically increases the level of copper in water. (Ironically, in an effort to ensure a safer water supply, many homeowners retrofitted their older, pre-1970s homes with copper piping to replace potentially corrosive lead.)

Humans evolved to metabolize organic forms of copper, and it is an essential food nutrient. However, inorganic copper is something brand new in our environment, and humans appear to be ill-equipped to metabolize it. Although inorganic copper has not conclusively been shown to cause Alzheimer's disease, the evidence is growing, and there is now ample reason for you to take some simple steps to avoid inorganic copper exposure.

Better Brain Action Steps to Avoid Inorganic Copper

1. Choose supplements with no copper ingredients or organic copper ingredients.

    Examples of organic copper ingredients are:

    - Copper glycinate
    - Copper bisglycinate
    - Copper amino acid chelates

    Examples of inorganic copper ingredients, which you should avoid, are:

    - Copper oxide
    - Copper sulfate (commonly used as a pesticide, but also very common in poor-quality supplements)
    - Copper carbonate

2. If you have copper plumbing in your home, get a reverse-osmosis filter to remove it from the water you use for

drinking and cooking. A reverse-osmosis filter is an easy way to achieve safe, dependable drinking water for your household. It will also remove chlorine, lead, fluoride, and other impurities. To be practical, don't fret over the whole house. Concentrate on the kitchen sink, your source of water for drinking, cooking, and food preparation.

3. Don't cook with copper-lined pots and pans. Copper cookware is popular because it is a superior heat conductor, but at the same time, heated copper can leach into foods it comes into contact with, especially acidic foods (such as tomato sauce). Copper cookware exteriors and bottoms are acceptable, but make sure pot and pan interiors are copper-free.

4. Get organic copper, which your body can process and use, from food. Eat more nuts, seeds, dark chocolate, mushrooms, and green leafy vegetables daily.

7. Pesticides

For years, studies have shown an association between pesticide exposure and an increased risk for dementia. As with tobacco and other carcinogens, pesticides' link to cancer is alarming enough—but research continues to prove that they are also extremely damaging to the brain.

In a study of 989 men and women at least seventy or older, scientists measured concentrations of blood pesticide levels and monitored those same subjects for ten years. Compared to those with low pesticide levels, those with the highest blood levels were 350 percent more likely to develop dementia. And a study in Taiwan found that even a single acute incident of poisoning with pesticides would double a person's lifetime risk for dementia.

Because of their prevalence in agriculture and manufacturing, it's impossible to totally eliminate pesticides—they are everywhere, including in our air and water. Yet you can significantly lower your exposure. The biggest source of pesticides isn't fruits and vegetables that have been sprayed with these toxins, but rather meat, poultry, and dairy products from animals that eat and drink pesticide-contaminated food and water. Estimates vary, but up to 80 percent of pesticide intake in

America comes from animal products, with fruits and vegetables providing only 10 percent. This is why it is so important to buy organically raised poultry, meat, and dairy.

Better Brain Action Steps to Avoid Pesticides

1. If you eat meat, poultry, dairy, or any other animal products, always choose organic. Pesticide residues accumulate in and are passed on through animal fat, so if you cannot access organic dairy such as milk or yogurt, choose nonfat varieties.

2. For produce, be aware that certain types are more heavily sprayed than others, such as strawberries, cherries, apples, celery, cucumbers, and bell peppers. Some foods, such as onions and avocados, are seldom or lightly treated with pesticides. The Environmental Working Group provides "Clean Fifteen" and "Dirty Dozen" produce lists, updated annually. For the latest ones, visit their website at www .ewg.org.

Do You Need to Detox?

If reviewing these common brain toxins has you concerned about your exposure, and you are thinking you need to both detox and avoid future exposures, here are some tips to get you started. Even if you don't think you are at high risk, everyone would likely benefit from a four-to-seven-day detox once or twice per year to help remove and process toxins we have stored over time.

Certain foods and supplements increase your ability to remove heavy metals and other compounds. Cruciferous vegetables (broccoli, cauliflower, Brussels sprouts, kale, bok choy, and cabbage) are high on the list, as they contain sulfuranes, which help your liver remove toxins from your system. To boost your detox power over the long term, aim to eat at least one cup of cruciferous vegetables daily. You'll notice that these vegetables are featured often in my recipes (see Chapter 10). For an even bigger dose of sulfuranes, consider broccoli sprouts, the greatest source of these detoxification compounds. During a brief detox, enjoy two cups of cruciferous vegetables every day.

Garlic, shallots, and onions are another source of potent detoxifying foods. They are loaded with sulfur, which helps you rid the body of toxins. Garlic in particular has been used for thousands of years to detox and improve health. To benefit, don't use deodorized garlic, as the garlic fragrance has the active agents. And avoid overcooking garlic, since it turns bitter when overcooked and loses its detoxification activity—best is to add it during the last one or two minutes of cooking on low heat. Onions and shallots retain much of their nutrient content with cooking, so you can use them any way you choose. Your goal should be to consume at least a quarter of a medium onion and/or one garlic clove daily. During a brief detox, I recommend two garlic cloves daily; try dicing raw garlic and adding it to a salad or side of vegetables, with a balsamic vinaigrette dressing.

During a four-to-seven-day detox, you should add these foods, but there are also some healthy foods that you should avoid. Nightshade plants can slow down some key aspects of liver detoxification: these include potatoes, tomatoes, eggplant, and peppers, including cayenne pepper. On a daily basis, you don't have to avoid nightshade plants, unless you have a specific intolerance to them, but during a detox, shun them.

Beyond foods, a partial intermittent fast will also help you detox. Fasting for fifteen hours generates ketones and shifts you to fat burning. (See the full discussion of partial intermittent fasting in Chapter 4.) When you burn fat, you release toxins stored in your fat tissue. During a brief detox, fast for fifteen hours each day. If you want to make that fast easier, you may drink organic coffee with organic ghee and MCT oil to start your day. (You may have coffee during a detox if it is organic.)

Avoid all alcohol during a detox. Recall that all forms of alcohol block liver detoxification. The last thing you want during a detox, when you are releasing toxins from your fat stores to your bloodstream, is to delay your ability to eliminate them.

Some supplements are excellent additions to a detox; take them during the detox and for at least one week afterward to help clear away any lingering toxins in your system. Curcumin has many health benefits, especially for the brain (see Chapter 5), and it also helps the liver remove toxins. To support your detox process, take a curcumin supplement with 1000 mg daily. Glucomannan (konjac root) is another supplement that is very helpful during a detox. It pulls toxins out of your system, acting like a sponge. (A commercial version of glucomannan is sold as PGX.) Not only does glucomannan help to eliminate poisons, but as a very viscous form of fiber, it also improves blood sugar control and enhances cholesterol profiles nicely. Ask your physician about taking 3 grams of glucomannan one to three times per day. If you can't find glucomannan, all forms of fiber are helpful to remove toxins.

Beyond food and supplements, sweating is another way to help remove toxins. Aim to sweat during a workout every day. And for added benefit, try sweating in a sauna or steam bath one to two times per week. Humans have used sweat lodges for tens of thousands of years to improve many aspects of health. It remains a great tradition. During a four-to-seven-day detox, schedule time for a sauna or steam bath, or enjoy a steamy hot bath.

During a detox, keep in mind that you are pulling toxins from bone and fat and eliminating them. Many people experience some short-term symptoms while they are eliminating toxins, as toxins are circulating in the bloodstream as they are removed. Common symptoms during a detox can include skin rashes, smelly stools and urine, congestion, headaches, and muscle aches. Despite these short-term issues, the benefits of removing toxins outweighs these discomforts. If your symptoms are severe, you might be more sensitive, or you might suffer from a heavier toxin load. If this applies to you, stop the detox, and talk to your doctor for guidance.

Avoiding brain toxins isn't easy, but if you are vigilant, you can significantly minimize your exposure to the most common toxins that can injure your brain. By doing so, you will protect your cognitive function and your overall health. Now let's shift toward creating a happier and better brain for the rest of your life.

CHAPTER 9

A Better (Happier) Brain for Life

The Better Brain Solution is designed to help prevent memory loss, protect brain health, and build and maintain mental sharpness for years to come. Still, particularly as we age, a handful of factors beyond those already discussed can impact cognitive performance as well as emotional well-being—and those two functions are intimately connected.

Some of these are normal changes that every healthy person will eventually experience. For instance, women and men both will have hormonal fluctuations across their lifetimes capable of impacting cognitive function. Other conditions and circumstances that can influence brain health, such as depression or social isolation, are not inevitable consequences of growing older.

Looking ahead, it is beneficial to understand precisely how factors as varied as these influence brain health and overall health. There are some aspects of aging we can't control, but the Better Brain Solution offers a pathway to lessen their negative impact, and inspiration to make choices that will keep us not just physically strong but intellectually engaged, emotionally connected, and happy.

Hormonal Changes and the Brain

Dressed alike, in shorts and with similar hairstyles, little girls and boys can be hard to tell apart. But eventually puberty transforms them into young women and men, with physical differences that are startlingly apparent. But then, as the decades pass and menopause or andropause sets in, once again the two genders start to look more alike than different. At an advanced age, dressed alike with the same hairstyles, it may once again be hard to tell females and males apart. After all, we have the same hormones; it is the balance of hormones that makes the genders different.

After puberty, boys clearly have more testosterone, while girls have more estrogen and progesterone. But as we age, these vast differences in hormone levels naturally diminish. Following menopause, women's estrogen and progesterone levels drop substantially; men, after andropause, experience a steady decline in testosterone levels.

Just as puberty is a time of dramatic change and sometimes frustration for boys and girls, menopause and andropause can challenge women and men and impact their quality of life, their ability to think sharply and clearly, their sleep, and their risk for depression and anxiety. Still, there are ways to manage these changes and, at the same time, protect brain function.

Menopause

Menopause is a normal stage in a woman's life: the cessation of menstruation. The diagnosis is usually made retrospectively after a woman has missed menses for twelve consecutive months and when the ovaries no longer release an egg each month. The average age for menopause is fifty-one, but it may occur anytime between forty and sixty. Symptoms vary greatly and may include insomnia, hot flashes, night sweats, decreased libido, and vaginal dryness. Cognitive dysfunction—or brain fog—is also a common symptom. One-third of women have minimal short-term issues, one-third have moderate symptoms that last one or two years, and up to one-third may have more severe symptoms that may last up to twenty years.

Perimenopause typically begins two or three years before menopause, as the ovaries produce less estrogen and progesterone, and cycles become more irregular as the ovaries fail to release an egg each month. Many menopause symptoms can occur with perimenopause, especially night sweats and hot flashes.

My own patients report that cognitive dysfunction and insomnia are the most disruptive menopause-related symptoms, as these have the biggest impact on the ability to function in a work setting day after day.

(Workday aside, living with these issues on a personal level is also difficult.) Insomnia—which can intensify the feelings of brain fog—can be made worse by night sweats (nighttime hot flashes). Because some of these symptoms are interdependent, successfully addressing one or two may have a positive domino effect on the others. Stop the night sweats, for example, and insomnia may improve. Get a good night's sleep, and the brain fog may go away.

Several lifestyle changes have been shown to alleviate menopause symptoms. Although they are not as powerful as hormone replacement therapy (HRT, such as estrogen, progesterone, and testosterone therapies), each can reduce menopause symptoms by 20 to 30 percent.

- For a woman who doesn't exercise, adding 30 minutes of aerobic activity four or five days per week, or yoga for one hour each day, will decrease menopause symptoms by 20 to 30 percent.
- Eating one or two servings of soy foods per day will decrease menopause symptoms by 25 percent, plus help to decrease breast cancer risk and improve bone density. (Choose organic soy products only.) However, up to 15 percent of people may be soy intolerant—if you don't tolerate soy, then avoid it.

If you are following the Better Brain Solution, then regular physical activity and eating foods containing soy (such as edamame) or fermented soy (found in natto, miso, and tempeh) may already be part of your plan. For those who have yet to reach perimenopause or menopause, the Better Brain Solution is an excellent way to reduce your risk of symptoms.

If you have significant menopause symptoms, in particular cognitive dysfunction, then you should speak to your physician about the benefits and risks of bioidentical hormone replacement options—specifically topical estradiol (commonly in patch, cream, or gel form), oral progesterone, and topical testosterone. (Bioidentical hormones have the exact same molecular structure as naturally occurring hormones produced by our bodies.) Though lifestyle changes can help reduce symptoms, hormone replacement therapy is still the most effective treatment.

Can Hormone Replacement Therapy Impact the Heart-Brain Connection?

Because brain and heart health are closely linked, it is important to note that estrogen therapy—a form of traditional hormone replacement therapy (HRT)—has been linked to heart disease. It has many benefits, but because of its potential cardiovascular risks, it is critical to get a personalized recommendation for it from your own physician.

In the 1980s and '90s, women were regularly advised to begin estrogen therapy once they reached menopause because it offered protective benefits to the heart. However, results from the Heart and Estrogen/Progestin Replacement Study (HERS) and the Women's Health Initiative showed otherwise. The data, published in the late 1990s, revealed that estrogen therapy seemed to be doing more harm to women's hearts than good, particularly for women who had been in menopause for more than ten years. And though HRT was highly effective in addressing a broad spectrum of menopause symptoms, the conclusion among experts was that the cardiovascular risks outweighed the benefits. Women were advised to stop estrogen therapy.

In the years that followed, researchers discovered that the *timing* of HRT was crucial, as were *the types of hormones* involved. Once again, the pros and cons of estrogen therapy are being re-evaluated by doctors and patients alike.

Here are the three things to keep in mind regarding HRT:

1. **Timing is critical.** Two studies have shown that during the first six to ten years of menopause, taking estrogen can lower your risk for heart attack or stroke. This is especially true if you use bioidentical hormones (see page 219). However, when you reach the ten-to-twelve-year window, estrogen can make your heart risk climb. If you continue therapy beyond this point, the increased risk must be weighed against other benefits you may be getting.

2. **The type of progesterone used is critical.** Typically, progesterone is taken along with estrogen. But what many women—and their doctors, unfortunately—don't realize is that the type of progesterone used is critical for how well a woman does on the therapy, no matter her age, and it can have heart health implications, as well.

   Medroxyprogesterone (MPA) is a synthetic form of progesterone *that should be avoided,* as it increases the risk of heart disease, memory loss, and breast cancer. Despite its dangers, it is still on the market and in use. Make sure you know which form of progesterone your doctor has prescribed.

   Beyond MPA, there are progestins, a class of pseudoprogesterone drugs. Since drug companies are unable to patent natural bioidentical progesterone, they tinker with it at the structural level to create "unique" compounds they can patent. Unfortunately, when you compare some of these near-clones to natural progesterone, the risk of side effects—including heart problems—goes up.

   I recommend *micronized bioidentical progesterone,* which has minimal adverse effects. If you are taking progesterone, talk to your doctor about switching to this form. Ask for oral rather than topical for the most reliable absorption.

3. **Bioidentical topical estrogen is best.** When it comes to estrogen, again I recommend bioidentical forms. Estradiol is the most popular, but *choose topical forms instead of oral.* (Traditionally, it has been taken in pill form.) According to one study, oral estradiol increased inflammation levels by 192 percent and blood clot risk by 400 percent when compared to topical estrogen. (Increased inflammation, as measured through hs-CRP levels, is a telltale marker of metabolic syndrome.) Because the pill form is so common, many doctors are not aware that the FDA has approved several topical estrogens—I recommend a patch, a gel, or a cream.

Ultimately, the choice of whether to embark on HRT is up to you and your doctor, but if you do so, there are clearly some decisions you can make to lower your cardiovascular risk and, by extension, protect your brain as well.

Andropause (Male Menopause)

After age forty, men experience a decrease in testosterone every year. A twenty-year-old male likely has a testosterone level of 1,100 ng/dL. Thirty years later testosterone levels for a normal fifty-year-old may vary from 300 to 800 ng/dL, with 500 being the average. Some men develop symptoms of low testosterone when their level drops below 400, and most men have symptoms if they fall below 300 ng/dL. Nearly 20 percent of men in their fifties have low levels, and these rates will worsen over time.

The signs of low testosterone vary and may include low energy, decreased drive (exercise, work, and libido), decreased mental sharpness, decreased sexual function (including erectile dysfunction), and difficulty with weight control characterized by a loss in muscle mass and a gain in fat mass—especially around the waist. In addition to these symptoms, low testosterone levels can lead to a drop in bone density and an increased fracture risk, as well as an increased risk for heart attack and stroke.

The total testosterone level is only part of the story, as the level of free (active) testosterone also plays a role in symptoms. Because of this factor, some men have symptoms when their testosterone levels are below 400 or 500, while others have minimal symptoms even when their levels fall close to 300. A substantial portion of total testosterone can be bound (stuck) to protein and not be available to stimulate tissues, so the percentage that is free is as important as total testosterone.

The benefits of testosterone therapy for a man with low levels are numerous. Testosterone therapy appears to:

- Improve energy, drive, and sexual function
- Increase mental sharpness
- Improve bone density
- Impact body composition, adding more muscle and decreasing waistline body fat

Also important is that testosterone therapy appears to decrease the risks for heart attacks and strokes, as documented by a large study that followed 83,000 men over fourteen years at VA hospitals. This cardiovascular benefit ultimately provides major protection for brain function.

If you have symptoms of low testosterone, talk to your doctor about testing and treatment options. Lifestyle changes will improve testosterone levels, but not nearly as effectively as hormone therapy. Still, men can increase their testosterone levels and decrease their low-testosterone symptoms by making the following changes, all of which are consistent with the recommendations in the Better Brain Solution:

- *Get enough sleep.* Most testosterone is made during the sleep cycle. If you are sleep deprived, you will experience a drop in testosterone production, too.
- *Lose body fat.* Fat cells convert testosterone to estrogen. Lose ten to twenty pounds, and you will see an increase in testosterone levels.
- *Eat more healthy fat.* Enjoy fat from avocados, nuts, olive oil, and seafood. Testosterone is made from fat, and people on low-fat diets have a drop in testosterone levels.
- *Get enough zinc.* Men who are zinc-deficient experience a drop in testosterone production; the body needs adequate zinc to generate testosterone. Good sources are oysters, dark chocolate, and a quality multivitamin. (Men with normal zinc intake will not make more testosterone by adding more zinc.)

In addition, aim to increase free testosterone. If testosterone is bound (stuck) to protein, it isn't free to stimulate testosterone receptors and activate testosterone activity.

- *Get enough vitamin D.* You need at least 1,500 to 2,000 IU daily. Adequate vitamin D lowers sex-hormone-binding globulin, which binds to testosterone.
- *Avoid eating sugar and refined carbs.* Avoid any source of flour or sugar, for that matter. A jump in blood sugar levels increases blood stickiness, binding testosterone to protein.

- *Do interval or burst exercise training.* Intense exercise increases free testosterone levels by releasing testosterone that is stuck to proteins.
- *Do strength training to build muscle mass.* Building mass increases free testosterone levels.

To unblock testosterone receptors:

- *Eat hormone-free dairy, poultry, and meats.* Estrogens block testosterone receptors, decreasing testosterone activity. Avoid consuming dietary hormones by choosing organic, free-range, or grass-fed animal protein.
- *Avoid plastic.* Avoid cooking and storing food in plastic. It contains estrogen-like compounds that block testosterone receptors.
- *Minimize drinking out of plastic bottles.* Soft plastic bottles release plastic compounds (estrogen-like molecules) into the liquid.
- *Avoid cans and containers lined with BPA.* It's toxic.

If you're following the Better Brain Solution, you're already doing many of these testosterone-boosting actions to improve and protect your brain. Now you have extra motivation to make these critical lifestyle changes.

Mood and Memory: How Depression Affects the Brain

The combination of chronic and high levels of stress, limited physical activity, and a diet low in essential nutrients is a perfect storm for causing depressed brain function, which leads to clinical depression. Because so many people, particularly those under stress, rush through their days with poor self-care habits, it is not surprising that depression is one of the most common medical problems that primary care physicians encounter on a daily basis. In addition to its paralyzing effects on emotional well-being, depression can take a serious toll on overall health, including everyday and long-term brain function.

Many of my patients confuse depression with bereavement. Bereavement is grieving appropriately over a loss, such as the death of a family member or dear friend, a divorce or the demise of a close relationship, or a dramatic life upheaval such as the ending of a career (be it unexpected or planned for) or moving out of a beloved home.

Such losses are painful, each in its own way, and we may grieve and shed tears. Bereavement is a normal coping mechanism and helps us to mourn our loss and deal with our pain. It doesn't always lead to depression, although up to half of people with a major loss may eventually fall into a clinical depression. With bereavement, typically a person has good times and bad times. They may have fun and laugh when something funny occurs, yet moments later be moved to tears when they remember their loss. Normally, bereavement gradually lessens over time, though it may be intense for at least three to six months. Gradually, the sadness begins to lift, with progressively more good times and fewer moments of grief. Still—and this is to be expected—it's natural for us to feel some pain from a significant loss for the rest of our lives.

Depression, however, is different. It may easily be triggered by the types of losses mentioned above, such as death, divorce, or the end of a significant era in one's life. But for my patients, I describe depression as a lingering state of depressed brain function. It impacts our physiological function, not just our mood, and it doesn't "get better" the way bereavement eventually loosens its grasp.

People suffering from true depression have abnormal sleep patterns (they sleep all the time or can't get to sleep), low energy, poor concentration and memory, and increased aches and pains, and they may simply feel like they can't move past their sadness. One of the most important signs of a real depression is anhedonia, the inability to find pleasure. A person with depression will seem functional in terms of completing daily tasks—the bills get paid, the dog gets walked—but they don't seem to enjoy anything the way they did in the past. There is a marked drop in drive as well—libido, exercise, work, and more.

With a real clinical depression, the brain lacks the neurotransmitters and nutrients needed for normal functioning, and there are no longer good days and bad days—just these enduring symptoms of depressed brain function. Still, it is possible to reverse and recover from depression. As people age, some may think depression is a normal state of mind, an inevitable passage everyone goes through. While some times of sadness are, in fact, normal (at any age), periods of unrelenting clinical depression are not. Depression is not a given as we age; nor should we accept it as inevitable, especially because of its link to dementia. There are steps we can take to prevent cognitive decline and clinical depression, but before addressing these actions, let's first clarify how depression and memory loss are intertwined.

Breaking the Chain of Depression and Memory Loss

Depression doesn't impact only your quality of life; it also increases your risk for Alzheimer's disease. Women with a history of depression have a 300 percent greater risk of suffering from dementia in the future. Men have a 400 percent greater risk.

However, clarifying how much dementia risk is associated with depression is complicated. Many of the same nutrient deficiencies that increase your risk for memory loss, such as low levels of vitamin B12 and mixed folates, also increase your risk for depression. High levels of unmanaged stress and low levels of activity and fitness also increase your risk for both depression and memory loss. Prolonged, unmanaged stress increases your risk for brain shrinkage and memory loss, in part because of high levels of cortisol, the stress hormone. Over time, stress depletes nutrients and brain chemicals that are essential for proper brain function. Deplete these neurotransmitters over time, and you will experience physical signs of depression (such as poor sleep; decreased concentration, drive, and energy; and anhedonia).

Another factor that makes this cause-and-effect picture complex is that depression is often a *symptom* of early memory loss. After all, early on you may not admit that you are losing your memory to your family, friends, and co-workers. But if you are losing your memory, you likely know it, and that is in itself depressing.

What about medication? Can it address the variety of factors that contribute to depression? Unfortunately, one myth about depression is that medications are highly effective treatments—but they are not a sure bet. While drug therapies do have some modest effect for those with diagnosed depression, they have fewer benefits than most people realize, especially over the long term. Antidepressants are even less effective in people who are inactive and have poor nutritional intake.

The good news is that the same lifestyle choices that improve brain function and prevent future memory loss also help prevent and reverse depression. In my medical training, I was taught to offer people antidepressants when they showed symptoms of depression, but I was never impressed with their improvement from drug therapy alone.

For several years now, I have been offering a thirty-day version of my Better Brain Solution not only to prevent and reverse memory loss and heart disease but also to treat depression. The improvements I've observed have been amazing. When I follow up at the thirty-day mark with patients who suffered from depression, the vast majority who followed these recommendations saw their depression symptoms melt away, and if they didn't improve, we still had the option of adding a medication.

As with addressing memory loss, the answer lies not in one approach but in a combination of approaches. Here are the recommendations I make for my patients with depression. You will notice that they are similar to the recommendations I make to improve cognitive function.

Nutrition (Don't Forget the Good Fats)

Nutrient deficiencies increase your risk of drifting from bereavement to depression, and from feeling chronically stressed to being clinically depressed. High on the list are long-chain omega-3 fats, vitamin B12, mixed forms of active folates, smart fats, and magnesium. Antidepressant medications won't work as well if you don't address these key nutrient needs; nor will your brain function well. (Note: The suggested types and amounts of nutrients here are consistent with the Better Brain supplement recommendations in Chapter 5.)

B vitamins are the primary tools for the body to create mood-lifting biochemicals. The full spectrum of B vitamins should be found in a good-quality multivitamin, but vitamin B12 and mixed folates (not just folic acid) are especially important. A longitudinal study at Rush University showed that higher levels of B6 (pyridoxine), B9 (folate), and B12 (methylcobalamin) were related to a decreased rate of depression over time, for at least twelve years of follow-up. I recommend mixed, active forms of folate, such as 400–800 mcg of 5-methylenetetrahydrofolate (5-MTHF), and at least an extra 100–500 mcg daily of vitamin B12 (preferably methylcobalamin) to ensure adequate blood levels.

The brain is made up of at least 60 percent fat by weight, and low-fat diets—particularly those lacking in nutritious smart fats—are associated with depression. Your brain needs **long-chain omega-3 fats.** Ensure that you get at least two servings of wild salmon or sardines per week, or 1,000 mg of EPA and DHA daily. Other beneficial fats are also important for balanced brain chemistry, so don't hesitate to eat more **smart fats,** including avocado, nuts, olive oil, and dark chocolate every day.

Minerals (found in a quality multivitamin) such as **zinc, iodine,** and **selenium** will also help prevent depression. **Magnesium,** too big a molecule to fit into a multivitamin, requires a source of its own. Consume at least 400 mg of magnesium daily. Though you can get a good amount from food (see "Magnesium Content in Food," page 137), it is a challenge for most people to reach that goal. If necessary, supplement with extra magnesium (choose protein-bound magnesium glycinate over other forms).

Physical Activity: Good for the Heart, Great for the Mind

Exercise is beneficial for any brain, but it is particularly essential and effective for a depressed, sluggish brain. Exercise not only improves brain speed and performance, but it helps boost a sense of well-being (the well-documented "runner's high"), and it releases the stress and anxiety that exacerbate depression. You need not be a hard-training marathon runner to get the brain and mood benefits of a runner's high. I recommend thirty minutes of aerobic activity each day, especially for my patients with depression.

Sleep Quality: Rest Your Brain

Depression can wreck the sleep cycle, causing sufferers to sleep far beyond what is normal or triggering insomnia and interrupted sleep. Sleeping less than seven hours or more than eight hours is associated with an increased risk not only for memory loss and weight gain but for depression as well. If you have sleep issues, revisit the recommendations in Chapter 7. A rested, relaxed, and happy brain and a rested body are interdependent. Meditation in particular can be very helpful for depression sufferers with sleep issues because it can help the brain achieve a settled, rested state. Regular meditators report that one of the most immediate benefits of meditation is a dramatic improvement in sleep quality.

Fun: The Finishing Touch

Having fun is like having fireworks go off within your brain circuitry, restoring healthy brain function. My patients are always surprised when I create their plan to reverse depression and include a directive to schedule at least a couple of fun activities each week. Like exercise and adequate sleep, taking time out for yourself is a stress-buster that offers protection against depression, but it also puts joy back into your life. For people who are depressed, however, being encouraged to have fun can feel like a tall order. This is when gentle peer pressure can provide an assist. If you make it a point to schedule pleasurable activities with a partner, relative, or friend and get something on your calendar—coffee or lunch, a museum, the movies—you're more likely to get out the door and make fun happen.

Why Every "Old Brain" Should Learn New Tricks

The classic happy retirement goes something like this: you leave behind the rat race, settle into a comfortable chair, and relax for the rest of your days.

That, of course, is the worst thing anyone can do. Even if your retirement is still decades away, to stay physically and emotionally fit and protect against memory loss, you need to work your brain and body *more* as you age, not less.

Just like your muscles, your brain needs to be exercised to function optimally. If you don't use your biceps, they will shrink. Likewise, your brain, without appropriate challenge, will shrink as well. German researcher Ulman Lindenberger, an expert on brain aging, has shown that cognitive training exercises in older adults can decrease brain shrinkage over time and improve cognitive abilities. The brain, in other words, needs a regular workout to stay strong.

The key to protecting your brain and improving cognitive performance is continuous new learning. It creates ever-expanding neuropathways and builds cognitive reserve. Does that mean you need to sign up for a structured "brain training" program? Or is it enough to read more challenging material, work harder problems and puzzles, and finally take up piano or learn Italian? And later in life, is it even possible to "get smarter"?

Let's look at what works.

High-Tech Brain Training: Keep it Challenging

One of the debates in the scientific community is whether brain training can only make you quicker and sharper or if it can actually make you more intelligent. In recent years, the majority of studies suggest that brain training can improve IQ by several points, perhaps a 2 to 8 percent improvement. Some of the first scientists to publish in this field were a Swiss couple, Dr. Susanne Jaeggi and Dr. Martin Buschkuehl. They have consistently shown how ultra-challenging computer games can improve fluid intelligence, which is the ability to solve problems and identify relationships and patterns.

Still, as encouraging as their research has been—that training on a computer program for thirty minutes four or five days per week improves brain IQ—what is more impressive is that you can enhance your cognitive function by following the Better Brain Solution. In my research, the men and women who followed my plan did just that and had a 25 percent jump in brain sharpness, allowing them to accomplish more every day.

For those who are curious about structured brain-training programs, perhaps the best known is Luminosity, one of the largest companies featuring brain-challenging games that subscribers can access on their home computers. In 2013 it released data showing that its training programs helped its 40 million users increase cognitive function, and that the benefits persisted for several weeks, although younger adults showed greater benefits than older adults. Luminosity also noted findings very similar to my own: that those who got at least seven hours of sleep (compared to sleeping less than that or more than eight hours), and those who had one or two alcoholic drinks per day (but not more and not less) had the best testing scores. In addition, they noted that the single most important lifestyle factor impacting cognitive function scores was regular exercise.

Luminosity claimed—falsely, as it turns out—it had proof that playing computer games for ten to twenty minutes per day several days per week would delay memory decline; protect against dementia and Alzheimer's disease; and improve school, work, and athletic performance. However, it did not have the data to support these claims, even though it could show short-term improvements in cognitive testing for young adults. Eventually the Federal Trade Commission fined Luminosity $2 million for deceptive marketing practices, and the creators and marketers agreed to settle.

Another company that provides computerized cognitive training is BrainHQ (www.BrainHQ.com). Brain HQ has published a variety of studies showing that their training programs can enhance brain function over time with online exercises focused on attention, brain speed, people skills, and intelligence.

Even the prestigious Mayo Clinic now recommends cognitive training to prevent memory loss. It studied cognitive function in 487 healthy people older than sixty-five who "brain-trained" on computers for one hour per day, five days per week over eight weeks. The results showed a 21 percent improvement in memory. (Unlike Luminosity, the Mayo Clinic did not make sweeping promises regarding Alzheimer's disease prevention or better work/school/athletic performance.)

The U.S. government has also embarked on computerized brain-training games. In 2014 the Intelligence Advanced Research Projects Activity (IARPA, part of the network of government intelligence agencies), announced a $12 million program called Strengthening Human Adaptive Reasoning and Problem Solving, or SHARP training. The goal is to help elite troops in all branches of the armed forces increase their working memory and cognitive performance.

Clearly, cognitive training has some benefits, but the catch with many of these programs is that you need to be constantly challenged in order to improve, and over time it's hard to maintain that challenge. Yes, you might get better over eight to twelve weeks, but how do you keep getting better, and how do you maintain that improvement? Take playing bridge, as an example. A beginner struggles to grasp what cards to play and where they lie. During functional MRI scanning, the brain lights up with activity as the novice player struggles to play her or his hand. However, an expert bridge player dealt the same hand will likely figure out how to play the hand easily—just find the queen and jack of spades, and the work is done. On a functional MRI scan, the expert hardly seems to be thinking.

The key to improving brain function is to *keep learning*. If you can win the most difficult Sudoku game every day, congratulations—but then move up to something that gives you more of a challenge. The same can be said for crossword puzzles as well. (And perhaps you are also seeing the parallel to exercise; you cannot increase your level of fitness unless you challenge yourself to go harder.) If you do sign up for a brain-training program, remember that it is effective only if you can keep pushing beyond your level of mastery. And there are other ways to challenge your brain without paying for a monthly subscription to computer games.

Low-Tech Learning: The Pay-off (and pleasure) of Being a Late Bloomer

Adults who decide to take up a second language gain much more than the ability to communicate in a foreign country on their next vacation. Learning a new language has been shown to help prevent memory loss. But learning it and using it regularly, not just brushing up on something you know already, is the key.

Researchers have found that adults in bilingual households and those who learn a new language later in life—that is, they become fluent in it—can delay the onset of Alzheimer's disease by four to five years. The effect was greatest for people who used the second language often. Delaying the onset of Alzheimer's by five years will decrease 50 percent of all cases, as it commonly occurs at the end of life. That is a very powerful reason to recommend that everyone learn another language and use it.

If learning a second or third language is not appealing, consider music, which also challenges the brain in a stimulating way. In medical school, I decided to start playing classical flute. I practiced for thirty to forty-five minutes every day and had a lesson once per week. I saved my most challenging science studying for immediately after my music session, as the music study seemed to make me more alert and help me retain more information.

Plenty of research links music education to improved cognitive performance. In London, children in a program called the Bridge Project were randomized to participate in music classes to learn instruments and singing. The children studying music had 18 percent better grades in math and literacy than those in the control group who didn't study music. In Toronto, Glenn Schellenberg and his research team randomized 144 six-year-olds to a drama group, a control group, and to music groups, both voice and piano. Those in the music group had greater IQ scores compared to those in drama and the control.

Doing a craft or artistic activity, such as needlework, painting, or making music, also seems to offer some protective brain benefits if done in midlife and continued into later years. In one study, people who engaged in such activities, combined with social interaction, had about a 50 percent decreased risk of mild cognitive impairment when they reached their eighties. It seems that the activities themselves maintain and stimulate neural growth, particularly when the brain is pushed to do a bit more.

Whether it is a new language, a musical instrument, computer software, landscape architecture, a puzzle or game, oil painting, or whatever appeals, learning something new as an adult—and then, after you've mastered it at a basic level, moving ahead and challenging yourself to get better—is a rewarding and pleasurable way to prevent and delay memory decline.

Connection (because your brain can't go it alone)

The same technology that brings us together through social media also isolates us from one another. We text and e-mail instead of speak, we settle for posted photos of friends and loved ones rather than visit in person, and we transact business on the Internet instead of personally. On top of that, phases of our lives end and others begin, as children grow up and move on, and as careers shift and relationships change. As our circumstances change, we need to do more to stay connected—not just for our emotional satisfaction but also because our brains crave connection. The benefits of developing loving and supportive relationships, and maintaining them, can last throughout our lifetimes.

Loving and being loved by a spouse, a partner, a parent, a child or other relative, or a friend is good for our brains and our bodies, beginning on a biochemical level. Stress raises cortisol, but oxytocin (the bonding hormone) reduces it. Any activity that increases oxytocin (including intimacy and sex) is great for stress reduction. But you don't have to be sexual to enjoy the benefits of this hormone. Caressing touch, a twenty-second hug, cuddling the new grandchild, and playful interactions with your children will help release it, too.

Pets are also a reliable and loving source of comfort and connection and often become like family members or cherished friends. Humans have enjoyed the loyal companionship of domesticated animals for thousands of years, and there are good reasons why. Research shows that the act of grooming, petting, and caring for an animal is a boon to human health, both physical and emotional, lowering stress levels and decreasing feelings of loneliness. Animals in need of regular exercise, such as dogs and horses, also give us an excellent motivation to stay active and be in nature. If you love animals and don't have a pet, consider welcoming one into your life.

Beyond loving and supportive relationships, we also benefit from being connected to our community. When we share our positive energy with others, we feel bound and supported in achieving our goals. That is why being involved with a religious group (church, synagogue, temple, or mosque) or being actively engaged in a charity we believe in can be so powerful. Besides, we reap rewards that we never expected when we give of our time and energy. We forge meaningful relationships, assist those in need, and create opportunities that had never existed before, all of which can even help us feel good about ourselves. Indeed, research has shown that an individual who lives a generous, altruistic life can discover deeper relationships, happiness, health, and even longevity.

When you have high levels of stress in your life, spend time with loved ones and community projects you believe in. For the greatest benefit, share random acts of love and kindness generously with others without seeking anything in return.

Some of the most common barriers to developing loving and satisfying relationships are traumas from our past. Sometimes we are unaware of how a traumatic event that occurred during childhood or young adulthood is impacting us decades later. A mental health therapist, psychologist, or psychiatrist can be incredibly insightful in showing us how these past events can create stress-filled personal relationships today. Many of us have forgotten the triggers that make us feel anxious or afraid, but working through them can enhance intimacy and soothe relationships.

It is possible to feel lonely even if you are in a relationship, particularly if you have issues that you haven't yet dealt with. Researchers have found that loneliness can cause an increase in chronic inflammation, which has been linked to so many devastating conditions, including dementia. All the more reason to counteract it with connection.

It is never too late to take steps to protect your cognitive function and your overall health, and to enjoy the added bonus of becoming mentally sharper and more physically fit. That's precisely what will happen if you follow the Better Brain Solution. Simple lifestyle changes are at the heart of this plan, including preparing and enjoying easy, delicious, and nutrient-packed meals designed to offer an array of brain benefits. Invite your friends and family into the kitchen and connect over flavorful food that will nourish you and your loved ones in mind, body, and spirit.

In the next chapter are my favorite recipes, designed for you, specifically for your brain.

CHAPTER 10

Getting Started: Recipes to Nourish Your Brain

I t's completely realistic that you will improve cognitive function and prevent or delay memory loss through the four strategies that make up the Better Brain Solution. Getting started with an exercise plan, incorporating high-quality supplements as needed, and practicing stress management might involve some obvious purchases or tasks, such as buying comfortable workout clothing, locating an excellent source for vitamins, or finding a yoga class. For most people, however, the biggest shift in their thinking and actions will involve food.

Having read this book, you know what to eat for a better brain. This chapter is dedicated to showing you how to do just that. The fifty recipes I've created to get you started offer a satisfying and realistic variety of ideas for breakfasts, snacks, lunch, or dinner entrées, and even desserts. There are vegetarian options as well as those featuring poultry, seafood, and meat. I have included recipes for sauces, broths, and condiments to complete your dishes. And if you happen to be gluten sensitive, *all* these recipes are gluten-free.

Here is a list of the recipes that can be found starting on page 255.

Breakfasts

1. *Steven's Morning Shake*
2. *Coffee (or Tea) with Organic Ghee and MCT Oil (for partial fasting)*
3. *Eggs Benedict with Smoked Salmon and Spinach*
4. *Frittata with Artichoke Hearts, Sun-dried Tomatoes, and Spinach*

5. Coconut and Almond Pancakes
6. Yogurt Berry Bowl

Snacks

7. Guacamole
8. Salmon Spread with Sliced Cucumber and Capers
9. Chicken Wings with Buffalo Sauce
10. White Bean, Cauliflower, and Hazelnut Dip
11. Smoked Salmon Spread with Endive

Soups

12. Avocado and Asparagus Soup
13. Black Bean Soup
14. Miso Soup

Entrées

VEGETARIAN OPTIONS

15. Garbanzo, Tomato, and Okra Curry
16. Thai Coconut Curry Soup
17. Spinach and Shiitake Mushroom Soufflé
18. Spicy Tofu and Pineapple with Stir-fry Vegetables
19. Pecan Nut Loaf

SEAFOOD OPTIONS

20. Almond-coated Tilapia
21. Shrimp with Thai Curry Sauce
22. Shrimp Kebabs
23. Sautéed Teriyaki-Pineapple Salmon
24. Broiled Scallops with Pesto

POULTRY OPTIONS

25. Italian Turkey Meatloaf
26. Chicken, Mushroom, and Broccoli Sauté

27. *Roasted Cornish Game Hens with Mediterranean Herbs and Butternut Squash*
28. *Chicken Curry*
29. *Duck with Cherry Sauce*
30. *Chicken Marsala*
31. *Turkey Tenders with Middle Eastern Spices*

MEAT OPTIONS

32. *Roasted Lamb and Vegetables*
33. *Sirloin, Peppers, and Onion with Mixed Salad*
34. *Pork Chops with Italian Herbs and Mushrooms*

Side Dishes

35. *Mixed Salad*
36. *Kale with Red Bell Pepper and Garlic*
37. *Spinach, Beet, and Goat Cheese Salad*
38. *Broccoli with Lemon Sauce*
39. *Curried Garbanzo Beans with Spinach*
40. *Steamed Artichokes with Lemon Shallot Dip*
41. *Lentil Salad*
42. *Green Beans, Rosemary, and Vinaigrette Dressing*

Desserts

43. *Pear, Chocolate, and Nut Delight*
44. *Fruit Crumble*
45. *Chocolate Mousse*

Sauces/Broths/Dressings

46. *Pesto Sauce*
47. *Hollandaise Sauce*
48. *Mushroom Gravy*
49. *Vegetable Broth*
50. *Masley House Vinaigrette Dressing*

Before you head to the kitchen, the first step is to ensure you have foods that will nourish and support your brain and that you have eliminated the obvious things that harm it. For most people, that means a Kitchen and Pantry Makeover to make room for the brain-boosting 12 Smart Foods, along with other ingredients and supplies that will make cooking and meal preparation fun and easy.

Kitchen and Pantry Makeover

It's time to toss out what you don't need and what your brain doesn't want. Get a box or a trash bag and go through your kitchen, refrigerator, freezer, and pantry and get rid of the foods that will damage your brain. Donate items to a local food bank if throwing away food seems wasteful. If you keep these foods around, you'll likely end up eating them and denying yourself the incredible cognitive and physical benefits that come with following the Better Brain Solution. The following items should be removed:

Start with Cooking Oils and Bad Fats

- Any food item containing hydrogenated or partially hydrogenated oil (read the ingredients list for those terms)
- Any oil that is expired or in a plastic bottle
- Corn oil or canola oil (except organic, expeller-pressed canola oil in a glass bottle)
- Nonorganic butter

Next, Get Rid of Any High Glycemic Load Foods

- See page 108 for the list of such foods. Products containing sugar and corn syrup (not just the obvious like soda but even condiments like some barbecue sauces, bottled salad dressings with sugar, and ketchups)
- Chips, crackers, pretzels, cereals (except rolled or steel-cut oats) and granola bars, cookies, breads, and other flour products, which act like sugar in your system

- Any packaged or prepared food item containing unhealthy added sugars. (Tip: If you're concerned about hidden sugars, see page 85 for a list of common names for added sugar; scan the ingredient lists for those terms.)
- Sweeteners (sugar substitutes). If you see packs of Splenda, Nutrasweet, Equal, or Sweet & Low, toss them. Sweeteners that you may keep include stevia, erythritol, and xylitol. (But excess use of erythritol and xylitol can cause crampy loose stools, so don't overindulge.)

If you have some special honey or maple syrup that you will use sparingly, keep it if you wish. But are you and your loved ones reserving it for special occasions or consuming it regularly? If you end up eating it day after day and have trouble controlling your cravings for something sweet, having these even healthier items readily available will make craving control harder. If fighting the desire for a "sweet fix" is an issue in your household, you are better off removing the honey and maple syrup.

Don't Forget to Throw Out Foods with Nitrosamines (brain toxins)

- Deli meats, bacon, sausages, ham, and hot dogs contain nitrosamines. You have the choice to replace some of these foods, but only with nitrosamine-free options.

What About Gluten?

- Products made with wheat, rye, or barley. If you suspect you are gluten sensitive, as you have had chronic health issues, including problems with your gut, brain, thyroid, joints, or skin, or unexplained weight gain, this would be a great time to go gluten-free for a month and see if that transforms your symptoms and your life. In this case, get rid of these products.

If you don't have unexplained, chronic health problems, then simply focus on cutting out the foods noted, and adding the foods in the next section to support your brain.

Grocery Shopping Guide

Create a shopping list, featuring the 12 Smart Foods (see Chapter 3). (If it's helpful and keeps you organized, use an app to do this.) Start by listing brain-boosting items that you and your family already enjoy or that you already know how to prepare. Include ingredients for some of the recipes in this chapter. (Peek ahead and choose some that you might want to try right away.) Over time add more variety and flavor to your shopping list with new items you don't recognize or ordinarily prepare.

For the most up-to-date list of vegetables and fruits that should be purchased as organic, download the Environmental Working Group's free shopping app for the "Dirty Dozen" and the "Clean Fifteen," at https://www.ewg.org/foodnews/. Or simply skip these items.

Here are the dozen core foods to buy and keep on hand, so that you can enjoy them every day.

- Green leafy vegetables, e.g., broccoli, kale, spinach, Brussels sprouts, salad greens, Swiss chard, and collard greens. Select the ones you like and buy them fresh or frozen. Frozen varieties are typically far less expensive and won't go bad in your refrigerator. Items currently on the EWG's "Dirty Dozen" list that should be bought organic include spinach and lettuce.
- Other vegetables, e.g., beets, carrots, butternut squash, green beans, fennel, peppers of any color, tomatoes, celery, artichoke hearts, and artichokes. Items currently on the EWG's "Dirty Dozen" list that should be bought organic include bell peppers and celery.
- Omega-3 rich wild seafood, e.g., wild salmon filets, sole, trout, mussels, oysters, clams. No doubt about it—wild, fresh seafood is expensive. Far more economical and easy to find would be canned wild salmon and sardines. Canned wild salmon (especially pink salmon) can be used in place of nearly any canned tuna recipe and makes a great spread. Wild salmon vacuum-packed frozen filets are also less expensive than fresh wild salmon. After thawing, I typically

rinse with tap water and then marinate wild seafood in orange juice for five to ten minutes to minimize any fishy flavor.

- Olive oil and other healthy cooking oils. I suggest that you stock at least two or four varieties of oil in your pantry for salads and cooking. Extra virgin olive oil is a must for dressings and sauces. For cooking, pick from among avocado oil, almond oil, macadamia nut oil, virgin olive oil, and ghee (clarified butter). You can also use sesame and coconut oil, just not at medium-high or high heat. An important reminder: Be sure you cook the right oil at the right temperature or you risk making a healthy oil toxic (such as extra virgin olive oil or even more delicate coconut oil). For details on oil smoke points, see Chapter 3 and visit my website: www.DrMasley.com.

Is Avocado Oil Expensive?

Be aware that prices vary greatly. We buy a one-liter bottle for less than $10 at Costco (only 5 cents per tablespoon serving), yet some grocery stores sell high-quality organic avocado oil in 500-ml fancy bottles for $17.99, nearly four times the price. Keep in mind that per serving, even the most expensive avocado oil products only cost about 50 cents per meal, so even when buying expensive oil in small bottles at your local grocery store, buying avocado oil won't break your budget over the long term. Overall, avocados are very clean, so you don't have to pay extra for organic avocados or avocado oil. A terrific resource for buying high-quality staples, such as avocado oil, at a great price is Thrive Market (see the resource section on my www.DrMasley.com/Resources website for a link), as you can find food products for prices 30 to 50 percent lower than those listed at a typical grocery store.

- Nuts and other healthy fats. My favorite nuts are almonds, pecans, walnuts, pistachios, hazelnuts, and macadamias. Buy the ones you like the most. Nuts can be salted or unsalted, in a can or jar. Typically they are less expensive if you buy them in bulk. Just keep them sealed airtight, or store them in the freezer in a sealed jar to keep them fresh. Don't forget to buy avocados, and look for BPA-free canned coconut milk.
- Berries and cherries, e.g., blueberries, strawberries, raspberries, blackberries, and cherries. Items that should be bought organic include blueberries, strawberries, and cherries. Consider buying them either in bulk or frozen from warehouse stores, such as Costco, Walmart, and Sam's Club.
- Cocoa and dark chocolate. Dark chocolate should be at least 70 percent cocoa, and 74 to 80 percent is even better for you. Most of my patients don't like 80 to 90 percent chocolate as it is somewhat bitter; 74 percent seems to be the most popular. If a label says dark chocolate, but the first ingredient listed is sugar, put it back; it isn't really dark. Brands that are less than 70 percent typically say dark chocolate but don't reveal the percentage of cocoa butter. For the brain benefits from drinking cocoa, select unsweetened, unprocessed cocoa. (For maximum flavonoid content, look for the words *natural* or *non-alkalized* and avoid "Dutch process" varieties.)
- Red wine. More expensive wines aren't healthier, so choose what you enjoy and can afford. Enjoy one to two servings with a meal daily, not more than three. If you don't drink wine, ensure you benefit from eating other purple/red pigments such as pomegranate, watermelon, cherries, plums, and blueberries.
- Caffeine sources, e.g., green tea and coffee. If you avoid caffeine, decaf options are good for your brain. I recommend organic coffee and tea, as the industry uses excessive pesticides on commercial production. Loose tea leaves are better than those that come in a tea bag. If you

drink coffee, all options have brain benefits in moderation, so you don't need to buy a specific roast.

- Herbs and spices. There are literally hundreds to choose from, and buying all of them would be impractical. Here are the ones I use most often in recipes for a variety of cooking styles:

  Italian herb seasoning
  fines herbes
  thyme
  dill weed
  ground paprika
  ground cayenne pepper
  whole black pepper
  curry spice (in a blend)
  cinnamon
  cardamom
  sea salt
  fresh garlic
  ginger (fresh gingerroot)

  Ideally, you will grow some fresh herbs in your garden or on your windowsill, in particular parsley, cilantro, basil, mint, and rosemary; you can buy these herbs fresh, but the convenience and price savings are worth the effort to grow them—as is the simple pleasure of planting and harvesting them!

- Beans, e.g., any beans you like; garbanzos, black, red, lentils, cannellini, butter, pinto, etc. If you buy them in cans, look for cans that are BPA-free, or cook them from scratch.

- Probiotic foods, e.g., organic yogurt and kefir, sauerkraut, pickles, miso, tempeh, kombucha, or natto. Natto, tempeh, and kombucha are not easy to find, and you may need to visit a health food or Asian food store. And most people won't appreciate natto or kombucha either, so if you are a picky eater, you have my permission to hold off on trying them right away.

Additional Considerations

- Protein options. Buy cage-free, organic-fed eggs and poultry products. If you buy red meat, be sure to find grass-fed and nitrosamine-free options. Frozen products may be less expensive.
- Other fresh fruits, especially citrus—you'll want to keep lemons, limes, and oranges on hand—as well as apples, pears, and melons. You can buy frozen sliced peaches (for smoothies), which are less expensive than fresh.
- Condiments. Consider red wine and balsamic vinegar, hot chili sauce, gluten-free tamari sauce, salsa, Dijon mustard, and vegetable broth or chicken stock.
- Flour. Instead of using standard wheat flour, almond flour (also called almond meal) makes an excellent substitution. It has similar fiber content as whole grain flour, but has an ultra-low glycemic load and is packed with nutrients. If you can't find almond flour/meal at your local grocery store, visit my resource page at www.DrMasley.com/resources for a link to Thrive Market. Or, prepare your own almond flour. Simply process 1¼ cups of raw almonds or dry roasted almonds in a food processor or blender to make 1 cup of almond flour; store in an airtight container for later use.
- Beverages. Consider unsweetened almond milk, organic soymilk, organic kefir, unsweetened tea, and water (still or bubbly). Choose glass or BPA-free cartons and cans. Ideally, you'd have a reverse-osmosis filter in your kitchen for water so you don't have to buy water for cooking and drinking.

Before You Leave Home for the Store

Glance through some recipes in this chapter. Pick a few you'd like to try over the next few days, and be sure you have the ingredients to try those that pique your interest.

If you're donating unwanted items to your local food bank, it's time to drop off the box and visit the grocery store. Keep in mind, grocery stores are designed to entice you to buy foods that you don't want or need. Focus on your shopping list. Don't be surprised if you spend more money on this first shopping trip than you usually do on groceries, perhaps even double what you normally spend. Extra spices, cooking oils, and condiments are expensive, but you won't be making these initial investments every time you shop.

If you are on a tight budget, here are some money-saving tips for purchasing healthy foods:

- Buy frozen foods in large quantities. Frozen berries, cherries, seafood, and vegetables are far less expensive than fresh and have the same nutritional content.
- Organic meat and poultry are more expensive, anywhere from 50 to 100 percent more. If you are on a budget, eat smaller portions and serve them with larger vegetable and side dish portions. If you have a freezer, buying organic meat in bulk is a big savings.
- Buy food in bulk from warehouse stores. Costco, Sam's Club, and Walmart are often less expensive if you stick to the key items on your shopping list. The challenge is not purchasing all the other items on display. In recent years, due to consumer demand, the big-box grocers have expanded their organic selections with competitive pricing.
- Subscribe to a CSA, short for community-supported agriculture. CSAs will deliver locally farmed produce, and in some cases grass-fed meat and dairy, to your home, or you can pick up your goods from a designated location. You might find prices lower. For more information and a list of CSAs that serve your area, visit www.localharvest .org. Or look into joining a food co-op if there is one in your community. You typically work for a few hours a week in exchange for discounts and access to a variety of fresh, organic foods.

Food Storage

How you store your food matters, as piling food from the store straight into the refrigerator can cause pesticide levels to build up over time. It's best to wash your fruits and vegetables in the kitchen sink under cold water with enough hand soap to generate bubbles. Then rinse away the soap. Place organic produce in the bath first, remove and rinse, and wash the nonorganic produce items last.

Berries, mushrooms, onions, and root vegetables shouldn't be washed and stored, as they easily get mildewed. Keep them in a separate bag/container, and wash individual servings before consuming.

Avoid plastic containers as much as possible. I prefer glass containers with plastic-sealing lids in the refrigerator for leftovers, soups, and sauces. Never cook with plastic, including in the microwave; transfer food to a glass or ceramic container for reheating.

Kitchen Equipment That Makes Cooking Easier

Cooking should be enjoyable, and having the right tools (and a few fun gadgets) makes food preparation much easier and quicker. Compare the list below—items you'll find in my own kitchen—with what you already have, and consider filling in the gaps.

1. Knives and scissors. More than any tool, I need a good quality chef's knife. Longer blades are better. I use both my 8-inch and 12.5-inch blades often. A small high-quality paring knife and pair of sturdy kitchen scissors are also essential.
2. Cutting boards. You should have at least two of them— and don't rely on a board that pulls out from a counter and wiggles when you chop. Pull the board out of its sleeve, place it on top of a dishtowel on the counter, and chop from a steady position. Wood and plastic have different advantages, and both are fine. Some people like glass for poultry, meat, or fish, as the surface can be easily disinfected and cleaned.
3. Sauté pans. You'll need medium and large. Avoid aluminum and cast-iron pans. Look for stainless-steel or anodized aluminum. Avoid pans with Teflon or other nonstick plastic linings.
4. Saucepans. You should have at least a small and a medium saucepan.

5. Big soup pot. It should have at least an 8-quart capacity. As with sauté and saucepans, it should be stainless steel, not aluminum.

6. Strainer and colander. Some cooks like salad spinners for washing and drying greens and fresh herbs.

7. Steamer. Use it for your saucepans.

8. Measuring spoons. I like to have a couple of sets so when one is dirty, I have a backup.

9. Glass measuring cups. Have one-, two-, and four-cup options.

10. Blender. These are great for making sauces and smoothies. Hand-held immersion blenders are also popular and clean up easily.

11. Food processor and egg beater. Especially if you don't like chopping vegetables, a good food processor is a must.

12. Wooden spoons and spatulas. A variety of sizes, materials, and shapes come in handy.

13. Peeler, cheese grater, or microplane for citrus zest. A mandoline for thin-sliced vegetables is also handy.

14. Ovenproof baking dish (9 by 13 inches). Get glass or ceramic, preferably at least two.

15. Baking sheets, some with rims. Rimmed sheets are especially good for roasting larger amounts of vegetables.

16. Glass storage containers with plastic lids. A variety of sizes is useful for storing leftovers. You can find brands that will go safely from freezer or fridge to oven.

17. Glass and metal mixing bowls. Get several sizes.

Mindful Eating

As important as the nutritional value of food is how you eat it. Some of the benefits of the Mediterranean diet have to do not with what you eat but with how. Mediterranean meals are typically served at a table, consumed in a leisurely fashion, and enjoyed with family and friends. Meals are not taken in front of a television or at the computer. Food is discussed, savored, and enjoyed. Some of my favorite tips for mindful eating include the following:

1. **Focus.** Don't multitask while you eat. Put aside your to-do list, turn off all screens, and focus on your eating! Do enjoy the company of friends and family, and talk about the flavors and the aromas of the food you are enjoying together. Eating in front of the TV (or while fiddling with a smartphone or computer) is either hypnotizing or mindless; people eat to great excess while watching TV and never seem satisfied because they are utterly unaware of what and how much they have consumed.

2. **Sit down at a table when you eat.** When you stand and eat, you distract yourself from the act of consuming the food, and you eat more than you should—similar to eating in front of the TV. In particular, don't eat while staring into the refrigerator or pantry, or standing at the kitchen counter. Serve your food on a plate and enjoy it while sitting at a table.

3. **Taste and enjoy each bite.** This will improve not only your digestion but also your appreciation for the food you have.

4. **Eat your favorite food last.** You will remember the last bit of food you ate the best. This prevents you from eating more later because the finest experience is still fresh in your mind.

Dining Out

Eating out should be fun. You have nothing to cook, nor kitchen and dishes to clean. You can just relax and enjoy the food and the company of your fellow diners. Ideally, you are in good enough health that on occasion, you can eat what you wish and not worry about the consequences. However, if you have significant health problems or if you eat out frequently (for business or personal reasons), it's especially important to order your food with care. Today, fortunately, it is much easier to modify a meal to match your needs than it was in the past, and savvy restaurants who want your business are frequently willing to honor your requests.

When I view a menu, I think of all the items offered as available options. You don't have to have the chicken Marsala with the recommended side of mashed potatoes. If you see grilled trout with a side of broccoli with lemon sauce, you should be able to request chicken Marsala with broccoli with lemon sauce if you desire.

Don't hesitate to ask how dishes are prepared. You should feel free to modify a sauce and change oils to a healthier option. I'll frequently ask what oil they use in a specific dish, and if I don't like their choice, I'll ask them to switch to olive oil and even make a request for extra herbs and garlic at the same time. When asking about the oil, also ask if they use a sweetener, and feel free to suggest they skip it at the same time.

The easiest way to order a meal that you can enjoy and that will also nourish your brain is to skip the bread basket and select a salad with vinaigrette dressing to start. Next, request the cleanest protein choice you would enjoy, double the portion of the vegetable-legume side dish, and skip the starch (typically a high glycemic load option such as potatoes, rice, bread, or pasta). Accompany your meal with a glass of nice wine, or a sparkling water with lemon, and skip the dessert, planning to enjoy some dark chocolate when you get home. If you really have something to celebrate, consider the bread (or starchy side dish) or the dessert—but it is preferable if you don't eat both. If you choose the bread, ask for olive oil for dipping, and if you choose dessert, split it with another person—it will still be plenty.

You should have little problem ordering like this at a casual spot or a high-end restaurant. If they can't accommodate these reasonable requests, then let the manager know you won't be back. Fast-food restaurants are likely the biggest challenge, because they don't have much room to modify your order. Usually your best bet with fast food is a salad with a protein on top and a vinaigrette dressing on the side.

If you are at a buffet, restaurants typically feature the starches at the beginning of the line. Buffet diners have a habit of loading up on what they see first. Be sure to take a tour of the entire buffet before you fill your plate. Identify the items you should be having, such as clean protein options and extra vegetable-legume side dishes. Then go fill your plate with the best choices in mind. If you happen to be preparing a buffet for your own guests, do them a very good turn and put the three healthiest items first in line, as that is the majority of what they will eat.

How to Involve Your Friends and Family

When you announce you're about to change your way of eating, friends and family usually respond in one of two scenarios.

In the first, they'll be right there with you, supporting your efforts all the way. If you've had health issues in the past or if they've expressed concern for your well-being, perhaps they've been asking you to make healthier lifestyle changes for a long time. Now they're thrilled that you're finally taking action. Tell them they were right all along, and you're ready to accept their help. (Your praise will make you golden.)

Then there's the second scenario: resistance. You're tossing out the chips and cookies. You aren't going to be eating your regular breakfast of cereal and toast, or having your usual meal together at the greasy burger joint that's a "tradition." You're *changing.* Some people, no matter how much they love you, will have a hard time with that.

If they resist, don't nag and preach. Instead, lead by example. As you embark on the Better Brain Solution, share how much better you feel. (They're likely to notice how much better you look.) Often the desire to make healthy lifestyle changes that get results are a good topic for a family meeting (but not over a meal, where they'll feel like you're judging what's on their plates). Share your goals, what you hope to achieve, and ask for their help and support, without telling them what they have to do. In this setting, loved ones are very likely to support you.

Make this about you and your brain health, not about their choices. Tell them that to succeed, you need to get the chips and candy out of the house because *you* end up eating them, not because they should be skipping them, too. Then make that request, letting them know that they can eat as they wish, but you don't want to be tempted by certain foods in the refrigerator and in the cabinets. If they are willing to try the food you'll be bringing home and preparing, that's wonderful—offer a taste if they're curious, but don't force them. Should they begin to come around to your side, invite them into the kitchen to cook with you, and you may find that you've quietly converted them to a better lifestyle.

If you have children, the 12 Smart Foods and all the recipes in this book are fantastic for kids. There is a myth that children need to be treated to cookies, cakes, candy, and soda regularly, almost as if sugar were a required part of childhood. But poor food choices are ruining the health and potential of our youth. Yes, let them eat cake at a birthday party, but they don't need sweets and junk day after day. I raised my own children on the foods I'm recommending to you. I'm delighted to say that I have two extremely healthy boys (with adventurous palates as a bonus) and that they enjoy eating this way. I want your children and grandchildren to grow up healthy and productive as well—and with strong, vital, healthy brains.

Beyond Food

Here is a quick look at the other three components of the Better Brain Solution, to help you get started and combine all four strategies—food, supplements, exercise, and stress management.

Supplements

When you follow the Better Brain Solution eating plan, you'll get many brain-saving vitamins, minerals, and other compounds from food. But because you cannot always get adequate amounts of these key nutrients from food, here are supplement options to enhance your diet. For details, see Chapter 5.

Step 1. Get the Essentials, Including:

- Vitamin D: 2,000 IU daily
- A daily multivitamin, with key ingredients:
  - Vitamin B12: at least 100 mcg
  - Folates: at least 400 mcg of mixed folates
  - Chromium: 400–800 mcg

- Long-chain omega-3 fats (fish oil): Eat fish 2–3 times per week or take 1000 mg of EPA and DHA from a high-quality fish oil supplement.
  - Vegetarians: Alternatively, take 500 mg of DHA from a seaweed supplement
  - If you have the ApoE4 genotype: I recommend 2,000 mg of EPA and DHA daily

- Probiotic source: Foods first, then supplement.
- Magnesium: at least 400 mg daily. Foods first, then supplement.
  - For people with mild cognitive impairment, discuss with your doctor about consuming 2,000 mg of Magtein Magnesium L-Threonate daily, which includes 144 mg of elemental magnesium

Step 2. Consider Some Additional Supplements, Including:

- Curcumin: 500 mg 1–2 times daily
- Resveratrol: 200–250 mg of trans-resveratrol, 1–2 times daily
- MCT oil: start with 10 grams daily, increase to 20 grams

Step 3. Learn More About Supplements for High-Risk Individuals, Including:

- Coenzyme Q10
- Phosphatidylserine
- Huperzine A
- Compounds designed to support mitochondrial function (alpha lipoic acid)

Exercise

Because everyone who begins the Better Brain Solution has a different level of fitness, it is important to identify one of three recommended steps to begin with. For details, see Chapter 6.

- If you currently get little daily activity, begin with Step 1.
- If you already have a regular exercise routine, you are probably ready for Step 2.
- If you are fit and active (you meet the benchmarks in Step 2), try Step 3.

Step 1: Get Moving

- Count your daily steps and build up to 10,000 steps 5–6 days per week (the equivalent of walking 4–5 miles). Once you've reached this level of activity, move to Step 2.

Step 2: Rev Up Your Heart Rate and Add Strength Training

- Figure out what aerobic level is right for you by determining your target heart rate. (I recommend that you do a workout with an exercise physiologist to find your target heart rate.) Whatever aerobic activity you choose (walking briskly, running, swimming), here are the three phases to work through:

  - *Phase 1.* Target heart rate 60–70 percent of your max, 20–30 minutes, 4–5 times per week.
  - *Phase 2.* Target heart rate 70–80 percent of your max, 30–40 minutes, 4–5 times per week.
  - *Phase 3.* Moderate aerobic workout, 2–3 days per week, combined with interval/burst training, at 80–90 percent of your max, 2–3 days per week.

- Add 1–2 strength training workouts per week, either on the same day as your aerobic workout or on your off days.

Step 3: Mix It Up for a Better Brain

- Work out a minimum of 4–5 days per week. (Take one rest day, though you can do low-impact exercise if you wish.) Do a combination of moderate aerobic activity 2–3 days per week, interval training 2–3 days, and an activity like Pilates for core strength and balance 1–2 times per week.

Stress Management

Add pleasure, fun, and social connection to create joy and reduce stress in your life. For details, see Chapter 7.

Step 1: Focus on What You Can Control—Your Lifestyle Choices

- Add daily exercise to release tension.
- Get a good night's sleep, 7–8 hours.
- Don't overuse stimulants like caffeine and alcohol and avoid all tobacco products.

Step 2: Unplug, Recharge, and Rest

- Schedule some peace and calm every day, like yoga or a hot bath by candlelight.

Step 3: Go Deeper to Get Calmer

- Try meditation, focused breathing, or a biofeedback program like HeartMath.

If You Have the ApoE4 Gene

Here is a quick look at four actions to focus on:

1. Follow a low glycemic load eating plan. Avoid sugar and refined carbs. Aim to eat the 12 Smart Foods daily to boost your brain and protect your cognitive function.
2. Keep to a modest intake of saturated fat from animal protein and dairy products. Because ApoE4 genotypes are less able to utilize MCT fats effectively as fuel, you have

     less reason to use MCT oil, coconut oil, and other coconut products.

3. Double your fish oil intake. Aim for 2,000 mg (2 grams) of DHA and EPA daily. People with the ApoE4 gene need extra fish oil.

4. Add daily exercise. While everyone benefits from exercise, those with the ApoE4 gene may derive even more brain benefits.

5. Partial intermittent fasting is popular in the ApoE4 community.

6. As people with the ApoE4 gene have more inflammation potential, consider taking supplements that lower inflammation, in particular fish oil and curcumin, and absolutely avoid tobacco products.

     For support, visit the website at https://www.apoe4 .info/wp/.

A Final Message

You can improve your brain function starting right now, and prevent or delay future memory loss, so get started and stick with it. The Better Brain Solution isn't just a fifteen- or thirty-day plan—it's designed as a lifestyle you can enjoy for the rest of your life.

Yes, your genes are fixed, but the messages encoded in them are not set in stone. You get to choose how you express them. Your current health is an expression of your genetic potential, but you are free to change your lifestyle and express your genes differently, through a life that is filled with health, fitness, emotional well-being, and purpose.

You can improve your mental sharpness and, at the same time, prevent and even reverse heart disease and decrease your risk for memory loss. You will get healthier, fitter, and sexier, and you'll start feeling better.

Better Brain Solution Recipes

Breakfast

STEVEN'S MORNING SHAKE

Here is the shake I enjoy several days a week. It includes many of the dozen brain-boosting foods, is quick and easy to make and drink, and tastes great. Except for the protein powder and a fluid (I prefer unsweetened almond milk), you can drop or substitute the ingredients freely.

PREP TIME: 2 minutes

Serves: 1

½ cup organic kefir (I prefer low fat)
1 cup frozen organic cherries
½ cup frozen spinach or kale
20 grams whey protein powder, vanilla or chocolate (or pea-rice protein if you avoid dairy)
8 ounces unsweetened almond milk

OPTIONAL
1 tablespoon unprocessed unsweetened cocoa powder

Combine all the ingredients in a blender. Purée until smooth. Enjoy.

CALORIES: 296
PROTEIN: 30 G
FAT: 7 G
CARBS: 25 G
FIBER: 5 G
SODIUM: 268 MG

TIP: Create your own smoothie-making station to make this prep go quickly every morning. I store a mix of frozen raw spinach and kale leaves together, next to a tub of frozen fruit. I keep the dry ingredients together in a cupboard next to my blender. There is never any searching for ingredients.

COFFEE (OR TEA) WITH ORGANIC GHEE AND MCT OIL

Drink this for breakfast if you are doing partial intermittent fasting. Adding fat without carbs or protein to extend the length of carb fasting and increase ketone body formation is an intriguing concept. For people who are dairy intolerant, the trace amount of protein in regular butter can cause undesirable symptoms. Ghee (clarified butter) is essentially free of dairy protein and is a better choice. Use caution as you increase the dosage of MCT (medium-chain triglycerides) oil. Many people have major GI symptoms if they start with 20 grams (1½ tablespoons) of MCT oil.

PREP TIME: 5 minutes

Serves: 1 (using 10 g MCT oil)

1 cup freshly brewed organic coffee
1½ tablespoons organic ghee (clarified butter)
5 to 20 grams MCT oil (which is about 1 teaspoon to 1½ tablespoons;
    start out with less and gradually increase over time; see pages 115–116)

While the coffee is brewing, pour hot water into a blender to warm the blender up. When the coffee is ready, pour out the water. Combine the hot coffee, ghee, and MCT oil in the blender; secure the lid tightly to avoid splattering. Blend and serve immediately.

CALORIES: 237
PROTEIN: 0.5 G
FAT: 27 G
CARBS: 0 G
FIBER: 0 G
SODIUM: 7 MG

EGGS BENEDICT WITH SMOKED SALMON AND SPINACH

I really like this breakfast because it tastes wonderful, and it's loaded with brain-healthy fats and plant pigments. If you don't have an egg poacher, having an assistant to help serve is useful.

PREP TIME: 25 minutes

Serves: 2

2 cups chopped frozen spinach, thawed
4 ounces smoked salmon, thinly sliced
4 large organic, cage-free eggs
2 teaspoons salt (if not using an egg poacher)
4 teaspoons white vinegar (if not using an egg poacher)
½ cup Hollandaise Sauce (page 313, or use store-bought)

Cook the spinach, drain well, and return to pan. Place the salmon in the pan next to the spinach.

If you have an egg poacher, follow the directions for poaching 4 eggs at once.

If you don't have an egg poacher, add enough water to two medium saucepans to fill them about 2 inches deep. Add 1 teaspoon of the salt and 2 teaspoons of the white vinegar to each pan and bring to a gently bubbling simmer. Meanwhile, crack 2 eggs into two separate small bowls, keeping the yolks intact. When the water is simmering, use the handle of a spatula or spoon to quickly swirl the water (one pan at a time) in one direction until the water is spinning in the pan. Gently drop 1 egg at a time into the center of the whirlpool—the swirling water will help prevent the white from feathering or spreading out in the pan. Cover and let the eggs poach, setting your timer for 5 minutes; leave the eggs untouched while poaching. Repeat for the second serving of eggs; this is why it's useful to have an extra pair of hands if you're making more than one serving.

While the eggs are poaching, gently warm the spinach, smoked salmon, and hollandaise sauce.

On two plates, divide the warm spinach into two mounds on each plate. Next add a layer of sliced salmon. When the eggs are ready, remove them from the water with a slotted spoon, place each poached egg on top of each spinach and salmon mound, and drizzle with the hollandaise sauce. Serve immediately.

CALORIES: 499
PROTEIN: 29 G
FAT: 41 G
CARBS: 4.5 G
FIBER: 1 G
SODIUM: 993 MG

FRITTATA WITH ARTICHOKE HEARTS, SUN-DRIED TOMATOES, AND SPINACH

This simple-to-make dish can be served at breakfast, lunch, or dinner. Artichokes are loaded with vitamins, fiber, and minerals, and the sour cream provides a dose of probiotic support as well. If you'd like this dairy free, skip the sour cream and cheese and garnish with fresh herbs.

PREP TIME: 15 minutes
BAKING TIME: 20 minutes

Serves: 4

2 tablespoons extra virgin olive oil, plus more for the baking dish
1 medium sweet onion, diced
½ teaspoon sea salt
½ teaspoon ground black pepper
1 teaspoon Italian herb seasoning
1 cup chopped artichoke hearts (in olive oil), drained
¼ cup sun-dried tomatoes, chopped
4 cups fresh spinach, chopped
8 large organic, cage-free eggs
¼ cup organic sour cream
½ cup grated organic Gruyère cheese

Preheat the oven to 375°F. Coat the inside of a medium-size ovenproof baking dish with olive oil.

Heat a sauté pan to medium heat. Add 2 tablespoons of oil, onion, salt, pepper, and Italian herbs and sauté for 2 to 3 minutes, stirring occasionally, until translucent. Add the artichoke hearts, tomatoes, and spinach, and heat for another 3 to 4 minutes, until the spinach has wilted. Remove the pan from the heat.

In a bowl, whisk the eggs with the sour cream. Then, combine the egg mixture and the vegetable mixture in the baking dish. Top with the grated cheese. Bake for 20 minutes, or until the eggs have set. Serve while hot, or allow to cool and then serve at room temperature or chilled.

CALORIES: 323
PROTEIN: 18 G
FAT: 23 G
CARBS: 10 G
FIBER: 3 G
SODIUM: 728 MG

COCONUT AND ALMOND PANCAKES

Here is an option for healthy pancakes without the sugar and typical flour. Almond flour (also sold as almond meal) is a gluten-free option that you can find in most well-stocked markets. Serve with fresh berries and, for an occasional treat, a dollop of whipped cream and/or maple syrup.

PREP TIME: 5 to 10 minutes
COOKING TIME: 5 to 10 minutes

Serves: 2 to 3 (makes about 6 medium pancakes)

1 cup almond flour/meal
¼ cup unsweetened coconut flakes
½ teaspoon aluminum-free baking powder
1/16 teaspoon sea salt
½ cup unsweetened almond milk
½ teaspoon pure vanilla extract
3 large organic, cage-free eggs, beaten
1 tablespoon organic ghee (clarified butter)
2 to 3 tablespoons almond butter
1 to 2 cups fresh berries of your choice

OPTIONAL
2 tablespoons maple syrup
2 tablespoons organic whipped cream

Combine the almond flour, coconut, baking powder, and salt in a large bowl. Combine the almond milk, vanilla, and beaten eggs in a separate bowl. Make a well in the dry ingredients and pour in the egg mixture, mixing well.

Heat a pan to medium heat. Add the ghee and melt. Ladle the pancake batter into the pan and cook for 3 to 5 minutes. Flip and cook for another 2 to 4 minutes, until golden.

Heat the almond butter until warm and drizzle a spoonful over each 2-stack of pancakes. Garnish with berries and serve. For a special treat, stir maple syrup into the almond butter as it melts, and/or a dollop of whipped cream as a garnish over the pancakes.

CALORIES: 478
PROTEIN: 18 G
FAT: 38 G
CARBS: 23 G
FIBER: 8 G
SODIUM: 151 MG

YOGURT BERRY BOWL

This is basic, but quick and tasty, and it can be eaten as a snack. Use whatever berries or nuts you prefer. The sweetener and coconut are optional.

PREP TIME: 5 minutes

Serves: 2

1 cup organic plain yogurt
1 cup fresh berries of your choice
¼ cup nuts, chopped

OPTIONAL
1 to 2 teaspoons xylitol (or stevia or, for an occasional treat, honey)
1 to 2 tablespoons unsweetened shredded coconut

Combine all the ingredients in a bowl and serve.

CALORIES: 201
PROTEIN: 8 G
FAT: 11 G
CARBS: 20 G
FIBER: 4 G
SODIUM: 76 MG

Snacks

GUACAMOLE

Guacamole doesn't store well, so prepare this just before serving. It is a fantastic dip served with sliced vegetables, but it can also be used as a spread when you would otherwise use mayonnaise. I prefer to use cilantro for a more authentic taste, but parsley will also work.

PREP TIME: 10 minutes

Serves: 2 or more

1 medium Hass avocado (or ½ Florida avocado)
2 tablespoons fresh lime juice
2 tablespoons diced sweet onion
2 tablespoons finely diced tomato
⅛ teaspoon sea salt
½ teaspoon ground paprika
⅛ teaspoon cayenne pepper (or to taste)
¼ cup fresh cilantro, chopped

FOR DIPPING
1 medium cucumber, thinly sliced into rounds
1 medium red bell pepper, cut lengthwise into ¾-inch-wide slices

Peel, pit, and mash the avocado. Combine the avocado and all the remaining ingredients except the cucumber and bell pepper slices and stir.

   If not serving immediately, squeeze additional lime juice over the surface and cover well (use an airtight container). The lime juice will slow the guacamole from browning. When ready to serve, use sliced cucumber rounds and bell pepper slices for dipping.

CALORIES: 161
PROTEIN: 2 G
FAT: 15 G
CARBS: 8 G
FIBER: 7 G
SODIUM: 140 MG

SALMON SPREAD WITH SLICED CUCUMBER AND CAPERS

This spread is full of flavor and ingredients that control blood sugar levels and nourish your brain. Canned salmon works well in this recipe.

PREP TIME: 5 to 10 minutes

Serves: 2 or more

3½ ounces cooked salmon (volume is the size of a deck of cards)
1 medium celery stalk, diced
¼ cup chopped fresh Italian parsley
¼ teaspoon ground black pepper
½ cup hummus

TO SERVE
1 medium cucumber, sliced into rounds
2 tablespoons capers, drained

Combine the salmon, celery, parsley, pepper, and hummus in a bowl. To serve, spread sliced cucumber on a plate. Spoon the salmon spread over each slice and garnish with the capers.

CALORIES: 219
PROTEIN: 19 G
FAT: 10 G
CARBS: 15 G
FIBER: 5 G
SODIUM: 539 MG

CHICKEN WINGS WITH BUFFALO SAUCE

Serve these wings at your next party or sports-themed event. The ingredients in this buffalo sauce support your brain with healthy fats, herbs, and plant pigments.

PREP TIME: 10 to 15 minutes
BAKING TIME: 45 to 55 minutes

Serves: 4

24 organic, cage-free chicken wings
1 tablespoon aluminum-free baking powder
½ teaspoon fine sea salt
¼ teaspoon ground black pepper
¼ cup extra virgin olive oil
½ cup tomato sauce
6 medium garlic cloves, crushed and minced
1 teaspoon Italian herb seasoning
1 teaspoon ground paprika
⅛ to ½ teaspoon cayenne pepper (to taste)

Preheat the oven to 400°F. In a bowl, combine the chicken with the baking powder, salt, and black pepper and place on a roasting tray. Bake for 35 to 40 minutes, until the chicken is browned.

Meanwhile, combine the oil, tomato sauce, garlic, Italian herbs, paprika, and cayenne in a separate large bowl.

Reduce oven heat to 350°F. Stir the browned chicken into the bowl of sauce until the wings are well covered. Return to the roasting tray and bake for another 12 minutes.

CALORIES: 523
PROTEIN: 32 G
FAT: 42 G
CARBS: 4 G
FIBER: 1 G
SODIUM: 549 MG

WHITE BEAN, CAULIFLOWER, AND HAZELNUT DIP

This dip pairs well with sliced vegetables. Canned beans make this even simpler to prepare (if you prepare your own, use 2 cups of cooked beans).

PREP TIME: 10 to 15 minutes
BAKING TIME: 30 minutes

Serves: 6 (makes 3 cups)

½ head cauliflower florets, cut into 1-inch pieces (about 2 cups)
2 tablespoons avocado oil
½ cup hazelnuts
4 medium garlic cloves, chopped
One 15-ounce can white beans, cooked, rinsed, and drained
2 tablespoons extra virgin olive oil
½ teaspoon sea salt
¼ cup low-sodium vegetable broth (or water)

Preheat the oven to 375°F. On a baking sheet, mix the cauliflower florets with the avocado oil. Bake for 20 minutes. After 20 minutes, reduce the oven heat to 350°F.

Add the hazelnuts to an ovenproof dish and bake for 10 minutes. At the same time, remove baking sheet with the cauliflower, stir in the garlic, and return to the oven for 10 minutes.

In a food processor, combine the roasted cauliflower, the hazelnuts, beans, olive oil, salt, and vegetable broth. Blend until smooth. Serve warm, or refrigerate and serve chilled.

CALORIES: 247
PROTEIN: 8 G
FAT: 16 G
CARBS: 20 G
FIBER: 5 G
SODIUM: 205 MG

SMOKED SALMON WITH ENDIVE

Here's another way to enjoy omega-3-rich salmon. You can also get additional nutrients, including DHA, if you use seaweed sheets (such as nori) to wrap the salmon instead of endive leaves.

PREP TIME: 15 minutes

Serves: 2

8 medium endive leaves (3 × 4-inch seaweed sheets)
½ pound smoked salmon, divided into 8 thin strips
1 medium Hass avocado, peeled, pitted, and cut into 8 slices
8 teaspoons organic sour cream
2 tablespoons chopped fresh Italian parsley

Separate the endive leaves and place on a serving plate. To each endive leaf, add a slice of the smoked salmon and a slice of the avocado, top with 1 teaspoon of the sour cream, and garnish with the parsley.

If using seaweed, spread the sheets on a work surface and stack the ingredients in the same order. Wrap or fold the seaweed as desired to form a salmon roll and transfer to a serving plate.

CALORIES: 412
PROTEIN: 32 G
FAT: 26 G
CARBS: 18 G
FIBER: 14 G
SODIUM: 1,400 MG

Soups

AVOCADO AND ASPARAGUS SOUP

This is a delicately flavored, light soup—loaded with brain-supporting fats, vitamin C, fiber, and healthy plant pigments. To make it into a complete meal, add 2 cups of cooked white beans when you add the avocado. This soup can be served hot or chilled.

PREP TIME: 15 minutes

Serves: 4

2 cups low-sodium vegetable broth
12 ounces fresh asparagus, tough ends trimmed away, cut into 1-inch
    pieces
½ medium white onion, chopped
1 teaspoon fresh lemon juice
½ teaspoon ground black pepper
¼ cup organic sour cream
2 medium Hass avocados, peeled, pitted, and cut into ½-inch cubes

Bring the vegetable broth to a gentle boil in a pot. Add the asparagus and onion, reduce the heat to medium, and simmer for 10 to 12 minutes, until the asparagus is tender. Meanwhile, divide the avocado cubes equally among soup bowls.

When the asparagus simmering time is complete, carefully transfer the hot soup to a blender. Add the lemon juice, pepper, and sour cream and blend until smooth. Pour the hot soup over the avocado cubes and serve immediately. To serve cold, prepare the soup and refrigerate for up to 24 hours. Cube the avocado right before serving, divide it into bowls, and pour in the chilled soup.

CALORIES: 207
PROTEIN: 4 G
FAT: 16 G
CARBS: 16 G
FIBER: 8 G
SODIUM: 197 MG

BLACK BEAN SOUP

This soup is especially good with home-cooked beans, although using canned beans is both quicker and easier. Some cooks get into the habit of making a batch of beans once or twice a week, so the beans are always on hand. With precooked beans, you can have this velvety soup on the table in less than thirty minutes. This soup is absolutely loaded with brain-supporting plant pigments, fiber, nutrients, and probiotics.

PREP TIME: 15 to 20 minutes
SIMMERING TIME: 10 minutes

Serves: 6

8 cups black beans (or four 15-ounce cans), cooked, rinsed, and drained
1 tablespoon avocado oil
1 medium sweet onion, chopped
2 medium celery stalks, diced
1 teaspoon sea salt
1 teaspoon dried oregano
1 teaspoon ground paprika
½ teaspoon red pepper flakes
1 medium red bell pepper, chopped
1 medium green bell pepper, chopped
4 medium garlic cloves, crushed and diced
15 ounces chopped tomatoes (about 2 cups)
2 cups low-sodium vegetable broth

GARNISH
2 tablespoons organic sour cream
2 tablespoons chopped fresh cilantro

When the beans are ready, heat a large pot to medium-high heat. Add the oil, onion, celery, salt, oregano, and paprika and sauté for 2 to 3 minutes, stirring occasionally, until the onion softens. Add the red pepper flakes and bell peppers, and heat for another 2 minutes, continuing to stir occasionally.

Add the garlic, tomatoes, vegetable broth, and beans to the pot and bring to a gentle boil. Reduce the heat to medium and simmer for 10 minutes. Divide among the soup bowls and garnish with the sour cream (1 teaspoon in each bowl) and cilantro.

CALORIES: 363
PROTEIN: 21 G
FAT: 4.5 G
CARBS: 62 G
FIBER: 21 G
SODIUM: 490 MG

MISO SOUP

This savory soup boosts immune function and is an excellent source of up to 120 probiotic strains. Light and salty, it works well as a first course for a meal. Yellow miso is sweet and creamy, while red miso is stronger and saltier—buy to match your taste preferences. Seaweed sheets come in a variety of types and sizes; choose what is convenient for you.

PREP TIME: 15 minutes

Serves: 2

3 cups water
1 cup shiitake mushrooms, sliced into bite-size slivers
2 medium garlic cloves, crushed and minced
One 4 × 4-inch seaweed sheet (such as kombu, wakame, or nori), cut into small strips or squares
¼ pound organic silken tofu, cut into ½-inch cubes
2 medium green onions, diced
2 tablespoons red or yellow miso paste

Bring the water and shiitake mushrooms to a boil in a saucepan. Reduce the heat to a simmer. Add the garlic, seaweed, tofu, and green onions, and simmer for 5 to 7 minutes, until the mushrooms are tender. Place the miso in a small bowl and set aside.

When the simmering is complete, with a ladle extract ¼ cup of liquid from the soup and whisk with the miso paste to fully dissolve. Return the miso mixture to the pot, stir well, turn off the heat, and serve.

CALORIES: 86
PROTEIN: 6 G
FAT: 1 G
CARBS: 12 G
FIBER: 3 G
SODIUM: 675 MG

Entrées

VEGETARIAN OPTIONS

GARBANZO, TOMATO, AND OKRA CURRY

This brightly flavored main dish features brain-supporting spices such as ginger, cinnamon, and curry, and it makes great leftovers. You can use fresh or frozen okra. (If you use frozen, thaw it before using, or allow a few extra minutes of simmering time.)

PREP TIME: 20 minutes

Serves: 4

2 tablespoons macadamia nut oil (or almond or avocado oil)
1 medium sweet onion, chopped
1-inch piece fresh ginger, peeled and sliced into matchsticks
2 tablespoons curry spice blend
½ teaspoon ground cinnamon
30 ounces (or two 15-ounce cans) tomatoes, chopped
4 medium garlic cloves, crushed and diced
30 ounces (or two 15-ounce cans) garbanzo beans, cooked, rinsed, and
    drained
4 cups okra (fresh or frozen), cut into 1-inch pieces

Heat a sauté pan to medium-high heat. Add the oil and onion and sauté for 2 minutes, stirring occasionally. Reduce the heat to medium and add the ginger, curry spice, cinnamon, tomatoes, garlic, garbanzo beans, and okra. Simmer for 7 to 10 minutes until the okra is tender. Serve immediately.

CALORIES: 157
PROTEIN: 5 G
FAT: 8 G
CARBS: 21 G
FIBER: 7 G
SODIUM: 22 MG

THAI COCONUT CURRY SOUP

This soup, with its distinctive flavors, can be served as a vegetarian dish with tofu, or chicken or shrimp can be substituted for the tofu. If you can locate fresh galangal (Thai ginger), use it in place of fresh ginger. If you can't find lemongrass, the dish is still very good without it. Use more, or less, red curry paste to reflect your tolerance for heat.

PREP TIME: 15 minutes
SIMMERING TIME: 20 minutes

Serves: 6

1 tablespoon avocado oil
2 medium shallots, diced
1½ cups sweet potato, peeled and cut into ½-inch cubes (about 1 small to
    medium sweet potato)
2 medium garlic cloves, crushed and diced
2 teaspoons red curry paste (to taste, depending on your preference for
    heat)
2 tablespoons tamari sauce
3 cups low-sodium vegetable broth
2 medium lemongrass stalks (3 to 4 inches), sliced lengthwise
One 1-inch cube fresh ginger (or galangal), peeled and sliced into
    1-inch-wide slices
1½ cups broccoli florets, cut into bite-size pieces
15 ounces canned coconut milk (from a BPA-free can, if possible)
Zest and juice of 1 medium organic lime
1 pound organic soft tofu, cut into ½-inch cubes
2 tablespoons chopped fresh basil (or Thai basil)

Heat a large saucepan to medium heat. Add the oil and shallots and sauté for 2 to 3 minutes. Next, add the sweet potato, garlic, curry paste, tamari sauce, vegetable broth, lemongrass, and ginger, and turn up the heat to bring to a boil. Once the mixture is bubbling, reduce the heat to a simmer and cook for 10 minutes. Add the broccoli and simmer for another 5 minutes, until the sweet potato and broccoli are tender but not soft.

Add the coconut milk, lime zest, lime juice, cubed tofu, and basil, and simmer for another 5 minutes. Remove the pieces of lemongrass and ginger and discard. Serve the soup in bowls.

CALORIES: 242
PROTEIN: 7 G
FAT: 18 G
CARBS: 15 G
FIBER: 2 G
SODIUM: 426 MG

SPINACH AND SHIITAKE MUSHROOM SOUFFLÉ

This is perhaps the easiest soufflé to make. The spinach provides structure, and although the soufflé won't rise as high as the classic version, the spinach keeps it from collapsing. It is critical to use brain-healthy organically fed, cage-free eggs for this dish. The almonds and clean egg yolks add brain-supporting fats, while the spinach also provides a blast of protective antioxidants and nutrients.

PREP TIME: 30 minutes
BAKING TIME: 30 to 35 minutes

Serves: 4

2 tablespoons almond oil, plus more for the dish
1 medium sweet onion, diced
½ pound (about 2 cups) shiitake mushrooms, stems discarded, tops finely diced
½ teaspoon sea salt
½ teaspoon ground black pepper
1 teaspoon Italian herb seasoning
10 ounces frozen spinach (about 1 box), thawed and drained well
2 tablespoons organic salted butter
½ cup almond flour/meal
1 cup dry white wine
¾ cup organic Comté (or Gruyère) cheese, grated
7 large organic, cage-free eggs

GARNISH
2 tablespoons grated Parmesan cheese
2 tablespoons almond slivers

Preheat the oven to 400°F. Coat the inside of a ceramic soufflé dish (1½-quart capacity—about 4 inches high and 9 inches in diameter) with almond oil.

Heat a sauté pan to medium-high heat. Add the oil and onion and stir occasionally for 2 minutes, until the onion softens. Add the mushrooms, salt, pepper, and Italian herbs. Continue to sauté, stirring occasionally, until the mushrooms soften, 3 to 4 minutes. Add the spinach to the mushrooms. Stir, and reduce the heat to simmer for 1 minute. Remove from the heat and set aside.

Heat a separate saucepan to medium heat. Add the butter and stir in the flour until the mixture is smooth and thickens. Reduce the heat to low. Add the white wine, bring to a simmer, and stir until the mixture thickens into a sauce. Stir in the Comté, remove from the heat, and combine with the vegetable mixture.

Carefully separate the eggs into whites and yolks. Don't allow any yolk to fall into the whites. Whisk the yolks and stir into the vegetable mixture.

Whip the egg whites with an egg beater or mixer at high speed until they are stiff and form peaks. Gently fold one-quarter of the egg whites into the vegetable mixture, making the mixture lighter and less sticky. Next, gently fold this vegetable mixture with the remaining egg whites, blending them together. It's fine to have a few lumps, so don't overmix or the air trapped in the egg whites will be lost and the soufflé won't rise.

Carefully pour the soufflé mixture into the oiled dish. Top with Parmesan cheese and almond slivers.

Bake for 30 to 35 minutes, until a long wooden skewer or a thin knife blade inserted into the center comes out clean. Serve immediately. The soufflé should be moist but not runny in the center. If it is runny, just pop it back into the oven for another 5 minutes. Slice into quarters and serve.

CALORIES: 511
PROTEIN: 24 G
FAT: 36 G
CARBS: 14 G
FIBER: 5 G
SODIUM: 603 MG

SPICY TOFU AND PINEAPPLE WITH
STIR-FRY VEGETABLES

Marinate tofu slices in a sweet-and-sour mixture for an extra burst of flavor. This recipe calls for 1 teaspoon of red curry sauce, but the amount is up to you; use more if you enjoy more heat. I also like to substitute Sriracha to change up the flavors. Don't overcook the vegetables, because they lend a satisfying crunch to this wholesome dish.

PREP TIME: 30 minutes
BAKING TIME: 40 minutes

Serves: 3

TOFU MARINADE
1 pound organic extra-firm tofu, sliced (slice a vertical block in half, then
    slice it widthwise into ¾-inch strips)
1 teaspoon red curry sauce (to taste, up to 1 tablespoon)
1 teaspoon ground paprika
1 tablespoon grated or minced fresh ginger, peeled
4 medium garlic cloves, crushed and minced
2 tablespoons tamari sauce
1 tablespoon rice vinegar
2 tablespoons toasted sesame oil
8 ounces pineapple chunks, drained (if canned, unsweetened)

STIR-FRY
2 tablespoons avocado oil
1 medium red onion, cut lengthwise into slivers
2 cups cauliflower florets, cut into bite-size pieces
1 medium yellow bell pepper, cut lengthwise into slivers
1 cup snow pea pods
1 teaspoon tamari sauce
¼ cup low-sodium vegetable broth (or water)
¼ teaspoon red pepper flakes (to taste, up to ½ teaspoon)
1 tablespoon sesame seeds

Preheat the oven to 350°F. Combine the sliced tofu with the red curry sauce, paprika, ginger, garlic, tamari sauce, vinegar, and sesame oil in a glass bowl. Marinate in the refrigerator for at least 30 minutes and up to 12 hours.

After marinating, place the tofu on a rimmed baking sheet. Drizzle the marinade with the garlic and ginger on top of the tofu. Bake for 30 minutes.

After 30 minutes, remove the baking sheet from the oven (the marinade should have dried but not burned). Add the pineapple to the baking sheet, stirring gently with the tofu strips and mixing the pineapple into the sauce. Return the tofu and pineapple to the oven and bake for 10 more minutes.

Meanwhile, heat a sauté pan to medium-high heat. Add the avocado oil and onion and sauté for 2 minutes, stirring occasionally, until the onion softens. Add the cauliflower and sauté for another 2 minutes. Add the bell pepper, snow peas, tamari sauce, vegetable broth, and red pepper flakes. Reduce the heat to medium, cover the pan, and simmer for another 4 to 5 minutes, until the vegetables are tender but not overcooked. Remove from the heat, serve with the tofu-pineapple mixture, and garnish with the sesame seeds.

CALORIES: 459
PROTEIN: 21 G
FAT: 27 G
CARBS: 34 G
FIBER: 7 G
SODIUM: 668 MG

PECAN NUT LOAF

This simple-to-prepare and elegant vegetarian entrée can be served alone or with Mushroom Gravy (page 314). You can substitute almonds or hazelnuts for the pecans or walnuts.

PREP TIME: 20 minutes
BAKING TIME: 25 to 30 minutes

Serves: 4

2 tablespoons almond oil (or avocado oil)
4 cups mushrooms, diced
1 medium sweet onion, diced
½ teaspoon sea salt
½ teaspoon ground black pepper
2 medium celery stalks, diced
¼ cup chopped fresh basil
¼ cup chopped fresh Italian parsley
1 teaspoon dried oregano
½ cup port wine
6 large organic, cage-free eggs, beaten
1 cup pecans or walnuts, finely chopped
1 cup grated organic Comté (or Gruyère) cheese

Preheat the oven to 400°F. Grease an 8 × 4-inch loaf pan with almond oil or line with parchment paper.

Heat the oil in a sauté pan over medium-high heat. Add the mushrooms, onion, salt, and pepper and cook for 3 to 4 minutes, stirring occasionally, until the onion is translucent and the mushrooms soften. Add the celery, basil, parsley, and oregano and cook for another 3 minutes, with occasional stirring. Reduce the heat to low, add the port, and simmer for another 2 to 4 minutes, until the port has mostly evaporated and the sauce thickens. Set aside.

Combine the eggs, nuts, and grated cheese in a bowl, then fold together with the mushroom mixture. Pour the mixture into the loaf pan. Bake for 25 to 30 minutes, until a toothpick inserted into the center comes out clean. Remove the loaf from the oven and let sit for 5 minutes prior to serving. Slice and serve like meatloaf. This dish goes well with mushroom gravy (page 314).

CALORIES: 521
PROTEIN: 22 G
FAT: 40 G
CARBS: 14 G
FIBER: 4 G
SODIUM: 476 MG

SEAFOOD OPTIONS

ALMOND-COATED TILAPIA

A crunchy crust of nuts works well on any type of fish, and adds an extra dose of brain-boosting fat. You can substitute sole, cod, halibut, or white fish for tilapia.

PREP TIME: 15 minutes
BAKING TIME: 20 minutes

Serves: 3

Avocado oil, for the dish
1 pound tilapia fillets (or other whitefish: sole, cod, catfish, flounder), rinsed
1 cup fresh orange juice
1 large organic, cage-free egg
½ cup almond flour/meal
¼ cup almond slivers (or finely chopped almonds)
½ teaspoon sea salt
¼ teaspoon ground black pepper
½ teaspoon Italian herb seasoning

Preheat the oven to 400°F. Grease an ovenproof baking dish with avocado oil.

Rinse the fish fillets, place in a bowl with the orange juice, and marinate for 5 minutes.

Meanwhile, while the fillets are marinating, beat the egg in a bowl and set aside. On a large plate, combine the almond flour, almond slivers, salt, pepper, and Italian herbs. Remove the fillets from the juice and pat dry with a paper towel. Dip the fillets in the egg, then coat with the almond flour mixture. Place the fillets in the baking dish and bake for 20 minutes, until the fillets flake. Serve immediately.

CALORIES: 478
PROTEIN: 45 G
FAT: 27 G
CARBS: 15 G
FIBER: 3 G
SODIUM: 482 MG

SHRIMP WITH THAI CURRY SAUCE

In a restaurant this would be served over rice, but with all the flavors here you won't miss it (nor will your brain miss its high glycemic load). You can easily substitute chicken, bay scallops, or tofu for shrimp and use any type of nut butter in the curry sauce. If using chicken, make sure it is fully cooked before adding it to the sauce.

PREP AND SIMMERING TIME: 30 minutes

Serves: 4

CURRY SAUCE
15 ounces canned coconut milk (from a BPA-free can, if possible)
2 tablespoons almond butter
2 tablespoons red chili sauce (to taste, 1 to 3 tablespoons; such as sriracha)
1 tablespoon fish sauce (or oyster sauce, or skip it if you don't have either)
2 tablespoons fresh lime juice
¾ cup fresh pineapple chunks (or 8-ounce can unsweetened, drained)
2 medium garlic cloves, crushed and minced
1 tablespoon chopped fresh basil (or Thai basil)
2 lemongrass stalks, cut 1 inch from the base into 2-inch pieces
½ cup low-sodium vegetable broth

SAUTÉ
2 tablespoons macadamia oil (or avocado, almond, or other nut oil)
2 pounds wild extra-large shrimp
¼ teaspoon sea salt
1 medium onion, slivered lengthwise
2 medium carrots, thinly sliced
½ cup low-sodium vegetable broth
2 cups sliced broccoli
1 medium red bell pepper, cut into bite-size pieces
1 cup snow pea pods

GARNISH
2 tablespoons chopped fresh cilantro

Whisk together the coconut milk, almond butter, chili sauce, fish sauce, lime juice, pineapple, garlic, basil, lemongrass, and vegetable broth in a saucepan. Bring to a gentle boil, then reduce the heat to a simmer to let the sauce thicken.

Meanwhile, heat a wok or large sauté pan to medium-high heat. Add the oil, shrimp, and salt and sauté for a few minutes, stirring often, until cooked through. Remove the shrimp from the wok and set aside.

To the same wok over medium-high heat, add onion and carrots and sauté for 2 to 3 minutes, until the onions soften. Add the vegetable broth mixture and broccoli, stirring occasionally, and sauté for another 3 minutes. Add the bell pepper and snow peas, continue to stir frequently, and cook until the vegetables are al dente. Remove the lemongrass stalks from the curry sauce and discard. Return the shrimp to the simmering curry sauce, reduce the heat to medium-low, and simmer for 3 to 4 minutes. Serve in bowls and garnish with fresh cilantro.

CALORIES: 647
PROTEIN: 53 G
FAT: 35 G
CARBS: 33 G
FIBER: 5 G
SODIUM: 871 MG

SHRIMP KEBABS

You can make easy-to-prepare kebabs with shrimp, chicken, or steak. Make some extras for a quick meal later in the week, because they are excellent leftovers. Cut the vegetables into generous bite-size pieces; aim to keep them roughly uniform in size to easily thread on skewers for grilling. Serve with the Masley House Vinaigrette (page 316) or use a store-bought balsamic vinaigrette.

PREP TIME: 15 to 20 minutes
MARINADE TIME: 20 minutes to 2 hours
GRILL TIME: 7 to 10 minutes

Serves: 2

1 pound large shrimp, uncooked, peeled and deveined, rinsed, and
    drained
1 medium sweet onion, cut into 1-inch squares
6 medium button mushrooms, cut in half (or quartered, if larger)
3 tablespoons extra virgin olive oil (or avocado oil)
3 tablespoons balsamic vinegar
¼ teaspoon sea salt
½ teaspoon ground black pepper
1 teaspoon Italian herb seasoning
4 medium garlic cloves, crushed and minced
1 medium green bell pepper, cut into 1-inch squares
1 medium red bell pepper, cut into 1-inch squares
8 ounces fresh spinach
3 tablespoons balsamic vinaigrette dressing (ready-made or see page 316)

In a large bowl, combine the shrimp, onion, mushrooms, oil, vinegar, salt, black pepper, Italian herbs, garlic, and bell peppers and marinate for at least 20 minutes and up to 2 hours. Stir occasionally.

Heat a grill to medium-high heat. Thread the shrimp and vegetable pieces onto skewers, alternating the pieces. Place the skewers on the grill and drizzle with a little additional marinade. Then discard any remaining marinade.

Grill the skewers for 6 to 8 minutes, until the shrimp are cooked through, turning the skewers every 3 to 4 minutes. Meanwhile, toss the spinach with the vinaigrette dressing and divide the salad among plates.

When the kebabs are done, slide the shrimp and vegetables off the skewers and onto the spinach salad.

CALORIES: 594
PROTEIN: 53 G
FAT: 32 G
CARBS: 28 G
FIBER: 6 G
SODIUM: 933 MG

SAUTÉED TERIYAKI-PINEAPPLE SALMON

Most people broil or grill salmon, but it is really easy, and quicker, to sauté it.
I typically prepare wild, frozen, vacuum-packed salmon, available year-round.
King (Chinook), red (sockeye), or silver (coho) salmon are my favorites, and all
are loaded with brain-nourishing omega-3 fats. If frozen, thaw the packs, rinse,
and marinate the fillets in orange juice for 5 to 10 minutes, which removes any
fishy flavor (even with fresh fish, you may prefer to soak the fillets). You can also
use pineapple juice.

PREP TIME: 20 minutes

Serves: 2

1 pound wild salmon fillet, cut into 1-inch-wide strips
1½ tablespoons tamari sauce
2 medium garlic cloves, crushed and minced
¼ teaspoon ground black pepper
1 tablespoon rice vinegar
1 cup pineapple chunks, cut into small pieces (if canned, 8 ounces,
    unsweetened and drained well)
1 tablespoon avocado oil

Soak the salmon strips for 5 minutes in orange or pineapple juice to
freshen, then discard the juice. Marinate the salmon strips in a bowl with
the tamari sauce, garlic, pepper, vinegar, and pineapple chunks for 20
minutes, turning occasionally. Remove the salmon, pat dry with paper
towels, and set aside. Reserve the marinade.

Heat a sauté pan to medium-high heat. Add the oil and then the
salmon. Spoon remaining marinade and pineapple on top of the fish.
Sauté on each side for 4 to 5 minutes, until lightly browned. Serve
immediately.

CALORIES: 473
PROTEIN: 49 G
FAT: 21 G
CARBS: 22 G
FIBER: 1 G
SODIUM: 848 MG

BROILED SCALLOPS WITH PESTO

Who said pesto goes only with pasta? This recipe is a great way to savor pesto and enjoy the healthy benefits of seafood at the same time. Of course, you can use frozen and thawed scallops if you can't locate fresh ones. For the pesto, I love to make my own from garden-fresh basil (see the recipe, page 312), but you can use a store-bought variety. A note on organic citrus: Anytime you use fresh zest (peel) from limes, lemons, or other citrus, choose organic to avoid pesticides that stay in the peel.

PREP TIME: 10 minutes
BROILING TIME: 8 minutes

Serves: 2

Avocado oil, for the dish
1 pound sea scallops rinsed and patted dry with paper towels
2 tablespoons Pesto Sauce (page 312 or store-bought)
2 tablespoons grated lemon zest (about 1 organic lemon)
2 tablespoons grated Parmesan cheese

Preheat the broiler. Grease a broiler-proof shallow baking dish with avocado oil.

Toss the scallops with the pesto in a bowl. Place the scallops in the baking dish. Sprinkle each scallop with the lemon zest and Parmesan cheese. Broil for about 8 minutes, until the scallops are lightly browned and cooked.

To serve, spoon the scallops over a bed of sautéed chopped kale or spinach, or fresh greens of your choice.

CALORIES: 296
PROTEIN: 42 G
FAT: 10 G
CARBS: 7 G
FIBER: 1 G
SODIUM: 577 MG

POULTRY OPTIONS

ITALIAN TURKEY MEATLOAF

It's often easier to find organic, cage-free ground turkey than grass-fed beef or pork, and the turkey tastes terrific in this recipe. Rolled oats offer a very nice gluten-free and low glycemic load alternative to bread crumbs.

PREP TIME: 15 minutes
BAKING TIME: 50 minutes

Serves: 4

1 tablespoon avocado oil, plus more for the pans
1 medium white onion, chopped
2 cups chopped mushrooms
1 pound organic, cage-free ground turkey
2 large organic, cage-free eggs
1 cup rolled oats
½ cup dry red wine
1 tablespoon Italian herb seasoning
4 medium garlic cloves, crushed and diced
½ teaspoon sea salt
1¼ cups marinara sauce
2 tablespoons grated Parmesan cheese

Preheat the oven to 375°F. Grease an 8 × 4-inch loaf pan with avocado oil.

Heat a sauté pan to medium-high heat. Add the oil, onion, and mushrooms and sauté, stirring occasionally, for about 2 to 3 minutes until the onions are translucent.

Meanwhile, in a large bowl, combine the ground turkey, eggs, oats, red wine, Italian herbs, garlic, salt, and ¼ cup of the marinara sauce, mixing well. Add the sautéed onion and mushrooms to the bowl and stir to combine. Pour the mixture into the loaf pan. Next, pour the remaining 1 cup marinara sauce over the mixture, then sprinkle with the Parmesan cheese. Bake for 50 minutes (the internal temperature should reach at least 165°F). Let sit for about 10 minutes before serving.

CALORIES: 436
PROTEIN: 31 G
FAT: 20 G
CARBS: 28 G
FIBER: 3 G
SODIUM: 814 MG

CHICKEN, MUSHROOM, AND BROCCOLI SAUTÉ

Chicken thighs are very good in this sauté. They are also less expensive and often more flavorful than chicken breast meat. Shiitake mushrooms are a bit more expensive, but they have more flavor and health benefits than regular white mushrooms.

PREP TIME: 20 minutes

Serves: 2

2 tablespoons organic ghee (clarified butter)
1 pound boneless organic, cage-free chicken thighs, cut into ¾-inch cubes
½ teaspoon sea salt
¼ teaspoon ground black pepper
1 teaspoon dried thyme
½ medium sweet onion, sliced into long strips
2 cups mushrooms, sliced (I prefer shiitake)
2 small yellow squash (or zucchini), chopped into cubes
2 cups sliced broccoli
½ cup chopped fresh Italian parsley
4 medium garlic cloves, crushed and diced

Heat a large sauté pan to medium-high heat. Add the ghee, chicken, salt, pepper, and thyme, and sauté for about 4 minutes, until the chicken is lightly browned. Add the onion, mushrooms, and squash. Cover the pan and cook for 2 to 3 minutes, until the onions and mushrooms start to soften. Add the broccoli, cover, and cook for another 2 to 3 minutes, stirring occasionally, until the broccoli is nearly al dente. Reduce the heat to a simmer, add the parsley and garlic, and cook, uncovered, for another 2 minutes, stirring occasionally. Serve immediately.

CALORIES: 457
PROTEIN: 51 G
FAT: 21 G
CARBS: 17 G
FIBER: 5 G
SODIUM: 767 MG

ROASTED CORNISH GAME HENS WITH MEDITERRANEAN HERBS AND BUTTERNUT SQUASH

When you cook whole birds, such as turkey, chicken, or these roasted game hens, look for cage-free poultry raised on an organic diet. This elegant combination is simple to prepare because you can roast the hens and the butternut squash—an outstanding source of vitamin A—at the same time. Olive oil and rosemary make this dish especially tasty and brain healthy.

PREP TIME: 10 minutes
ROASTING TIME: 60 minutes

Serves: 2

2 medium organic, cage-free Cornish game hens
2 tablespoons extra virgin olive oil
2 tablespoons Italian herb seasoning, dried
1 tablespoon diced fresh rosemary
½ teaspoon sea salt
½ teaspoon ground black pepper
1 medium butternut squash, sliced in half lengthwise, seeds removed
2 tablespoons organic butter
½ teaspoon ground cinnamon

Preheat the oven to 395°F. Rub the game hens with the oil, Italian herbs, rosemary, ¼ teaspoon of the salt, and the pepper. Place the hens in a roasting pan. Bake for 50 to 60 minutes, until the skin is browned and the internal temperature reaches at least 165°F. Transfer to a carving board. Allow the hens to rest for 10 minutes before carving.

The squash can be prepared at the same time. Place the halves in a baking dish, skin side down. For each half, add 1 tablespoon butter to the cavity and sprinkle with cinnamon and the remaining ¼ teaspoon salt. Bake the butternut squash until tender but not overcooked, about 60 minutes.

CALORIES: 604
PROTEIN: 51 G
FAT: 34 G
CARBS: 26 G
FIBER: 2 G
SODIUM: 700 MG

CHICKEN CURRY

The aromatic spices in this chicken curry will protect your brain while the flavors will please your palate. You may use almond or avocado oil if you don't have macadamia nut oil. Cilantro is more traditional, but Italian parsley will work, too.

PREP TIME: 30 minutes

Serves: 2

2 tablespoons macadamia nut oil (or almond or avocado oil)
1 pound boneless organic, cage-free chicken thighs, cut into strips
½ medium red onion, cut into long, thin slices
2 tablespoons curry powder
1 teaspoon ground paprika
¼ teaspoon cayenne pepper (to taste)
1 teaspoon ground ginger (or 1 tablespoon peeled and grated fresh ginger)
¼ teaspoon sea salt
¼ teaspoon ground black pepper
½ medium cauliflower, cut into bite-size pieces
1 cup peas (frozen or fresh, shelled)
½ cup organic, low-sodium chicken stock
1 cup organic plain yogurt
¼ cup fresh cilantro or Italian parsley, chopped

Heat a large sauté pan to medium-high heat. Add 1 tablespoon of the oil and the chicken and sauté, stirring occasionally, for about 5 minutes, until all sides are lightly browned. Remove the chicken from the pan and place in a holding bowl. Add the remaining 1 tablespoon oil to the sauté pan and sauté the onion with the curry powder, paprika, cayenne, ginger, salt, and black pepper for 2 minutes, stirring occasionally. Add the cauliflower, cover, and cook for another 3 to 4 minutes, until the cauliflower is al dente. Reduce the heat to medium-low. Stir in the chicken, peas, and chicken stock, and simmer for 4 to 5 minutes, until the chicken is cooked through. Turn off the heat, stir in the yogurt, and serve, garnished with cilantro.

CALORIES: 583
PROTEIN: 58 G
FAT: 25 G
CARBS: 33 G
FIBER: 10 G
SODIUM: 816 MG

DUCK WITH CHERRY SAUCE

People seem to shy away from duck, perhaps because they think of it as difficult to prepare and therefore more of a restaurant specialty. In truth, it is not hard to make at home and is quite healthy. This recipe, featuring cherries, bursts with rich flavors and is a nice change from chicken and turkey.

PREP TIME: 20 minutes

Serves: 2

Two 7-ounce organic, cage-free duck breast halves
¼ teaspoon sea salt
¼ teaspoon ground black pepper
2 teaspoons avocado oil
½ medium sweet onion, finely chopped
⅓ cup organic, low-sodium chicken stock (or low-sodium veggie broth)
18 organic red cherries, halved and pitted (fresh or frozen, thawed)
3 tablespoons port wine
1 tablespoon balsamic vinegar

Using a sharp knife, for each duck breast half, score a ¾-inch diamond pattern into the skin (do not cut into the flesh). Pat dry with paper towels and season with salt and pepper.

Heat a large skillet to medium-high heat. Add the oil, then the duck, skin side down. Cover and cook until the skin is lightly browned and crisp, 4 to 6 minutes. Turn over the duck breasts, reduce the heat to medium, and cook until browned and cooked through, 4 to 6 minutes. The breasts should reach an internal temperature of 165°F. Transfer to a cutting board, cover with aluminum foil to keep warm, and let rest for 10 minutes.

Meanwhile, add the onion to the pan with the juices and heat, stirring occasionally, for 2 minutes. Next add the chicken stock, cherries, port, and vinegar. Increase the heat to medium-high and allow to bubble, stirring often, until the sauce thickens, 5 to 7 minutes.

Thinly slice the duck. Fan slices out onto plates or a serving platter. Spoon the sauce over the duck and serve.

CALORIES: 396
PROTEIN: 41 G
FAT: 13 G
CARBS: 14 G
FIBER: 2 G
SODIUM: 119 MG

CHICKEN MARSALA

This is a take on classic chicken marsala, but made with chicken thighs for more flavor, and with almond flour to keep this gluten-free and have a lower glycemic index than the traditional dish made with wheat flour.

PREP TIME: 10 minutes
COOKING TIME: 20 minutes

Serves: 2

½ cup almond flour/meal
1 teaspoon ground paprika
½ teaspoon sea salt
¼ teaspoon ground black pepper
¼ teaspoon cayenne pepper
1 teaspoon dried thyme
1 teaspoon dried oregano
1 pound boneless organic, cage-free chicken thighs
1 tablespoon avocado oil
2 tablespoons organic ghee (clarified butter)
3 cups mushrooms (shiitake, if available), halved and sliced
⅔ cup marsala wine
¼ cup organic, low-sodium chicken stock
2 medium garlic cloves, crushed and minced
¼ cup fresh herbs for a garnish (parsley and chives), finely chopped

In a shallow bowl or plate, combine the almond flour, paprika, salt, black pepper, cayenne, thyme, and oregano. Roll the chicken in the flour-seasoning mixture, shaking to remove any excess flour. Set aside the remaining flour mixture.

Heat a large skillet to medium-high heat. Add the oil and 1 tablespoon of the ghee, then cook the chicken until golden brown on both sides, about 3 minutes per side. Transfer the partially cooked chicken to a plate.

Add the remaining 1 tablespoon ghee to the skillet, then add the mushrooms, stirring frequently until the mushrooms have released their liquid and are lightly browned. Add 1 to 2 tablespoons of the seasoned flour and stir for 1 to 2 minutes. Add the marsala, bring to a gentle boil, and stir to thicken. When the wine is reduced by half, after about 3 minutes, add the chicken stock and cook for another 3 to 4 minutes, until the sauce thickens. Lower the heat to medium and add the partially cooked chicken and the garlic to the skillet. Cook until the chicken is done and the internal temperature reaches 165°F, 5 to 6 minutes. Garnish with fresh herbs before serving.

CALORIES: 689
PROTEIN: 54 G
FAT: 42 G
CARBS: 12 G
FIBER: 4 G
SODIUM: 825 MG

TURKEY TENDERS WITH MIDDLE EASTERN SPICES

Turkey is a flavorful alternative to chicken, and is quite affordable, but we tend to pass it by and reach for chicken, out of habit. This combination of spices lowers brain inflammation and improves blood sugar control.

MARINATING TIME: 20 to 60 minutes
PREP AND COOKING TIME: 15 minutes

Serves: 2

1 pound organic, cage-free turkey tenders, sliced into 1-inch-thick strips
2 tablespoons avocado oil
2 tablespoons fresh lemon juice
¼ teaspoon ground cardamom
½ teaspoon ground cumin
½ teaspoon ground turmeric
¼ teaspoon ground cinnamon
¼ teaspoon sea salt
¼ teaspoon ground black pepper
2 medium garlic cloves, crushed and diced
¼ cup fresh mint, chopped

Marinate the turkey strips with 1 tablespoon of the oil, lemon juice, spices, salt, pepper, garlic, and all but 1 tablespoon of the mint for 20 to 60 minutes.

Heat a sauté pan to medium-high heat. Add the remaining 1 tablespoon oil, then the turkey, and sauté until lightly browned on each side, turning every few minutes until fully cooked. Remove from the pan, garnish with the remaining tablespoon of mint, and serve immediately.

CALORIES: 456
PROTEIN: 43 G
FAT: 30 G
CARBS: 2 G
FIBER: 0 G
SODIUM: 935 MG

MEAT OPTIONS

ROASTED LAMB AND VEGETABLES

Look for organic, grass-fed lamb that has been pasture-raised. For this recipe you will want a French-cut lamb chop; "frenching" refers to the process of removing extra meat and cartilage from the rib bones so they appear as handles. You can do this yourself, or ask the butcher to do it for you.

PREP TIME: 15 minutes
BAKING TIME: 40 minutes

Serves: 3

1 pound lamb chops (preferably French cut)
1 tablespoon ghee (clarified butter), at room temperature
2 tablespoons fresh rosemary, thyme, and sage (or a similar combination),
    finely chopped
½ teaspoon sea salt
¼ teaspoon ground black pepper
½ medium sweet onion, chopped into chunks
1 medium fennel bulb, chopped into 1-inch chunks
2 medium carrots, chopped into 1-inch chunks
2 medium beets, peeled and chopped into ¾-inch chunks
1 tablespoon avocado oil

Preheat the oven to 350°F. Rub the lamb first with the ghee, then the herbs, salt, and pepper. Set aside.

In a roasting pan, mix the chopped vegetables with the oil. Place the lamb, fat side up, in the center of the roasting pan with the vegetables surrounding it. As beets bleed red juice, either roast them in a separate ovenproof container or place them to the side of the roasting pan. Roast for 40 to 50 minutes on the medium rack. (The USDA recommends for health safety that the final internal temperature of lamb should reach at least 145°F for medium to well-done, although those who prefer it medium-rare would stop at a temperature of 130° to 135°F.) When the internal temperature is 5 degrees less than your desired temperature, turn the heat to broil, cooking for another 2 to 3 minutes to render the fat crispy. Remove from the oven, transfer to a serving platter, cover with aluminum foil, and allow to rest for 5 to 10 minutes. Serve on a platter or individual plates with vegetables circling the lamb chops.

CALORIES: 467
PROTEIN: 48 G
FAT: 24 G
CARBS: 15 G
FIBER: 5 G
SODIUM: 572 MG

SIRLOIN, PEPPERS, AND ONION WITH MIXED SALAD

Choose organic, grass-fed beef for this easy-to-make dish. Bell peppers (in all colors) provide crisp flavors as well as a healthy dose of vitamins C and A. I suggest a red bell pepper here for a nice contrast with the green, but you can use yellow or orange, in any combination you desire.

PREP TIME: 25 minutes

Serves: 2

1 tablespoon organic ghee (clarified butter)
¾ pound sirloin steak
1 teaspoon dried oregano
½ teaspoon sea salt
½ teaspoon ground paprika
½ teaspoon ground cumin
¼ teaspoon ground black pepper
1 medium sweet onion, cut into slivers
1 medium red bell pepper (or any bright color), cut into slivers
1 medium green bell pepper, cut into slivers
2 tablespoons extra virgin olive oil
1 tablespoon balsamic vinegar
4 cups mixed greens

Heat a sauté pan to high heat. Add the ghee and sprinkle half of the oregano, salt, paprika, cumin, and black pepper over the steak. Sear the steak in the sauté pan, turning it until both sides are gently browned. Reduce the heat to medium-high, and cook through as desired. Remove the steak from the pan, cover the steak, and set aside. To the same sauté pan, add the onion and the remaining oregano, salt, paprika, cumin, and black pepper and sauté for 2 minutes, stirring occasionally.

Remove the pan from the heat, add the olive oil and vinegar and mix with the cooked vegetables, ghee, and meat drippings. Slice the steak across the grain into ¼- to ½-inch slices. To serve, toss the mixed greens with the vegetables and sauce. Place the steak strips over the salad.

CALORIES: 537
PROTEIN: 71 G
FAT: 21 G
CARBS: 14 G
FIBER: 4 G
SODIUM: 686 MG

PORK CHOPS WITH ITALIAN HERBS AND MUSHROOMS

It is increasingly easy to find pasture-raised pork that has been fed an organic diet—free of pesticides and hormones. Use white button or brown mushrooms, such as cremini or baby portobellos, in this hearty but simple dish. Serve with a green vegetable of your choice, and for a probiotic boost, sauerkraut. You don't have to overcook pork, it can be slightly pink; just make sure you heat the center of the pork to at least 145°F.

PREP TIME: 15 minutes

Serves: 2

Two 6- to 8-ounce organic, pasture-raised pork chops
2 tablespoons almond oil (or avocado oil)
1 tablespoon Italian herb seasoning
1 teaspoon ground paprika
½ teaspoon sea salt
¼ teaspoon ground black pepper
½ medium sweet onion, sliced thinly
2 cups mushrooms, sliced
2 tablespoons low-sodium vegetable broth (or organic, low-sodium
    chicken stock, white wine, or water)
¾ cup organic sour cream

Pat dry the pork chops with paper towels. Rub 1 tablespoon of the oil, the Italian herbs, paprika, salt, and pepper into the chops. Heat a sauté pan to medium-high heat. Add the remaining 1 tablespoon oil to the pan. Add the chops and sauté for about 3 to 4 minutes on each side, until golden and the internal temperature reaches 145°F.

Remove the chops from the pan and cover with aluminum foil. In the same pan, reduce the heat to medium, add the onion and mushrooms with the vegetable broth, and sauté for 3 to 4 minutes, until the onion is soft. Stir the sour cream into the sauce. Spoon the onion and mushrooms with the sauce over the chops on a platter and serve.

CALORIES: 613
PROTEIN: 71 G
FAT: 32 G
CARBS: 7 G
FIBER: 2 G
SODIUM: 709 MG

Side Dishes

MIXED SALAD

Here is a salad that will go with almost any meal, and one that you adjust with your own mix of vegetables and greens. For instance, instead of the carrot, garbanzo beans, and artichoke hearts, use 2 to 3 cups of any vegetable combination you enjoy (try a mix of broccoli, cucumber, capers, cauliflower, or celery). Serve with Masley House Vinaigrette Dressing (page 316), or extra virgin olive oil and your favorite vinegar.

PREP TIME: 10 minutes

Serves: 2

SALAD
4 cups mixed organic greens
1 small carrot, grated
½ cup garbanzo beans, cooked, rinsed, and drained
½ cup chopped artichoke hearts

DRESSING
2 tablespoons extra virgin olive oil
1½ tablespoons red wine vinegar
1 small garlic clove, crushed and minced
⅛ teaspoon sea salt
⅛ teaspoon ground black pepper

GARNISH
4 medium cherry tomatoes, quartered
½ to 1 medium avocado, peeled, pitted, and sliced
2 tablespoons sliced almonds

Combine the greens, carrot, garbanzo beans, and artichoke hearts in a salad bowl. Combine the dressing ingredients and toss with the salad. Garnish with the tomatoes, avocado, and almonds and serve.

CALORIES: 381
PROTEIN: 9 G
FAT: 28 G
CARBS: 30 G
FIBER: 14 G
SODIUM: 466 MG

KALE WITH RED BELL PEPPER
AND GARLIC

Nutrient-rich kale is very good cooked, particularly when paired with mushrooms and bell peppers. You can make this recipe with spinach or Swiss chard, as well.

PREP TIME: 10 to 15 minutes

Serves: 2

1 tablespoon extra virgin olive oil
2 cups sliced mushrooms (such as baby portobellos)
1 teaspoon Italian herb seasoning
¼ teaspoon sea salt
1 medium red bell pepper, sliced
4 cups kale, chopped
2 medium garlic cloves, crushed and minced
¼ cup low-sodium vegetable broth (or water)

Heat a large sauté pan to medium heat. Add the oil, mushrooms, Italian herbs, and salt, and sauté for 3 minutes, stirring occasionally, until the mushrooms soften. Add the bell pepper and cook for an additional 2 minutes. Then add the kale, garlic, and vegetable broth and cover. Remove from the heat when the kale has wilted, 2 to 3 minutes. Serve immediately.

CALORIES: 172
PROTEIN: 8 G
FAT: 8 G
CARBS: 23 G
FIBER: 5 G
SODIUM: 400 MG

SPINACH, BEET, AND
GOAT CHEESE SALAD

*The beets improve blood flow to your brain; the spinach and walnuts provide
additional cognitive benefits—and taste great with the beets and goat cheese.*

PREP TIME: 15 minutes
BAKING TIME: 40 minutes

Serves: 4

4 medium beets, unsightly skin peeled, cut into ¾-inch cubes
4 tablespoons extra virgin olive oil
¼ teaspoon fine sea salt
¼ teaspoon ground black pepper
1 teaspoon Italian herb seasoning
4 cups raw, pre-rinsed, and drained baby spinach
2 teaspoons balsamic vinegar
4 ounces organic goat cheese
2 ounces walnuts, shelled, toasted

Preheat the oven to 375°F. Toss the beets with 2 tablespoons of the oil, the
salt, pepper, and Italian herbs in an ovenproof baking dish and roast for
about 40 minutes, until the beets are tender but not overcooked.

When the beets are cooked, remove them from the oven and let cool a
few minutes. Toss the spinach with the remaining 2 tablespoons oil and
the vinegar and spoon onto individual serving plates. To each portion,
add beets, then garnish with the goat cheese and walnuts.

CALORIES: 360
PROTEIN: 10 G
FAT: 32 G
CARBS: 12 G
FIBER: 4 G
SODIUM: 367 MG

BROCCOLI WITH LEMON SAUCE

This is a flavorful way to get in a serving of brain-beneficial green vegetables. It is best with fresh broccoli, but in a pinch you can use frozen. Rather than use florets, cut the broccoli lengthwise into cross sections, about a half inch thick. The tangy lemon sauce in this recipe can be used with a variety of other side dishes or served with fish.

PREP TIME: 5 minutes
COOKING TIME: 5 minutes

Serves: 2

4 cups sliced broccoli (cut into long, ½-inch-thick slices)
1 tablespoon organic salted butter
1 tablespoon extra virgin olive oil
1 teaspoon fines herbes (or Italian herb seasoning)
Zest and juice of ½ organic lemon
¼ teaspoon sea salt

Steam the broccoli for 3 to 5 minutes, until tender but still al dente. Meanwhile in a small saucepan over medium-low heat, combine the butter, oil, herbs, lemon zest, lemon juice, and salt and cook for 2 minutes, until the butter has blended with the oil and zest. Place the broccoli in a bowl and toss with the lemon sauce before serving.

CALORIES: 176
PROTEIN: 5 G
FAT: 13 G
CARBS: 13 G
FIBER: 5 G
SODIUM: 368 MG

CURRIED GARBANZO BEANS
WITH SPINACH

These garbanzo beans (also called chickpeas) make a fragrant vegetarian meal on their own, or are an easy side dish. You can use prepared curry powder, or create your own blend with ground cumin, coriander, cardamom, turmeric, cinnamon, and chili powder—freshly ground spices are the most aromatic and release maximum flavor. I prefer low-fat yogurt, but if it is organic, you can use any fat percentage you prefer.

PREP TIME: 15 minutes

Serves: 2

1 tablespoon avocado oil
½ medium sweet onion, diced
⅓ teaspoon sea salt
15 ounces garbanzo beans, cooked, rinsed, and drained (1 can or 2 cups homemade)
1 tablespoon peeled and grated fresh ginger
1 to 2 tablespoons curry powder (to taste)
1½ cups cooked spinach (about 20 ounces frozen), drained
½ cup organic plain yogurt

Heat a saucepan to medium-high heat. Add the oil, onion, and salt, and sauté for 2 to 3 minutes. Reduce the heat to medium. Add the garbanzo beans, ginger, and curry powder, and simmer for 4 to 5 minutes, stirring occasionally. Add the spinach and cook for 2 to 3 minutes, until it wilts. Remove from the heat, stir in the yogurt, and serve.

CALORIES: 463
PROTEIN: 26 G
FAT: 14 G
CARBS: 67 G
FIBER: 21 G
SODIUM: 632 MG

STEAMED ARTICHOKES WITH LEMON SHALLOT DIP

Artichokes are loaded with fiber and nutrients, plus they are fun to eat. Look for firm, heavy, medium-green artichokes with compact center leaves. If you make your own mayonnaise, prepare it with a healthy fat such as avocado oil or almond oil. Artichoke steaming time depends on how large the artichoke is— the larger it is, the longer it takes to cook.

PREP TIME: 5 minutes
STEAMING TIME: 25 to 45 minutes (15 to 20 minutes in a pressure cooker)

Serves: 2

2 whole fresh artichokes (look for firm, heavy, medium-green artichokes with compact center leaves)
1 cup water, plus extra as needed
½ teaspoon whole peppercorns
½ teaspoon sea salt

DIP
¼ cup organic or homemade mayonnaise
1 tablespoon fresh lemon juice
2 teaspoons Dijon mustard
1 small shallot, finely diced (or 1 tablespoon diced fresh chives)
⅛ teaspoon sea salt

Rinse the artichokes and, optionally, trim off any thorny leaf ends. Slice off the stems at the base and remove any small leaves from the base.

Combine the water, peppercorns, and ½ teaspoon salt in a pot (or pressure cooker) with a steamer basket. Add water to reach the bottom of the steamer basket, if needed.

Place the artichokes, base down, into the steamer.

Cover and bring to a gentle boil for 25 to 45 minutes (15 to 20 minutes in a pressure cooker), until the lower leaves pull away easily and the artichoke bases are fork tender. Add water as needed to continue steaming.

Meanwhile, combine the mayonnaise, lemon juice, mustard, shallot, and ⅛ teaspoon salt. Adjust seasonings to taste and set aside in the refrigerator for the flavors to develop while the artichokes cook.

CALORIES: 267
PROTEIN: 4 G
FAT: 22 G
CARBS: 15 G
FIBER: 7 G
SODIUM: 437 MG

Artichokes may be served hot or cold. To eat the flesh on the leaves, pull off the outer leaves one at a time. Dip the base of the petal into the sauce. Put the base of the leaf in your mouth and pull it through your teeth to remove the soft, pulpy portion of the leaf. Discard the remaining leaf. To eat the heart, spoon out the fuzzy center at the base and discard, then enjoy the base of the artichoke, cutting it into pieces.

LENTIL SALAD

Lentils are an excellent source of fiber, protein, and mixed folates, and eating them improves blood sugar control. They cook quickly and don't require pre-soaking, unlike some larger beans and legumes. Make sure to look them over while rinsing, and remove any small stones that creep in during harvesting. Tip: When using celery, don't discard the leaves when you trim the stalks. Instead, treat these delicate greens like a fresh herb: chop finely and add to the dish for an extra layer of flavor.

PREP TIME: 15
SIMMERING TIME: 25

Serves: 4

1 tablespoon avocado oil
½ medium sweet onion, finely diced
1 medium carrot, diced
2 medium celery stalks, diced (divided into stems and leaves)
1 teaspoon Italian herb seasoning
¼ teaspoon cayenne pepper (to taste)
1 cup dried green lentils
2 medium garlic cloves, crushed and diced
2 cups low-sodium vegetable broth (see page 315, or organic, low-sodium chicken stock)
2 medium tomatoes, chopped

DRESSING
2 tablespoons extra virgin olive oil
1 tablespoon organic lemon zest
2 tablespoons fresh lemon juice
½ cup fresh Italian parsley, diced (combine with celery leaves from above)

In a large saucepan, heat the avocado oil over medium heat. Add the onion, carrot, celery stems, Italian herbs, and cayenne and sauté for 3 to 4 minutes, until the onion is translucent. Set aside.

Meanwhile, rinse the lentils well in water, picking them over to remove any rare small stones, and drain. Add the lentils, garlic, and vegetable broth to the saucepan with the sautéed vegetables. Bring to a gentle boil, cover, then simmer until the lentils are tender but not soft, 20 to 35 minutes, adding extra broth or water if the bottom of the pan turns dry. With a strainer, drain away any excess liquid, and transfer the cooked lentils and vegetables to a serving bowl. Stir in the chopped tomatoes.

As the lentils are simmering, in a small bowl whisk together the olive oil, lemon zest, lemon juice, and parsley. Gently combine the dressing with the lentil salad. Serve immediately, or refrigerate and serve chilled.

CALORIES: 276
PROTEIN: 12 G
FAT: 12 G
CARBS: 34 G
FIBER: 9 G
SODIUM: 309 MG

GREEN BEANS, ROSEMARY, AND VINAIGRETTE DRESSING

Here is an easy side dish that features fresh green beans and goes well with nearly any entrée. Green beans work well in a dish like this, but they can also be lightly steamed or blanched instead. Serve them with a squeeze of lemon juice, some olive oil, and sea salt, or add them to a cool garden salad.

PREP TIME: 15 minutes

Serves: 4

1 tablespoon avocado oil
1 medium sweet onion, sliced into long slivers
½ teaspoon sea salt
4 cups green beans, stems removed
1 tablespoon diced fresh rosemary
4 large garlic cloves, crushed and diced
2 tablespoons low-sodium vegetable broth (or water)
1 tablespoon extra virgin olive oil
1 tablespoon balsamic vinegar

Heat a sauté pan to medium-high heat. Add the avocado oil, onion, and salt, and sauté for 2 minutes, until the onion softens. Stir in the green beans and rosemary and cover, stirring occasionally, for 2 minutes more, until the green beans are nearly done. Reduce the heat to medium-low. Add the garlic and vegetable broth, stir, and cook for about 2 minutes, until the green beans are tender.

In a serving bowl, toss the green bean mixture with the olive oil and balsamic vinegar and serve.

CALORIES: 112
PROTEIN: 2.5 G
FAT: 7 G
CARBS: 12 G
FIBER: 4 G
SODIUM: 292 MG

Desserts

PEAR, CHOCOLATE, AND NUT DELIGHT

This dessert is good for your brain—a simple combination of dark chocolate, nuts, and fruit. I love this combo, but experiment with your own flavor favorites.

PREP TIME: 10 to 15 minutes

Serves: 4

4 ounces dark chocolate (at least 74% cacao)
2 tablespoons organic unsalted butter
2 ounces almonds
2 ounces pecans
2 medium Bosc pears, cut into ¾-inch cubes
2 medium apples, cut into ¾-inch cubes

Heat a small saucepan to medium-low heat. Add the chocolate and butter and stir until melted and blended. Remove from the heat. Meanwhile, in a sauté pan over medium heat, toast the almonds and pecans until warm and fragrant. Remove from the heat and set aside.

Place the almonds, pecans, pears, and apples on a plate. Drizzle the chocolate sauce over the nuts and fruit, then allow to cool before serving.

CALORIES: 458
PROTEIN: 7 G
FAT: 32 G
CARBS: 44 G
FIBER: 10 G
SODIUM: 2 MG

FRUIT CRUMBLE

Here is a dessert I look forward to serving. You can combine a variety of fruits (apples, pears, peaches, and berries), and it is loaded with brain-promoting pigments, fiber, and fat, yet it still has a low glycemic load. Be sure to pick organic fruit if they are on the Environmental Working Group's "Dirty Dozen" list (see page 212).

PREP TIME: 20 minutes
BAKING TIME: 15 minutes

Serves: 4

¼ cup port wine
¼ cup fresh lemon juice
1 tablespoon organic lemon zest
2 tablespoons quick-cooking tapioca
¼ teaspoon ground cinnamon
2 medium organic apples, cut into small cubes
2 medium pears, cut into small cubes
2 cups organic blueberries (frozen or fresh)
½ cup sliced almonds

Preheat the oven to 350°F. Combine the port, lemon juice, lemon zest, tapioca, and cinnamon in a saucepan over medium heat and bring to a gentle boil. Add the apples and pears. Stir occasionally for 5 minutes, add the blueberries, remove from the heat, and pour into a pie plate.

While the fruit is cooking, heat a sauté pan to medium heat. Toast the sliced almonds until warm and fragrant, but stop before they brown. Top the fruit mixture in the pie plate with the sliced almonds. Bake for 15 minutes. Serve in small bowls.

CALORIES: 253
PROTEIN: 4 G
FAT: 6 G
CARBS: 47 G
FIBER: 8 G
SODIUM: 3 MG

CHOCOLATE MOUSSE

Here is one of my wife's desserts, and my favorite. It is packed with brain-boosting cocoa and coffee, which give it a rich, delicious taste. Use unprocessed cocoa for greater flavonoid content. Note: Avoid consuming multiple servings as this contains xylitol; consuming excess xylitol can cause gastrointestinal distress.

PREP TIME: 15 minutes
CHILL TIME: 1 to 24 hours

Serves: 6

½ cup freshly brewed organic coffee (espresso or filtered, decaf or regular)
⅓ cup xylitol
⅛ teaspoon sea salt
4 ounces dark chocolate chips (at least 74% cacao, or use a dark chocolate bar)
½ cup unprocessed unsweetened cocoa powder
12 ounces organic silken tofu
3 tablespoons Grand Marnier (or brandy)
3 tablespoons grated orange zest

Heat the coffee, xylitol, and salt in a saucepan, until gently bubbling. Meanwhile, in a food processor, process the chocolate chips and cocoa until finely chopped, almost powdered. With the processor running, slowly pour in the hot coffee mixture and process until the chocolate has melted. Turn off the processor. Add the tofu, Grand Marnier, and 2 tablespoons of the orange zest and process until smooth. Pour into six serving containers, and garnish with the remaining orange zest. Chill in the refrigerator for at least 1 hour and up to 24 hours before serving.

CALORIES: 180
PROTEIN: 5 G
FAT: 8 G
CARBS: 17 G
FIBER: 3 G
SODIUM: 48 MG

Sauces/Broths/Dressings

PESTO SAUCE

I use pesto sauce on seafood, with poultry, and on vegetables. It stores well for 1 to 2 weeks in the refrigerator or up to 3 months in the freezer. Just make sure to pack it into a glass storage container, pour a thin layer of extra virgin olive oil on the top, and seal. You can substitute various nuts, including walnuts and pecans. Dry the fresh basil well in a salad spinner or pat dry with paper towels. Use high-quality Parmesan cheese for the best flavor.

PREP TIME: 15 minutes

Makes: 24 servings

¼ cup pine nuts
¼ cup almonds, preferably skinned
3 cups packed fresh basil leaves (stems removed)
4 large garlic cloves, peeled and smashed
½ teaspoon ground black pepper
½ cup extra virgin olive oil
½ cup grated Parmesan cheese (about 1¾ ounces)
⅛ to ¼ teaspoon fine sea salt (to taste)

Place the pine nuts and almonds in a food processor; pulse for 15 seconds. Add the basil, garlic, and pepper and process for another 15 seconds. With the food processor running, slowly pour in the oil until the pesto is thoroughly mixed. Add the Parmesan cheese and salt and pulse until the pesto is smooth, about 1 minute. Add salt to taste.

CALORIES: 70
PROTEIN: 2 G
FAT: 7 G
CARBS: 1 G
FIBER: 0 G
SODIUM: 54 MG

Note: Glass storage containers can break in your freezer. To avoid breakage, always use straight-sided containers, leave plenty of room at the top of the jar to allow for the contents to expand, and cool hot jars in the fridge before placing them in the freezer.

HOLLANDAISE SAUCE

This warm sauce elevates simple green vegetables such as broccoli with its rich but clean flavor. Use it all at one meal because it won't keep well.

PREP TIME: 5 minutes

Makes: ½ cup

¼ cup organic salted butter
2 large organic, cage-free egg yolks
¼ teaspoon Dijon mustard
1 tablespoon fresh lemon juice

In a double boiler, heat the butter until melted. (If you don't have a double boiler, heat a small saucepan over low heat.) Whisk in the remaining ingredients until smooth. Keep the sauce warm until ready to serve.

CALORIES: 289
PROTEIN: 3 G
FAT: 28 G
CARBS: 11 G
FIBER: 0.5 G
SODIUM: 188 MG

MUSHROOM GRAVY

This is a dish we enjoy serving over the holidays, and it goes nicely with the Pecan Nut Loaf (page 278). Leftovers freeze very well for up to one month; however, refrigerated mushroom gravy should be consumed within a couple of days. I like to use shiitake or baby portobello mushrooms, but you can make this gravy with any mushroom.

PREP TIME: 20 minutes

Serves: 6

2 tablespoons organic ghee (clarified butter)
1 medium sweet onion, chopped
4 cups sliced mushrooms (such as baby portobellos)
1 teaspoon Italian herb seasoning
2 tablespoons almond flour/meal
⅓ cup marsala wine (or any dry wine)
4 medium garlic cloves, crushed and diced
1 tablespoon tamari sauce
2 cups low-sodium vegetable broth

Heat a large sauté pan to medium-high heat. Add the ghee, onion, and mushrooms, stirring occasionally, until the onion turns translucent and the mushrooms soften, 3 to 4 minutes. Reduce the heat to medium, stir in the Italian herbs and almond flour, and heat for another 2 minutes. Add the marsala, garlic, and tamari sauce, and stir. Allow to simmer for 2 to 3 minutes. Add the vegetable broth, turn up the heat, and bring to a gentle boil. Reduce the heat and simmer for 5 minutes. Remove from the heat. Carefully transfer to a blender and puree until smooth. Serve immediately, store in the refrigerator for not more than 2 to 3 days, or freeze for up to a month.

CALORIES: 89
PROTEIN: 3 G
FAT: 5 G
CARBS: 7 G
FIBER: 1 G
SODIUM: 267 MG

VEGETABLE BROTH

I save onion skins and trimmed vegetable stems for preparing my own low-sodium vegetable broth, which I use in many recipes.

PREP TIME: 20 minutes
SIMMERING TIME: 1 to 4 hours

Makes: 2 quarts

2 medium onions, chopped
2 cups sliced mushrooms (such as button or crimini)
1 cup small red potatoes (or sweet potatoes), cut into 1-inch pieces
2 medium celery stalks, chopped
2 medium carrots, chopped
1 cup tomatoes, chopped
1 tablespoon Italian herb seasoning
1 tablespoon sea salt
½ teaspoon ground black pepper
2 quarts filtered water

Combine all the ingredients in a large pot. Bring to a gentle boil, then simmer for 1 to 4 hours. Skim off any foam that forms on the surface. When it is ready, pour the mixture through a screen, saving the liquid. Discard the vegetable contents. Use immediately, or store in a glass dressing container for a few days in the refrigerator, or for months in the freezer.

CALORIES: 5
PROTEIN: 0 G
FAT: 0 G
CARBS: 0 G
FIBER: 0 G
SODIUM: 402 MG

Note: Glass storage containers can break in your freezer. To avoid breakage, always use straight-sided containers, leave plenty of room at the top of the jar to allow for the contents to expand, and cool hot jars in the fridge before placing them in the freezer.

MASLEY HOUSE VINAIGRETTE DRESSING

Here is the quick, easy, and flavorful dressing I use at home most of the time. You can also use walnut or pistachio oil with a light vinegar.

Makes: 3 servings

3 tablespoons extra virgin olive oil
1 tablespoon balsamic vinegar (or red wine or champagne vinegar)
1 tablespoon dry white wine
1 medium garlic clove, crushed and minced
1 teaspoon Italian herb seasoning (or 1 tablespoon fresh herbs finely diced—parsley, thyme, basil, rosemary)
¼ teaspoon sea salt
¼ teaspoon ground black pepper

Combine all the ingredients in a covered glass jar, shake, and serve. Store in the refrigerator for not more than 2 to 3 days if it includes garlic and fresh herbs; just oil and vinegar will store refrigerated for months, but allow 20 minutes to warm at room temperature before tossing with salad.

CALORIES: 129
PROTEIN: 0 G
FAT: 14 G
CARBS: 1 G
FIBER: 0 G
SODIUM: 178 MG

Heart Rate (HR) Targets by Age

AGE	TARGET HR ZONE, 60–85%	AVERAGE MAXIMUM HR, 100%
20–29 years	120–170 beats per minute	200 beats per minute
30–34 years	114–162 beats per minute	190 beats per minute
35–39 years	111–157 beats per minute	185 beats per minute
40–44 years	108–153 beats per minute	180 beats per minute
45–49 years	105–149 beats per minute	175 beats per minute
50–54 years	102–145 beats per minute	170 beats per minute
55–59 years	99–140 beats per minute	165 beats per minute
60–64 years	96–136 beats per minute	160 beats per minute
65–69 years	93–132 beats per minute	155 beats per minute
70–74 years	90–128 beats per minute	150 beats per minute
75–79 years	87–123 beats per minute	145 beats per minute
80-plus years	84–119 beats per minute	140 beats per minute

Curcumin Absorption

Curcumin has very poor absorption. Some nutraceutical companies have added black pepper (bioperine) in supplement form to curcumin to enhance its absorption; however, black pepper may have some modest negative gastrointestinal side effects, and the level to which it increases absorption is controversial, with some scientists claiming it has only a minimal effect.

Combining curcumin with medium-chain triglycerides and lecithin has been shown to increase its absorption dramatically compared to a dry standard form of curcumin. Some studies suggest a nearly thirtyfold increase in absorption. Visit www.DrMasley.com/resources for product details.

ACKNOWLEDGMENTS

Numerous people have made this book possible, and I am deeply grateful for their assistance.

Many thanks to my literary agent, Celeste Fine, and her colleague John Mass; they were inspirational in selecting this topic and guided me throughout the production of this book.

I owe a special thanks to Victoria Wilson, my senior editor at Knopf, who appreciated this book from the beginning, has provided superb guidance, and has endeavored to ensure this book provides a powerful and important message. I also feel fortunate to have worked with Becky Cabaza, a talented and experienced writer, who helped me organize complex information and technical concepts into an easy-to-read and lively discussion.

I am grateful to Karen Roth and Rachelle Benzarti, the medical library staff at Morton Plant Hospital in Clearwater, Florida, for helping me to research thousands of articles that were seminal for the writing of this book.

My extended support team has been a wonderful source of ideas and support for this book. Special thanks to JJ Virgin, Karl Krummenacher, Alan Christianson, Leanne Ely, Ellyne Lonergan, Alan Foster, and members within my JJ Virgin Mastermind and Mindshare Summit community.

Several medical colleagues scheduled interviews with me to discuss material related to this book. I'd especially like to thank David Perlmutter, MD; Daniel Amen, MD; Anna Cabecca, DO; Pedram Shojai, OMD; Emeran Mayer, MD; and David Asprey.

During the last twenty years, my research has been supported by numerous organizations, including the American College of Nutrition, the American Heart Association, Morton Plant Hospital, and Group Health Cooperative, as well as had collaboration from medical colleagues, including: Richard Roetzheim, MD; Douglas Schocken, MD; Tom Gualtieri, MD; Lucas Masley, BS; and Angie Presby, BS. I am grateful for their time and consideration.

I have also been assisted by a group who tested and reviewed many of the recipes in this book. First and foremost is my wife, Nicole, who tested every recipe in this book. I would also like to thank my sons, Marcos and Lucas Masley; Brooke Masley; Evelyn Odegaard; Susan Thomas; Peggy and Arpad Masley; Joseph Pellicer; Kelvie Johnson; Patti Razor; and Burck Schultz, for their feedback and help in cooking and tasting various recipes.

I would also like to extend a special thanks to my patients. Not only have they agreed to participate in studies at my clinic, providing me with invaluable data, but they have also helped me convert this technical information into everyday words that empower people along a path to being mentally sharper; their struggles and triumphs continue to be my inspiration. My current medical team at the Masley Optimal Health Center has been very supportive in creating this manuscript, with special thanks to Angie Presby, Jessica Maguire, Claudia Marin, Michael Bologna, and Nicole Masley, plus extra thanks to my office coordinator, Kim Escarraz, who has had an invaluable role in supporting everything I do.

Last, thanks to my loving wife, Nicole. Not only has she aided my research, patient care, and recipe writing, but she has supported me in every aspect of my life.

BETTER BRAIN RESOURCES

As promised, here is my list of resources and sites to make it easier for you to improve your brain performance and prevent memory loss.

Website

To receive updated information and to join my online community, please visit www.DrMasley.com and enter your name and e-mail—it's free.

Masley Optimal Health Center
900 Carillon Parkway, Suite 201
St. Petersburg, FL 33716
www.clinic.DrMasley.com
Toll-free: 844-300-2973

Information Tools

For information related to carotid intimal media thickness (IMT) testing, oil smoke points, gluten testing, curcumin, strength training, fitness testing, mercury and chelation therapy, meditation, and HeartMath—please visit www .DrMasley.com/resources.

Products and Supplements

For educational products and high-quality supplements, visit www.DrMas leyStore.com.

Food and Shopping Sources
For links to:

- Thrive Market—discount healthy food items and condiments, such as almond flour, avocado oil, extra virgin olive oil, herbs, and spices
- Vital Choice Seafood—a wonderful source of clean seafood
- ButcherBox—a source of clean animal protein

—please visit www.DrMasley.com/resources.

Chapter 1: Origins of Memory Loss

8   **The intervention group, however, improved:** S. C. Masley et al., "Efficacy of Exercise and Diet to Modify Markers of Fitness and Wellness," *Alternative Therapies in Health and Medicine* 14 (2008): 24–29.

14 **People who are vaccinated:** R. Verrealt et al., "Past Exposure to Vaccines and Subsequent Risk of Alzheimer's Disease," *Canadian Medical Association Journal* 165 (2001): 1495–98; and A. C. Voordouw et al., "Annual Revaccination Against Influenza and Mortality Risk in Community-Dwelling Elderly Persons," *Journal of the American Medical Association* 292 (2004): 2089–95.

17 **a condition called insulin resistance:** R. Williamson, A. McNeilly, and C. Sutherland, "Insulin Resistance in the Brain: And Old-Age or New-Age Problem?" *Biochemical Pharmacology* 84 (2012): 737–45; and S. Cetinkalp, I. Y. Simsir, and S. Ertek, "Insulin Resistance in Brain and Possible Therapeutic Approaches," *Current Vascular Pharmacology* 12 (2014): 553–64.

17 **those with the highest levels of insulin:** A. A. Willette et al., "Association of Insulin Resistance with Cerebral Glucose Uptake in Late Middle-Aged Adults at Risk for Alzheimer disease," *JAMA Neurology* 72 (2015): 1013–20. See also L.D. Baker et al., "Insulin Resistance Is Associated with Alzheimer-like Reductions in Regional Cerebral Glucose Metabolism for Cognitively Normal Adults with Pre-Diabetes or Early Type 2 Diabetes," *Archives of Neurology* 68 (2011): 51–57; and T. Matsuzaki et al., "Insulin Resistance Is Associated with the Pathology of Alzheimer's Disease," *Neurology* 75 (2010): 764–70.

18 **uncontrolled blood sugar:** P. K. Crane et al., "Glucose Levels and Risk of Dementia," *New England Journal of Medicine* 369 (2013): 540–48; and E. Ronnemaa et al., "Impaired Insulin Secretion Increases the Risk of Alzheimer Disease," *Neurology* 71 (2008): 1065–71.

19 **Melissa Schilling:** M. A. Schilling, "Unraveling Alzheimer's: Making Sense of the Relationship between Diabetes and Alzheimer's Disease," *Journal of Alzheimer's Disease* 51 (2016): 961–77.

20 **The Maastricht Aging Study:** P. J. Spauwen et al., "Effects of Type

2 Diabetes on 12-Year Cognitive Change," *Diabetes Care* 36 (2013): 1554–61.

21 **In animal studies:** S. M. De la Monte, "Type 3 Diabetes Is Sporadic Alzheimer's Disease: Mini-Review," *European Neuropsychopharmacology* 24 (2014): 1954–60; and S. M. De la Monte and J. R. Wands, "Alzheimer's Disease Is Type 3 Diabetes—Evidence Reviewed," *Journal of Diabetes Science and Technology* 2 (2008): 1101–13.

22 **Metabolic syndrome reflects:** See J. Bajerska et al., "Eating Patterns Are Associated with Cognitive Function in the Elderly at Risk of Metabolic Syndrome from Rural Areas," *European Review for Medical and Pharmacological Sciences* 18 (2014): 3234–45; B. Misiak, J. Leszek, and A. Kiejna, "Metabolic Syndrome, Mild Cognitive Impairment and Alzheimer's Disease—The Emerging Role of Systemic Low-Grade Inflammation and Adiposity," *Brain Research Bulletin* 89 (2012): 144–49; G. M. Pasinetti and J. Eberstein, "Metabolic Syndrome and the Role of Dietary Lifestyles in Alzheimer's Disease," *Journal of Neurochemistry* 106 (2008): 1503–14; and C. Raffaitin et al., "Metabolic Syndrome and Risk for Incident Alzheimer's Disease or Vascular Dementia," *Diabetes Care* 32 (2009): 169–74.

23 **Kaiser Permanente study:** P. E. Casey et al., "Controlling High Blood Pressure," *Permanente Journal* 10 (2006): 13–16.

23 **Honolulu-Asia Aging study:** L. J. Launer et al., "Midlife Blood Pressure and Dementia: The Honolulu-Asia Aging Study," *Neurobiology of Aging* 21 (2000): 49–55.

23 **The landmark Rotterdam Study:** R. F. De Bruijn et al., "The Potential for Prevention of Dementia Across Two Decades: The Prospective, Population-Based Rotterdam Study," *BMC Medicine* 13 (2015): 132.

23 **follow-up studies:** A. Ott et al., "Association of Diabetes Mellitus and Dementia: The Rotterdam Study," *Diabetologia* 39 (1996): 1392–97.

24 **Our clinic database:** S. C. Masley, L. V. Masley, and T. Gualtieri, "Cardiovascular Biomarkers and Carotid IMT Scores as Predictors of Cognitive Function," *Journal of the American College of Nutrition* 33 (2014): 63–69.

Chapter 2: How Sharp Is Your Brain?

33 **Sample questions include:** For a full list of the questions, see http://www.dementiatoday.com/wp-content/uploads/2012/06/MiniMental StateExamination.pdf.

41 **patients in their seventies and eighties:** Sandra Levy, "Study: Concussions Lead to Increased Dementia Risk in Older Adults," *HealthLine*, October 29, 2014.

44   **In 2014, I published a paper:** S. C. Masley, L. V. Masley, and T. Gualtieri, "Cardiovascular Biomarkers and Carotid IMT Scores as Predictors of Cognitive Function," *Journal of the American College of Nutrition* 33 (2014): 63–69.

48   **The ApoE2 genotype:** R. Chouinard-Watkins and M. Plourde, "Fatty Acid Metabolism in Carriers of Apolipoprotein E Epsilon 4 Allele: Is It Contributing to Higher Risk of Cognitive Decline and Coronary Heart Disease?" *Nutrients* 6 (2014): 4452–71. See also J. Dose et al., "ApoE Genotype and Stress Response—A Mini Review," *Lipids in Health and Disease* 15 (2016): n.p.; and S. Egert, G. Rimbach, and P. Huebbe, "ApoE Genotype: From Geographic Distribution to Function and Responsiveness to Dietary Factors," *Proceedings of the Nutrition Society* 71 (2012): 410–24.

50   **controlling blood sugar:** A. Hofman et al., "Atherosclerosis, Apolipoprotein E, and Prevalence of Dementia and Alzheimer's Disease in the Rotterdam Study," *Lancet* 349 (1997): 151–54; and M.A. Schilling, "Unraveling Alzheimer's: Making Sense of the Relationship Between Diabetes and Alzheimer's Disease," *Journal of Alzheimer's Disease* 51 (2016): 961–77.

50   **simply delaying its onset:** R. Brookmeyer, S. Gray, and C. Kawas, "Projections of Alzheimer's Disease in the United States and the Public Health Impact of Delaying Disease Onset," *American Journal of Public Health* 88 (1998): 1337–42.

Part II: The Better Brain Solution

54   **The FINGER study from Finland:** T. Ngandu et al., "A 2 Year Multidomain Intervention of Diet, Exercise, Cognitive Training, and Vascular Risk Monitoring Versus Control to Prevent Cognitive Decline in At-Risk Elderly People (FINGER): A Randomised Control Panel," *Lancet* 385 (2015): 2255–63.

55   **Dr. Bredesen's program:** D. E. Bredesen, "Reversal of Cognitive Decline: A Novel Therapeutic Program," *Aging* 9 (2014): 707–17.

55   **a varied approach shows the most promise:** M. Baumgart et al., "Summary of the Evidence on Modifiable Risk Factors for Cognitive Decline and Dementia," *Alzheimer's and Dementia* 11 (2015): 718–26.

55   **food choices that are heart-healthy:** "Prevention and Risk of Alzheimer's and Dementia," Alzheimer's Association (n.d.), http://www.alz.org /research/science/alzheimers_prevention_and_risk.asp#exercise.

Chapter 3: Boost Your Brain with 12 Smart Foods

61　**a study performed in Australia:** E. L. Wightman et al., "Dietary Nitrate Modulates Cerebral Blood Flow Parameters and Cognitive Performance in Humans: A Double-Blind, Placebo-Controlled, Crossover Investigation," *Physiology and Behavior* 149 (2015): 149–58.

62　**greater long-chain omega-3 intake correlates:** V. A. Andreeva et al., "Cognitive Function After Supplementation with B Vitamins and Long-Chain Omega-3 Fatty Acids: Ancillary Findings from the SU.FOL.OM3 Randomized Trial," *American Journal of Clinical Nutrition* 94 (2011): 278–86; E. Y. Chew et al., "Effect of Omega-3 Fatty Acids, Lutein/Zeaxanthin, or Other Nutrient Supplementation on Cognitive Function," *JAMA* 314 (2015): 791–801; L. K. Lee et al., "Docosahexaenoic Acid-Concentrated Fish Oil Supplementation in Subjects with Mild Cognitive Impairment (MCI): A 12-Month Randomised, Double-Blind, Placebo-Controlled Trial," *Psychopharmacology* 225 (2013): 605–12; M. C. Morris et al., "Fish Consumption and Cognitive Decline with Age in a Large Community Study," *Archives of Neurology* 62 (2005): 1849–53; K. A. Page et al., "Medium-Chain Fatty Acids Improve Cognitive Function in Intensively Treated Type 1 Diabetic Patients and Support in Vitro Synaptic Transmission During Acute Hypoglycemia," *Diabetes* 58 (2009): 1237–44; B. Qin et al., "Fish Intake Is Associated with Slower Cognitive Decline in Chinese Older Adults," *Journal of Nutrition* 144 (2014): 1579–85; K. W. Shepard and C. L. Cheatham. "Omega-6 to Omega-3 Fatty Acid Ratio and Higher-Order Cognitive Functions in 7- to 9-Year-Olds: A Cross-Sectional Study," *American Journal of Clinical Nutrition* 98 (2013): 659–67; L. Shinto et al., "A Randomized Placebo-Controlled Pilot Trial of Omega-3 Fatty Acids and Alpha Lipoic Acid in Alzheimer's Disease," *Journal of Alzheimer's Disease* 38 (2014): n.p.; J. Thomas et al., "Omega-3 Fatty Acids in Early Prevention of Inflammatory Neurodegenerative Disease: A Focus on Alzheimer's Disease," *BioMed Research International* 2015 (2015): n.p.; H. Tokuda et al., "Low Doses of Long-Chain Polyunsaturated Fatty Acids Affect Cognitive Function in Elderly Japanese Men: A Randomized Controlled Trial," *Journal of Oleo Science* 64 (2015): 633–44; O. Van de Rest et al., "ApoE4 and the Associations of Seafood and Long-Chain Omega-3 Fatty Acids with Cognitive Decline," *Neurology* 86 (2016): 2063–70; A. V. Witte et al., "Long-Chain Omega-3 Fatty Acids Improve Brain Function and Structure in Older Adults," *Cerebral Cortex* 24 (2013): 3059–68; and Y. Zhang et al., "Intake of Fish and Polyunsaturated Fatty Acids and Mild-to-Severe Cognitive Impairment

Risks: A Dose-Response Meta-Analysis of 21 Cohort Studies," *American Journal of Clinical Nutrition* 103 (2016): 330–40.

63 **Higher-quality pure supplements:** D. Swanson, R. Block, and S. A. Mousa, "Omega-3 Fatty Acids EPA and DHA: Health Benefits Throughout Life," *Advances in Nutrition* 3 (2012): 1–7; N. Sinn et al., "Effects of n-3 Fatty Acids, EPA v. DHA, on Depressive Symptoms, Quality of Life, Memory and Executive Function in Older Adults with Mild Cognitive Impairment: A 6-Month Randomised Controlled Trial," *British Journal of Nutrition* 107 (2012): 1682–93; and J. Allaire et al., "Randomized, Crossover, Head-to-Head Comparison of EPA and DHA Supplementation to Reduce Inflammation Markers in Men and Women: The Comparing EPA to DHA Study," *American Journal of Clinical Nutrition* (2016): n.p.

64 **children appear to benefit:** W. Stonehouse, "Does Consumption of LC Omega-3 PUFA Enhance Cognitive Performance in Healthy School-Aged Children and Throughout Adulthood? Evidence from Clinical Trials," *Nutrients* 6 (2014): 2730–58.

64 **Predimed-Navarra study:** E. H. Martinez-Lapiscina et al., "Mediterranean Diet Improves Cognition: The PREDIMED-NAVARRA Randomized Trial," *BMJ* 84 (2012): online.

67 **with or without walnuts:** S. M. Poulose, M.G. Miller, and B. Shukitt-Hale, "Role of Walnuts in Maintaining Brain Health with Age," *Journal of Nutrition* 144 (2014): 561S–65; and P. Pribis et al., "Effects of Walnut Consumption on Cognitive Performance in Young Adults," *British Journal of Nutrition* 107 (2012): 1393–401.

68 **Feeding children blueberry-rich:** A. R. Whyte et al., "Cognitive Effects Following Acute Wild Blueberry Supplementation in 7- to 10-Year-Old Children," *European Journal of Nutrition* 55 (2016): 2151–62.

68 **older adults showed:** R. Krikorian et al., "Blueberry Supplementation Improves Memory in Older Adults," *Journal of Agricultural and Food Chemistry* 58 (2010): 3996–4000.

68 **blueberries have been shown to reduce:** Y. Zhu et al., "Blueberry Opposes B-Amyloid Peptide-Induced Microglial Activation via Inhibition of p44/42 Mitogen-Activation Protein Kinase," *Rejuvenation Research* 11 (2008): 891–901.

68 **cocoa intake improves:** Ibid.

68 **eight weeks of daily cocoa:** D. Mastroiacovo et al., "Cocoa Flavanol Consumption Improves Cognitive Function, Blood Pressure Control, and Metabolic Profile in Elderly Subjects: The Cocoa, Cognition, and Aging (CoCoA) Study—A Randomized Controlled Trial," *American Journal of Clinical Nutrition* 101 (2015): 538–48.

68   **Dark, unprocessed cocoa:** M. Alonso-Alonso, "Cocoa Flavanols and Cognition: Regaining Chocolate in Old Age?" *American Journal of Clinical Nutrition* 101 (2015): 423–24.

69   **Physicians' Health Study:** C. Matsumoto et al., "Chocolate Consumption and Risk of Diabetes Mellitus in the Physicians' Health Study," *American Journal of Clinical Nutrition* 101 (2015): 362–67.

70   **Caffeine increases information:** S. Haller et al., "Acute Caffeine Administration Effect on Brain Activation Patterns in Mild Cognitive Impairment," *Journal of Alzheimer's Disease* 41 (2014): 101–12.

70   **a J-shaped-curve relationship:** L. Wu, D. Sun, and Y. He, "Coffee Intake and the Incident Risk of Cognitive Disorders: A Dose-Response Meta-Analysis of Nine Prospective Cohort Studies," *Clinical Nutrition* 36 (2016): 730–36.

70   **in Japan, a study:** K. Sugiyama et al., "Association Between Coffee Consumption and Incident Risk of Disabling Dementia in Elderly Japanese: The Ohsaki Cohort 2006 Study," *Journal of Alzheimer's Disease* 50 (2016): 491–500.

70   **women display less cognitive:** M. N. Vercambre et al., "Caffeine and Cognitive Decline in Elderly Women at High Vascular Risk," *Journal of Alzheimer's Disease* 35 (2013): 413–21; and L. Arab, F. Khan, and H. Lam, "Epidemiologic Evidence of a Relationship Between Tea, Coffee, or Caffeine Consumption and Cognitive Decline," *Advances in Nutrition* 4 (2013): 115–22.

70   **Even decaf coffee:** D. A. Camfield, "A Randomised Placebo-Controlled Trial to Differentiate the Acute Cognitive and Mood Effects of Chlorogenic Acid from Decaffeinated Coffee," *PLoS One,* December 9, 2013: online.

70   **If you like drinking coffee:** For more information, see L. F. Araujo et al., "Inconsistency of Association Between Coffee Consumption and Cognitive Function in Adults and Elderly in a Cross-Sectional Study (ELSA-Brasil)," *Nutrients* 7 (2015): 9590–601; F. L. Dodd et al., "A Double-Blinded, Placebo-Controlled Study Evaluating the Effects of Caffeine and L-Theanine Both Alone and in Combination on Cerebral Blood Flow, Cognition and Mood," *Psychopharmacology* 232 (2015): 2563–76; and Q. P. Liu et al., "Habitual Coffee Consumption and Risk of Cognitive Decline/Dementia: A Systematic Review and Meta-Analysis of Prospective Cohort Studies," *Nutrition* 32 (2016): 628–36.

71   **97 mg of L-theanine:** T. Giesbrecht et al., "The Combination of L–theanine and Caffeine Improves Cognitive Performance and Increases Subjective Alertness," *Nutritional Neuroscience* 13 (2010): 283–90. See also S. J. Einother and V. E. Martens, "Acute Effects of Tea Consump-

tion on Attention and Mood," *American Journal of Clinical Nutrition* 98 (2013): 1700S–85; and D. J. White et al., "Anti-Stress, Behavioural and Magnetoencephalography Effect of an L-Theanine-Based Nutrient Drink: A Randomised, Double-Blind, Placebo-Controlled, Crossover Trial," *Nutrients* 8 (2016): 53.

72 **slow caffeine metabolizers' results:** *JAMA* and *Archives Journals,* "Coffee Consumption Linked to Increased Risk of Heart Attack for Persons with Certain Gene Variation," *Science Daily* (2006): online.

74 **those who consume alcohol:** M. A. Collins et al., "Alcohol in Moderation, Cardioprotection, and Neuroprotection: Epidemiological Considerations and Mechanistic Studies," *Alcoholism: Clinical and Experimental Research* 33 (2009): 206–19.

74 **New York City residents:** Y. Gu et al., "Alcohol Intake and Brain Structure in a Multiethnic Elderly Cohort," *Clinical Nutrition* 33 (2014): 662–67.

74 **In Australia, researchers:** O. P. Almeida et al., "Alcohol Consumption and Cognitive Impairment in Older Men," *Neurology* 82 (2014): 1038–44.

74 **A study in the Netherlands:** A.C.J. Nooyens et al., "Consumption of Alcoholic Beverages and Cognitive Decline at Middle Age: The Doestinchem Cohort Study," *British Journal of Nutrition* 111 (2014): 715–23.

75 **In France, researchers:** E. Kesse–Guyot et al., "A Healthy Dietary Pattern at Midlife Is Associated with Subsequent Cognitive Performance," *Journal of Nutrition* 142 (2012): 909–15.

77 **Garlic:** V. B. Gupta, S. S. Indi, and K.S.J. Rao, "Garlic Extract Exhibits Antiamyloidogenic Activity on Amyloid-Beta Fibrillogenesis: Relevance to Alzheimer's Disease," *Phytotherapy Research* 23 (2009): 111–15.

77 **Cinnamon:** B. Qin, K. S. Panickar, and R. A. Anderson, "Cinnamon: Potential Role in the Prevention of Insulin Resistance, Metabolic Syndrome, and Type 2 Diabetes," *Journal of Diabetes Science and Technology* 4 (2010): 685–93.

79 **They have the highest:** H. Wang et al., "Oxygen Radical Absorbing Capacity of Anthocyanins," *Journal of Agricultural and Food Chemistry* 45 (1997): 304–9. See also D. Li et al., "Purified Anthocyanin Supplementation Reduces Dyslipidemia, Enhances Antioxidant Capacity, and Prevents Insulin Resistance in Diabetic Patients," *Journal of Nutrition* 145 (2015): 742–48.

79 **eating legumes can even improve:** D. J. Jenkins et al., "Rate of Digestion of Foods and Postprandial Glycaemia in Normal and Diabetic Subjects," *BMJ* 281 (1980): 14–17; and V. Mohan et al., "Effects of Brown Rice, White Rice, and Brown Rice with Legumes on Blood Glucose and

Insulin Responses in Overweight Asian Indians: A Randomized Controlled Trial," *Diabetes Technology and Therapeutics* 16 (2014): 317–25.

80 **the gut microbiome:** See, for example, B. Caracciolo et al., "Cognitive Decline, Dietary Factors and Gut-Brain Interactions," *Mechanisms of Ageing and Development* 136 (2014): 59–69.

80 **weight gain:** A.V. Hart, "Insights into the Role of the Microbiome in Obesity and Type 2 Diabetes," *Diabetes Care* 38 (2015): 159–65.

81 **stomach acid is essential:** http://www.medscape.com/viewarticle /858909; and C. Bavishi and H. L. Dupont, "Systematic Review: The Use of Proton Pump Inhibitors and Increased Susceptibility to Enteric Infection," *Alimentary Pharmacology and Therapeutics* 34 (2011): 11–12.

88 **Martha Clare Morris:** M. C. Morris et al., "MIND Diet Slows Cognitive Decline with Aging," *Alzheimer's and Dementia* 11 (2015): 1015–22.

89 **when you combine saturated fat:** A. Chait and F. Kim, "Saturated Fatty Acids and Inflammation: Who Pays the Toll?" *Arteriosclerosis, Thrombosis, and Vascular Biology* 30 (2010): 692–93; M. Funaki, "Saturated Fatty Acids and Insulin Resistance," *Journal of Medical Investigation* 56 (2009): 88–92; and M.A.R. Vinolo et al., "Regulation of Inflammation by Short Chain Fatty Acids," *Nutrients* 3 (2011): 858–76.

89 **Veterans Affairs Medical Center:** A. J. Hanson et al., "Effect of Apolipoprotein E Genotype and Diet on Apolipoprotein E Lipidation and Amyloid Peptides," *JAMA Neurology* 70 (2013): 972–80.

90 **eating more saturated fat:** D. D. Wang et al., "Association of Specific Dietary Fats with Total and Cause-Specific Mortality," *JAMA Internal Medicine* 176 (2016): 1134–45; and S. J. Nicholls et al., "Consumption of Saturated Fat Impairs the Anti-Inflammatory Properties of High-Density Lipoproteins and Endothelial Function," *Journal of the American College of Cardiology* 48 (2006): 715–20.

93 **the Mediterranean diet:** Y. Gu et al., "Mediterranean Diet and Brain Structure in a Multiethnic Elderly Cohort," *Neurology* (October 21, 2015): online; Y. Gu et al., "Mediterranean Diet, Inflammatory and Metabolic Biomarkers, and Risk of Alzheimer's Disease," *Journal of Alzheimer's Disease* 22 (2010): 483–92; A. Knight, J. Bryan, and K. Murphy, "Is the Mediterranean Diet a Feasible Approach to Preserving Cognitive Function and Reducing Risk of Dementia for Older Adults in Western Countries? New Insights and Future Directions," *Ageing Research Reviews* 25 (2016): 85–101; A. Knight et al., "A Randomised Controlled Intervention Trial Evaluating the Efficacy of a Mediterranean Dietary Pattern on Cognitive Function and Psychological Well-being in Healthy Older Adults: The Medley Study," *BMC Geriatrics* 15 (2015): 55; M. Luciano et al., "Mediterranean-Type Diet and Brain

Structural Change from 73 to 76 Years in Scottish Cohort," *Neurology* 88 (2017): 1–7; C. Samieri et al., "Mediterranean Diet and Cognitive Function in Older Age: Results from the Women's Health Study," *Epidemiology* 24 (2013): 490–99; C. Valls-Pedret et al., "Mediterranean Diet and Age-Related Cognitive Decline: A Randomized Clinical Trial," *JAMA Internal Medicine* 175 (2015): 1094–103; H. Wengreen et al., "Prospective Study of Dietary Approaches to Stop Hypertension and Mediterranean-Style Dietary Patterns and Age-Related Cognitive Change: The Cache County Study on Memory, Health and Aging," *American Journal of Clinical Nutrition* 98 (2013): 1263–71; and X. Ye et al., "Mediterranean Diet, Health Eating Index–2005, and Cognitive Function in Middle-Aged and Older Puerto Rican Adults," *Journal of the Academy of Nutrition and Dietetics* 113 (2013): 276–81.

Chapter 4: More Ways to Feed Your Brain

98 **middle-aged, overweight women:** D. J. Lamport et al., "A Low Glycaemic Load Breakfast Can Attenuate Cognitive Impairments Observed in Middle Aged Obese Females with Impaired Glucose Tolerance," *Nutrition, Metabolism and Cardiovascular Diseases* 24 (2014): 1128–36; and A. Nilsson, K. Radeborg, and I. Bjorck, "Effects of Differences in Postprandial Glycaemia on Cognitive Functions in Healthy Middle-Aged Subjects," *European Journal of Clinical Nutrition* 63 (2009): 113–20. See also S. Seetharaman et al., "Blood Glucose, Diet-Based Glycemic Load and Cognitive Aging Among Dementia-Free Older Adults," *Journals of Gerontology. Series A, Biological Sciences and Medical Sciences* 70 (2015): 471–79.

100 **blood sugar responses can vary:** N. R. Matthan et al., "Estimating the Reliability of Glycemic Index Values and Potential Sources of Methodological and Biological Variability," *American Journal of Clinical Nutrition* (2016): online.

110 **partial intermittent fasting:** I. Amigo and A. J. Kowaltowski, "Dietary Restriction in Cerebral Bioenergetics and Redox State," *Redox Biology* 2 (2014): 296–304.

110 **intermittent fasting in mice:** M. P. Mattson, W. Duan, and Z. Guo, "Meal Size and Frequency Affect Neuronal Plasticity and Vulnerability to Disease: Cellular and Molecular Mechanisms," *Journal of Neurochemistry* 84 (2003): 417–31; and Amigo and Kowaltowski, "Dietary Restriction"; and G. Pani, "Neuroprotective Effects of Dietary Restriction: Evidence and Mechanisms," *Seminars in Cell and Developmental Biology* 40 (2015): 106–14.

110 **this method of alternating fasting:** M. P. Wegman et al., "Practicality of Intermittent Fasting in Humans and Its Effect on Oxidative Stress and Genes Related to Aging and Metabolism," *Rejuvenation Research* 18 (2015): 162–72.

111 **Those on the very-low-carb diet:** R. Krikorian et al., "Dietary Ketosis Enhances Memory in Mild Cognitive Impairment," *Neurobiology of Aging* 33 (2012): 425.e19–425.e27.

114 **Samuel Henderson:** S. T. Henderson and J. Poirier, "Pharmacogenetic Analysis of the Effects of Polymorphisms in APOE, IDE and IL1B on a Ketone Body Based Therapeutic on Cognition in Mild to Moderate Alzheimer's Disease: A Randomized, Double-Blind, Placebo-Controlled Study," *BMC Medical Genetics* 12 (2011): 137; and S.T. Henderson et al., "Study of the Ketogenic Agent AC-1202 in Mild to Moderate Alzheimer's Disease: A Randomized, Double-Blind, Placebo-Controlled, Multicenter Trial," *Nutrition and Metabolism* (London) 6 (2009): 31.

118 **The primary oil component:** Y. Nonaka et al., "Lauric Acid Stimulates Ketone Body Production in the KT-5 Astrocyte Cell Line," *Journal of Oleo Science* 65 (2016): 693–99.

118 **Coconut oil generally:** W.M.A.D.B. Fernando et al., "The Role of Dietary Coconut for the Prevention and Treatment of Alzheimer's Disease: Potential Mechanisms of Action," *British Journal of Nutrition* 114 (2015): 1–14.

Chapter 5: Key Nutrients for Brain Health

125 **low vitamin D levels are:** J. W. Miller et al., "Vitamin D Status and Rates of Cognitive Decline in a Multiethnic Cohort of Older Adults," *JAMA Neurology* 72 (2015): 1295–303. See also C. Annweiler et al., " 'Vitamin D and Cognition in Older Adults': Updated International Recommendations," *Journal of Internal Medicine* 277 (2015): 45–57; and A. K. Gangwar et al., "Role of Vitamin-D in the Prevention and Treatment of Alzheimer's Disease," *Indian Journal of Physiology and Pharmacology* 59 (2015): 94–99.

125 **larger brains:** B. Hooshmand et al., "Vitamin D in Relation to Cognitive Impairment, Cerebrospinal Fluid Biomarkers, and Brain Volumes," *Journals of Gerontology. Series A, Biological Sciences and Medical Sciences* 69 (2014): 1132–38.

129 **treating adults with vitamin B12:** N. L. Van der Zwaluw et al., "Results of 2-Year Vitamin B Treatment on Cognitive Performance," *Neurology* 83 (2014): 2158–66. See also E. L. Doets et al., "Vitamin B12 Intake Status and Cognitive Function in Elderly Patients," *Epidemiologic Reviews*

35 (2013): 2–21; S. J. Eussen et al., "Effect of Oral Vitamin B-12 with or without Folic Acid on Cognitive Function in Older People with Mild Vitamin B-12 Deficiency: A Randomized, Placebo-Controlled Trial," *American Journal of Clinical Nutrition* 84 (2006): 361–70; C. Castillo-Lancellotti et al., "Serum Folate, Vitamin B12 and Cognitive Impairment in Chilean Older Adults," *Public Health Nutrition* 18 (2015): 2600–8; D. Moorthy et al., "Status of B-12 and B-6 but Not of Folate, Homocysteine, and the Methylenetetrahydrofolate Reductase C677T Polymorphism Are Associated with Impaired Cognition and Depression in Adults," *Journal of Nutrition* 142 (2012): 1554–60; R. Clarke et al., "Effects of Homocysteine Lowering with B Vitamins on Cognitive Aging: Meta-Analysis of 11 Trials with Cognitive Data on 22,000 Individuals," *American Journal of Clinical Nutrition* 100 (2014): 657–66; and M. S. Morris, "The Role of B Vitamins in Preventing and Treating Cognitive Impairment and Decline," *Advances in Nutrition* 3 (2012): 801–12.

133 **Consuming rancid fish oil:** B. B. Albert et al., "Fish Oil Supplements in New Zealand Are Highly Oxidised and Do Not Meet Label Content of n-3 PUFA," *Scientific Reports* 5 (2014): n.p.

136 **magnesium L-threonate daily:** G. Liu et al., "Efficacy and Safety of MMFS–01, a Synapse Density Enhancer, for Treating Cognitive Impairment in Older Adults: A Randomized, Double-Blind, Placebo-Controlled Trial," *Journal of Alzheimer's Disease* 49 (2016): 971–90. See also U. Grober, J. Schmidt, and K. Kisters, "Magnesium in Prevention and Therapy," *Nutrients* 7 (2015): 8199–226.

141 **Dr. Katherine Cox:** K.H.M. Cox, A. Pipingas, and A. B. Scholey, "Investigation of the Effects of Solid Lipid Curcumin on Cognition and Mood in a Healthy Older Population," *Journal of Psychopharmacology* 29 (2015): 642–51.

141 **giving curcumin decreased:** S. J. Kim et al., "Curcumin Stimulates Proliferation of Embryonic Neural Progenitor Cells and Neurogenesis in the Adult Hippocampus," *Journal of Biological Chemistry* 283 (2008): 14497–505. See also L. Baum et al., "Six-Month Randomized, Placebo-Controlled, Double-Blind, Pilot Clinical Trial of Curcumin in Patients with Alzheimer Disease," *Journal of Clinical Psychopharmacology* 28 (2008): 110–13; N. Brondino et al., "Curcumin as a Therapeutic Agent in Dementia: A Mini Systemic Review of Human Studies," *Scientific World Journal* 2014 (2014): n.p.; D. Chin et al., "Neuroprotective Properties of Curcumin in Alzheimer's Disease—Merits and Limitations," *Current Medicinal Chemistry* 20 (2013): 3955–85; R. A. DiSilvestro et al., "Diverse Effects of a Low Dose Supplement of Lipidated Curcumin

in Healthy Middle Aged People," *Nutrition Journal* 11 (2012): 79; and K. G. Gooze et al., "Examining the Potential Clinical Value of Curcumin in the Prevention and Diagnosis of Alzheimer's Disease," *British Journal of Nutrition* 115 (2016): 449–65.

141 **no memory benefit:** J. M. Ringman et al., "Oral Curcumin for Alzheimer's Disease: Tolerability and Efficacy in a 24-Week Randomized, Double-Blind, Placebo-Controlled Study," *Alzheimer's Research and Therapy* 4 (2012): 43.

142 **prolonged calorie restriction:** G. Pani, "Neuroprotective Effects of Dietary Restriction: Evidence and Mechanisms," *Seminars in Cell and Developmental Biology* 40 (2015): 106–14.

142 **impact of taking resveratrol:** E. L. Wightman et al., "Effects of Resveratrol Alone or in Combination with Piperine on Cerebral Blood Flow Parameters and Cognitive Performance in Human Subjects: A Randomised, Double-Blind, Placebo-Controlled, Cross-Over Investigation," *British Journal of Nutrition* 112 (2014): 2013–213. See also G. M. Pasinetti et al., "Roles of Resveratrol and Other Grape-Derived Polyphenols in Alzheimer's Disease Prevention and Treatment," *Biochimica Biophysica Acta* 1852 (2015): 1202–8; and A. V. Witte et al., "Effects of Resveratrol on Memory Performance, Hippocampal Function Connectivity, and Glucose Metabolism in Healthy Older Adults," *Journal of Neuroscience* 34 (2014): 7862–70.

142 **only one small study:** R. S. Turner et al., "A Randomised, Double-Blind, Placebo-Controlled Trial of Resveratrol for Alzheimer Disease," *Neurology* 85 (2015): 1383–91.

144 **this compound as it relates:** D. L. Moran et al., "Effects of a Supplement Containing Apoaequorin on Verbal Learning in Older Adults in the Community," *Advances in Mind/Body Medicine* 30 (2016): 4–11.

146 **Coenzyme Q10 (CoQ10, also called):** Y. Momiyama, "Serum Coenzyme Q10 Levels as a Predictor of Dementia in a Japanese General Population," *Atherosclerosis* 237 (2014): 433–34; and L. V. Schottlaender et al., "Coenzyme Q10 Levels Are Decreased in the Cerebellum of Multiple-System Atrophy Patients," *PLoS One* (February 9, 2016): online.

147 **small study conducted in China:** Y. Y. Zhang, L. Q. Yang, and L. M. Geo, "Effect of Phosphatidylserine on Memory in Patients and Rates with Alzheimer's Disease," *Genetics and Molecular Research* 14 (2015): 9325–33. See also M. I. More, U. Freitas, and D. Rutenberg, "Positive Effects of Soy Lecithin–Derived Phosphatidylserine Plus Phosphatidic Acid on Memory, Cognition, Daily Functioning, and Mood in Elderly Patients with Alzheimer's Disease and Dementia," *Advances in Therapy* 31 (2014): 1247–62.

148 **controversy with phosphatidylserine:** B. L. Jorissen et al., "The Influence of Soy-Derived Phosphatidylserine on Cognition in Age-Associated Memory Impairment," *Nutrition Neuroscience* 4 (2001): 121–34.

148 **Huperzine A:** J. Y. Jia et al., "Phase I Study on the Pharmacokinetics and Tolerance of ZT-1, a Prodrug of Huperzine A, for the Treatment of Alzheimer's Disease," *Acta Pharmacologia Sinica* 34 (2013): 976–82.

149 **A twelve-week randomized study:** Z. Q. Xu et al., "Treatment with Huperzine A Improves Cognition in Vascular Dementia," *Cell Biochemistry and Biophysics* 62 (2012): 55–58.

149 **A review of twenty randomized:** G. Yang et al., "Huperzine A for Alzheimer's Disease: A Systematic Review and Meta-Analysis of Randomized Clinical Trials," *PLoS One* (September 23, 2013): online.

Chapter 6: How to Move Your Body for a Better Brain

151 **exercise and brain function:** J. R. Best et al., "Long-Term Effects of Resistance Exercise Training on Cognition and Brain Volume in Older Women," *Journal of the International Neuropsychological Society* 21 (2015): 745–56; R.T.H. Ho et al., "A 3-Arm Randomized Controlled Trial on the Effects of Dance Movement Intervention and Exercises on Elderly with Early Dementia," *BMC Geriatrics* 15 (2015): 127; O. Iyalomhe et al., "A Standardized Randomized 6-Month Aerobic Exercise-Training Down-Regulated Pro-Inflammatory Genes, but Up-Regulated Anti-Inflammatory, Neuron Survival and Axon Growth-Related Genes," *Experimental Gerontology* 69 (2015): 159–69; and L. F. Ten Brinke et al., "Aerobic Exercise Increases Hippocampal Volume in Older Women with Probable Mild Cognitive Impairment: A 6-Month Randomized Controlled Trial," *British Journal of Sports Medicine* 49 (2015): 248–54.

151 **In research I conducted:** S. C. Masley, R. Roetzheim, and T. Gualtieri, "Aerobic Exercise Enhances Cognitive Flexibility," *Journal of Clinical Psychology* 16 (2009): 186–93.

152 **daily activity:** N. T. Lautenschlager et al., "Effect of Physical Activity on Cognitive Function in Older Adults at Risk for Alzheimer Disease," *JAMA* 300 (2008): 1027–37.

153 **Exercise gets your blood pumping:** J. N. Barnes, "Exercise, Cognitive Function and Aging," *Advances in Physiology Education* 39 (2015): 55–62.

153 **preventing a loss in muscle:** J. M. Burns et al., "Lean Mass Is Reduced in Early Alzheimer's Disease and Associated with Brain Atrophy," *Archives of Neurology* 67 (2010): 428–33.

154 **exercise might affect brain size:** L. F. Ten Brinke et al., "Aerobic Exercise Increases Hippocampal Volume in Older Women with Probable

Mild Cognitive Impairment," *British Journal of Sports Medicine* 49 (2015): 248–54.

154 **My own most recent:** S. C. Masley et al., "Lifestyle Markers Predict Cognitive Function," *Journal of the American College of Nutrition.* Date and volume pending.

156 **In a study in Australia:** M.A.F. Singh et al., "The Study of Mental and Resistance Training (SMART) Study-Resistance Training and/or Cognitive Training in Mild Cognitive Impairment: A Randomized, Double-Blind, Double-Sham Controlled Trial," *JAMDA* 15 (2014): 873–80.

160 **research conducted by my clinic:** S. C. Masley, L. V. Masley, and T. Gualtieri, "Cardiovascular Biomarkers and Carotid IMT Scores as Predictors of Cognitive Function," *Journal of the American College of Nutrition* 33 (2014): 63–69.

161 **Two large national studies:** T. S. Church et al., "Effects of Aerobic and Resistance Training on HgbA1C in Type 2 Diabetics," *JAMA* 304 (2010): 2253–62; and R. J. Sigal et al., "Effects of Aerobic Training, Resistance Training, or Both on Glycemic Control in Type 2 Diabetes," *Annals of Internal Medicine* 147 (2007): 357–69.

165 **interval training improves blood sugar:** S. M. Madsen et al., "High Intensity Interval Training Improves Glycaemic Control and Pancreatic Beta Cell Function of Type 2 Diabetes Patients," *PLoS One* (2015): online; and I. Almenning et al., "Effects of High Intensity Interval Training and Strength Training on Metabolic, Cardiovascular, and Hormonal Outcomes in Women with Polycystic Ovary Syndrome," *PLoS One,* September 25, 2015: online.

165 **A study in the United Kingdom:** S. O. Shepherd et al., "Low-Volume, High-Intensity Interval Training in a Gym Setting Improves Cardiometabolic and Psychological Health," *PLoS One,* September 24, 2015: online.

168 **Dr. Teresa Liu-Ambrose:** J. R. Best et al., "Long-Term Effects of Resistance Exercise Training on Cognition and Brain Volume in Older Women," *Journal of International Neuropsychological Society* 21 (2015): 745–56.

172 **tai chi has been shown:** M. H. Nguyen and A. Kruse, "A Randomized Controlled Trial of Tai Chi for Balance, Sleep Quality and Cognitive Performance in Elderly Vietnamese," *Clinical Interventions in Aging* 7 (2012): 185–90.

Chapter 7: Calm Your Brain

178 **people with insomnia:** J. C. Chen et al., "Sleep Duration, Cognitive Decline, and Dementia Risk in Older Women," *Alzheimer's and Demen-*

tia 12 (2016): 21–33; and K. Yaffe et al., "Connections Between Sleep and Cognition in Older Adults," *Lancet Neurology* 13 (2014): 1017–28.

191 **Meditation can lower:** K. E. Innes et al., "Effects of Meditation Versus Music Listening on Perceived Stress, Mood, Sleep, and Quality of Life in Adults with Early Memory Loss: A Pilot Randomized Controlled Trial," *Journal of Alzheimer's Disease* 52 (2016): 1277–98; N. Wahbeh, E. Goodrich, and B. S. Oken, "Internet Mindfulness Meditation for Cognition and Mood in Older Adults: A Pilot Study," *Alternative Therapies in Health and Medicine* 22 (2016): 44–53; R. E. Wells et al., "Meditation's Impact on Default Mode Network and Hippocampus in Mild Cognitive Impairment: A Pilot Study," *Neuroscience Letters* 556 (2013): 15–19; and M. Pratzlich et al., "Impact of Short-Term Meditation and Expectation on Executive Brain Functions," *Behavioural Brain Research* 297 (2016): 268–76.

Chapter 8: Protecting Your Brain from Toxins

196 **two hundred chemicals:** From a report by Sanjay Gupta, a neurosurgeon and CNN's chief medical correspondent.

196 **BPA has also been shown:** Anahad O'Connor, "BPA in Cans and Plastic Bottles Linked to Quick Rise in Blood Pressure," *New York Times,* December 8, 2014.

201 **excessive amounts:** L. A. Hoffman, A. L. Sklar, and S. J. Nixon, "The Effects of Acute Alcohol on Psychomotor, Set-Shifting, and Working Memory Performance in Older Men and Women," *Alcohol* 49 (2015): 185–91; and A. M. Day, "Executive Functioning in Alcohol Use Studies: A Brief Review of Findings and Challenges in Assessment," *Current Drug Abuse Reviews* 8 (2015): 26–40.

201 **Dr. Suzanne de la Monte:** M. Tong et al., "Nitrosamine Exposure Causes Insulin Resistance Diseases: Relevance to Type 2 Diabetes Mellitus, NASH, and Alzheimer's Disease," *Journal of Alzheimer's Disease* 17 (2009): 827–44.

202 **harm associated with tobacco:** E. Yalcin and S. de la Monte, "Tobacco Nitrosamines as Culprits in Disease," *Journal of Physiology and Biochemistry* 72 (2016): 107–20.

203 **a DDT residue:** Robin Reese, "Potential Risk Factor for Alzheimer's: DDT Exposure," *Emory News Center,* January 30, 2014; and J. R. Richardson et al., "Elevated Serum Pesticide Levels and Risk for Alzheimer Disease," *JAMA Neurology* 71 (2014): 284–90.

205 **In 2012 my colleagues and I:** S. C. Masley, L. V. Masley, and T. Gualtieri, "Effect of Mercury Levels and Seafood Intake on Cognitive Function in Middle-Aged Adults," *Integrative Medicine* 11 (2012): 32–40.

211 **blood pesticide levels:** D. H. Lee et al., "Association Between Background Exposure to Organochlorinpesticides and the Risk of Cognitive Impairment," *Environment International* 89–90 (2016): 179–84.

211 **a study in Taiwan:** J. N. Lin et al., "Increased Risk of Dementia in Patients with Acute Organophosphate and Carbamate Poisoning," *Medicine* 94 (2015): e1187.

Chapter 9: A Better (Happier) Brain for Life

216 **menopause and andropause:** T. C. Castanho et al., "The Role of Sex and Sex-Related Hormones in Cognition, Mood and Well-Being in Older Men and Women," *Biological Psychology* 103 (2014): 158–66; C. E. Gleason et al., "Effects of Hormone Therapy on Cognition and Mood in Recently Postmenopausal Women: Findings from the Randomized, Controlled KEEPS-Cognitive and Affective Study," *PLoS Medicine,* June 2, 2015: n.p.; Y. Hara, "Estrogen Effects on Cognitive and Synaptic Health over the Lifecourse," *Physiological Reviews* 95 (2015): 785–807; A. McCarrey and S. M. Resnick, "Postmenopausal Hormone Therapy and Cognition," *Hormones and Behavior* 74 (2015): 167–72; H. Pintana, N. Chattipakorn, and S. Chattipakorn, "Testosterone Deficiency, Insulin-Resistant Obesity and Cognitive Function," *Metabolic Brain Disorders* 30 (2015): 853–76.

218 **Two studies have shown:** J. E. Manson and A. M. Kaunitz, "Menopause Management—Getting Clinical Care Back on Track," *New England Journal of Medicine* 374 (2016): 803–6; and H. N. Hodis et al., "Vascular Effects of Early Versus Late Postmenopausal Treatment with Estradiol," *New England Journal of Medicine* 374 (2016): 1221–31.

219 **oral estradiol increased:** S. Masley, "The Truth About Estrogen Therapy After Menopause," *Healthier Talk,* April 14, 2016.

220 **Testosterone therapy appears:** R. Sharma et al., "Normalization of Testosterone Level Is Associated with Reduced Incidence of Myocardial Infarction and Mortality in Men," *European Heart Journal* 36 (2015): 2706–15.

225 **study at Rush University:** K. A. Skarupski et al., "Longitudinal Association of Vitamin B-6, Folate, and Vitamin B-12 with Depressive Symptoms Among Older Adults over Time," *American Journal of Clinical Nutrition* 92 (2010): 330–35.

227 **German researcher:** S. Kühn et al., "Playing Super Mario Induces Structural Brain Plasticity: Gray Matter Changes Resulting from Training with a Commercial Video Game," *Molecular Psychiatry* 19 (2014): 265–71.

228   **Dr. Susanne Jaeggi:** S. M. Jaeggi et al., "The Role of Individual Differences in Cognitive Training and Transfer," *Memory and Cognition* 42 (2014): 464–80.

230   **Researchers have found that adults in bilingual households:** Judith F. Kroll, Susan C. Bobb, Noriko Hoshino, "Two Languages in Mind. Bilingualism as a Tool to Investigate Language, Cognition, and the Brain," *Sage Journals* 23, no. 3 (2014); D. Perani, J. Abutalebi, "Bilingualism, Dementia, Cognitive and Neural Reserve," *Current Opinion in Neurology* 28 (2015): 618–25; http://www.alzheimers.net/12-11-14 -bilingualism-delays-alzheimers/; and http://www.alzheimers.net/2013 -11-11/speaking-two-languages-delays-dementia/.

231   **craft or artistic activity:** R. O. Roberts et al., "Risk and Protective Factors for Cognitive Impairment in Persons Aged 85 Years and Older," *Neurology* 84 (2015): 1854–61.

231   **Whether it is a new language:** L. C. Lam et al., "Intellectual and Physical Activities, but Not Social Activities, Are Associated with Better Global Cognition: A Multi-Site Evaluation of the Cognition and Lifestyle Activity Study for Seniors in Asia (CLASSA)," *Age and Ageing* 44 (2015): 835–40.

Allen, M., et al. "Cognitive-Affective Neural Plasticity Following Active-Controlled Mindfulness Intervention." *Journal of Neuroscience* 32 (2012): 15601–610.

Ballesteros, S., et al. "Maintaining Older Brain Functionality: A Targeted Review." *Neuroscience and Biobehavioral Reviews* 55 (2015): 453–77.

Beilharz, J. E., J. Maniam, and M. J. Morris. "Diet-Induced Cognitive Deficits: The Role of Fat and Sugar, Potential Mechanisms and Nutritional Interventions." *Nutrients* 7 (2015): 6719–38.

Bellavia, A., et al. "Differences in Survival Associated with Processed and with Nonprocessed Red Meat Consumption." *American Journal of Clinical Nutrition* 100 (2014): 924–29.

Beydoun, M. A., et al. "Epidemiologic Studies of Modifiable Factors Associated with Cognition and Dementia: Systemic Review and Meta-Analysis." *BMC Public Health* 14 (2014): 643.

Beydoun, M. A., et al. "Dietary Antioxidant Intake and Its Association with Cognitive Function in an Ethnically Diverse Sample of US Adults." *Psychosomatic Medicine* 77 (2015): 68–82.

Clare, L., et al. "The Agewell Trial: A Pilot Randomised Controlled Trial of a Behavior Change Intervention to Promote Healthy Ageing and Reduce Risk of Dementia in Later Life." *BMC Psychiatry* 15 (2015): 25.

Cederholm, T. N. Salem, Jr., and Jan Palmblad. "W-3 Fatty Acids in the Prevention of Cognitive Decline in Humans." *Advanced Nutrition* 4 (2013): 672–76.

Cheng, P. F., et al. "Do Soy Isoflavones Improve Cognitive Function in Postmenopausal Women? A Meta-Analysis." *Menopause* 22 (2015): 198–206.

Cooper, C., et al. "Modifiable Predictors of Dementia in Mild Cognitive Impairment: A Systematic Review and Meta-Analysis." *American Journal of Psychiatry* 172 (2015): 323–34.

Cooper, J. K. "Nutrition and the Brain: What Advice Should We Give?" *Neurobiology of Aging* 35 (2014): 579–83.

Creegan, R., et al. "Diet, Nutrients and Metabolism: Cogs in the Wheel Driving Alzheimer's Disease Pathology?" *British Journal of Nutrition* 113 (2015): 1499–517.

De la Monte, S. M., et al. "Epidemiological Trends Strongly Suggest Exposures as Etiologic Agents in the Pathogenesis of Sporadic Alzheimer's Disease, Diabetes Mellitus, and Non-Alcoholic Steatohepatitis." *Journal of Alzheimer's Disease* 17 (2009): 519–29.

De la Monte, S. M., and M. Tong. "Brain Metabolic Dysfunction at the Core of Alzheimer's Disease." *Biochemical Pharmacology* 88 (2014): 548–59.

Eshkoor, S. A. "Mild Cognitive Impairment and Its Management in Older People." *Clinical Interventions in Aging* 10 (2015): 687–93.

Galasko D. R., et al. "Antioxidants for Alzheimer's Disease. A Randomized Clinical Trial with Cerebrospinal Fluid Biomarker Measures." *Archives of Neurology* 69 (2012): 836–41.

Gano, L. B., M. Patel, and J. M. Rho. "Ketogenic Diets, Mitochondria, and Neurological Diseases." *Journal of Lipid Research* 55 (2014): 2211–28.

Gil, S. S., and D. Seitz. "Lifestyles and Cognitive Health, What Older Individuals Can Do to Optimize Cognitive Outcomes." *Journal of the American Medical Association* 314 (2015): 774–75.

Gillette-Guyonnet, S., M. Secher, and B. Vellas. "Nutrition and Neurodegeneration: Epidemiological Evidence and Challenges for Future Research." *British Journal of Clinical Pharmacology* 75 (2013): 738–55.

Gleason, C. E., et al. "Cognitive Effects of Soy Isoflavones in Patients with Alzheimer's Disease." *Journal of Alzheimer's Disease* 47 (2015): 1009–19.

Guyot, E., et al. "Evidence of a Cumulative Effect of Cardiometabolic Disorders at Midlife and Subsequent Cognitive Function." *Age and Ageing* 44 (2015): 648–54.

Harcombe, Z., et al. "Evidence from Randomised Controlled Trials Did Not Support the Introduction of Dietary Fat Guidelines in 1977 and 1983: A Systematic Review and Meta-Analysis." *Open Heart* 2 (2015): n.p.

Hazzouri, A.Z.A., and K. Yaffe. "Arterial Stiffness and Cognitive Function in the Elderly." *Journal of Alzheimer's Disease* 42 (2014): s503–s514.

Hermanussen, M. "Stature of Early Europeans." *Hormones* 175 (2003): 175–78.

Hermida, A. P., et al. "The Association Between Late-Life Depression, Mild Cognitive Impairment and Dementia: Is Inflammation the Missing Link?" *Expert Review of Neurotherapeutics* 12 (2012): 1339–50.

Howes, M.J.R., and M.S.J. Simmonds. "The Role of Phytochemicals as Micronutrients in Health and Disease." *Current Opinion* 17 (2014): 558–66.

Jiao, J., et al. "Effect of n-3 PUFA Supplementation on Cognitive Function Throughout the Life Span from Infancy to Old Age: A Systematic Review and Meta-Analysis of Randomized Controlled Trials." *American Journal of Clinical Nutrition* 100 (2014): 1422–36.

Kantor, E. D., et al. "Lifestyle Factors and Inflammation: Associations by Body Mass Index." *PloS One* (July 2, 2013).

Kean, R. J., et al. "Chronic Consumption of Flavanone-Rich Orange Juice

Is Associated with Cognitive Benefits: An 8-Week, Randomized, Double-Blind, Placebo-Controlled Trial in Healthy Older Adults." *American Journal of Clinical Nutrition* 101 (2015): 506–14.

Kelly, J., et al. "Effects of Short-Term Dietary Nitrate Supplementation on Blood Pressure, O_2 Uptake Kinetics, and Muscle and Cognitive Function in Older Adults." *American Journal of Physiology-Regulatory, Integrative and Comparative Physiology* 304 (2013): 73–83.

Kesse-Guyot, E., L. Fezeu, C. Jeandel, et al. "French Adults' Cognitive Performance After Daily Supplementation with Antioxidant Vitamins and Minerals at Nutritional Doses: A Post Hhoc Analysis of the Supplementation in Vitamins and Mineral Antioxidants (SU.VI.MAX) Trial." *American Journal of Clinical Nutrition* 94 (2011): 94: 892–899.

Kim, D. H., et al. "Seafood Types and Age-Related Cognitive Decline in the Women's Health Study." *Journals of Gerontology. Series A, Biological Sciences and Medical Sciences* 68 (2013): 1255–62.

Knopman, D. S. "Go to the Head of the Class to Avoid Vascular Dementia and Skip Diabetes and Obesity." *Neurology* 71 (2008): 1046–47.

Langa, K. M., et al. "A Comparison of the Prevalence of Dementia in the United States in 2000 and 2012." *JAMA Internal Medicine* 177 (2016): 51–58.

Langa, K. M., and D. A. Levine. "The Diagnosis and Management of Mild Cognitive Impairment: A Clinical Review." *JAMA* 312 (2014): 2551–61.

Lara, J., et al. "A Proposed Panel of Biomarkers of Healthy Ageing." *BMC Medicine* 13 (2015): 222.

Lau, F. C., B. Shukitt-Hale, and J. A. Joseph. "Nutritional Intervention in Brain Aging: Reducing the Effect." *Sub-Cellular Biochemistry* 42 (2007): 299–318.

Lautenschlager, N. T., and O. P. Almeida. "Physical Activity and Cognition in Old Age." *Current Opinion in Psychiatry* 19 (2006): 190–93.

Lavialle, M., et al. "An (n-3) Polyunsaturated Fatty Acid-Deficient Diet Disturbs Daily Locomotor Activity, Melatonin Rhythm, and Striatal Dopamine in Syrian Hamsters." *Journal of Nutrition* 138 (2008): 1719–24.

Lin, F., et al. "Fatigability Disrupts Cognitive Processes' Regulation of Inflammatory Reactivity in Old Age." *American Journal of Geriatric Psychiatry* 22 (2014): 1544–54.

Lomagno, K. A., et al. "Increasing Iron and Zinc in Pre-Menopausal Women and Its Effects on Mood and Cognition: A Systematic Review." *Nutrients* 6 (2014): 5117–41.

Magrone, T., G. Marzulli, and E. Jirillo. "Immunopathogenesis of Neurodegenerative Diseases: Current Therapeutic Models of Neuroprotection with Special Reference to Natural Products." *Current Pharmaceutical Design* 18 (2012): 34–42.

McCaddon, A., and J. W. Miller. "Assessing the Association Between Homocysteine and Cognition: Reflections on Bradford Hill, Meta-Analyses, and Causality." *Nutrition Reviews* 73 (2015): 723–35.

McNeill, G., et al. "Effect of Multivitamin and Multimineral Supplementation on Cognitive Function in Men and Women Aged 65 Years and Over: A Randomised Controlled Trial." *Nutrition Journal* 6 (2007): 10.

Millan, M. J. "The Epigenetic Dimension of Alzheimer's Disease: Causal, Consequence, or Curiosity?" *Dialogues in Clinical Neuroscience* 16 (2014): 373–93.

Morris, M. C., et al. "Association of Seafood Consumption, Brain Mercury Level, and APOE e4 Status with Brain Neuropathology in Older Adults." *JAMA* 315 (2016): 489–97.

Na, L., et al. "Mangiferin Supplementation Improves Serum Lipid Profiles in Overweight Patients with Hyperlipidemia: A Double-Blind Randomized Controlled Trial." *Scientific Reports* 5 (2015): n.p.

Newport, M. T., et al. "A New Way to Produce Hyperketonemia: Use of Ketone Ester in a Case of Alzheimer's." *Alzheimer's and Dementia* 11 (2015): 99–103.

Nilsson, A., et al. "A Diet Based on Multiple Functional Concepts Improves Cognitive Performance in Healthy Subjects." *Nutrition and Metabolism* 10 (2013): 49.

Philip, D., et al. "Dihydrofolate Reductase 19-bp Deletion Polymorphism Modifies the Association of Folate Status with Memory in a Cross-Sectional Multi-Ethnic Study of Adults." *American Journal of Clinical Nutrition* 109 (2015): 1279–88.

Pinto, C., and A. Subramanyam. "Mild Cognitive Impairment: The Dilemma." *Indian Journal of Psychiatry* 51 (2009): s44–s51.

Presse, N., et al. "Vitamin K Status and Cognitive Function in Healthy Older Adults." *Neurobiology of Aging* 34 (2013): 2777–83.

Raji, C. A., et al. "Hot Topics in Research: Preventative Neuroradiology in Brain Aging and Cognitive Decline." *American Journal of Neuradiology* 36 (2015): 1803–9.

Reitz, C. "Genetic Diagnosis and Prognosis of Alzheimer's Disease: Challenges and Opportunities." *Expert Review of Molecular Diagnosis* 15 (2015): 339–48.

Roberts, R. O., et al. "Risk and Protective Factors for Cognitive Impairment in Persons Aged 85 Years and Older." *Neurology* 84 (2015): 1854–61.

Rodakowski, J., et al. "Non-Pharmacological Interventions for Adults with Mild Cognitive Impairment and Early Stage Dementia: An Updated Scoping Review." *Molecular Aspects of Medicine* 43–44 (2015): 38–53.

Sadehi, A., et al. "The Effect of Diabetes Mellitus on Apoptosis in Hippocampus: Cellular and Molecular." *International Journal of Preventive Medicine* 7 (2016): 57.

Sartori, A. C., et al. "The Impact of Inflammation on Cognitive Function in

Older Adults: Implications for Health Care Practice and Research." *Journal of Neuroscience Nursing* 444 (2012): 206–17.

Shah, S. H., et al. "Branched-Chain Amino Acid Levels Are Associated with Improvement in Insulin Resistance with Weight Loss." *Diabetologia* 55 (2012): 321–30.

Shepard, K. W., and C. L. Cheatham. "Executive Functions and the w-6-to-w-3 Fatty Acid Ratio: A Cross-Sectional Study." *American Journal of Clinical Nutrition* 105 (2017): 32–41.

Shinto, L., et al. "A Randomized Placebo-Controlled Pilot Trial of Omega-3 Fatty Acids and Alpha Lipoic Acid in Alzheimer's Disease." *Journal of Alzheimer's Disease* 38 (2014): n.p.

Sink, K. M., et al. "Effect of a 24-Month Physical Activity Intervention vs Health Education on Cognitive Outcomes in Sedentary Older Adults." *JAMA* 314 (2015): 781–90.

Smit, R.A.J., et al. "Higher Visit-to-Visit Low-Density Lipoprotein Cholesterol Variability Is Associated with Lower Cognitive Performance, Lower Cerebral Brain Flow, and Greater White Matter Hyperintensity Load in Older Subjects." *Circulation* 134 (2016): n.p.

Taniguchi, Y., et al. "Nutritional Biomarkers and Subsequent Cognitive Decline Among Community-Dwelling Older Japanese: A Prospective Study." *Journals of Gerontology, Series A: Biological Sciences and Medical Sciences* 69 (2014): 1276–83.

Torres, S. J., et al. "Dietary Patterns Are Associated with Cognition Among Older People with Mild Cognitive Impairment." *Nutrients* 4 (2012): 1542–51.

Traba, J., et al. "Fasting and Refeeding Differentially Regulate NLRP3 Inflammasome Activation in Human Subjects." *Journal of Clinical Investigation* 125 (2015): 4592–600.

Van de Rest, O., et al. "Dietary Patterns, Cognitive Decline, and Dementia: A Systematic Review." *Advances in Nutrition* 6 (2015): 154–68.

Vega, J. N., and P. A. Newhouse. "Mild Cognitive Impairment: Diagnosis, Longitudinal Course, and Emerging Treatments." *Current Psychiatry Reports* 16 (2014): 490.

Xu, R. B., et al. "Longitudinal Association Between Fasting Blood Glucose Concentrations and First Stroke in Hypertensive Adults in China: Effect of Folic Acid Intervention." *American Journal of Clinical Nutrition* (in press).

Yin, Y., Y. Fan, Y. Lin, et al. "Nutrient Biomarkers and Vascular Risk Factors in Subtypes of Mild Cognitive Impairment: A Cross-Sectional Study." *Journal of Nutrition, Health, and Aging* 19 (2015): 39–47.

Zhu, N., et al. "Cognitive Function in a Middle-Aged Cohort Is Related to Higher Quality Dietary Pattern 5 and 25 Years Earlier: The Cardia Study." *Journal of Nutrition, Health, and Aging* 19 (2015): 33–38.